AṢṬADAḶA YOGAMĀLĀ

AṢṬADAḶA YOGAMĀLĀ

(COLLECTED WORKS)

B.K.S. IYENGAR

Volume 3

Articles, lectures, messages

ALLIED PUBLISHERS PVT. LIMITED
NEW DELHI MUMBAI KOLKATA CHENNAI NAGPUR
AHMEDABAD BANGALORE HYDERABAD LUCKNOW

ALLIED PUBLISHERS PRIVATE LIMITED

Regd. Off. : 15 J.N. Heredia Marg, Ballard Estate, Mumbai 400001
Prarthna Flats (2nd Floor), Navrangpura, Ahmedabad 380009
3-2-844/6 & 7 Kachiguda Station Road, Hyderabad 500027
16-A Ashok Marg, Patiala House, Lucknow 226001
5th Main Road, Gandhinagar, Bangalore 560009
1/13-14 Asaf Ali Road, New Delhi 110002
17 Chittaranjan Avenue, Kolkata 700072
81 Hill Road, Ramnagar, Nagpur 440010
751 Anna Salai, Chennai 600002

First Published 2002

ISBN 81-7764-361-4

Cover design : The Author
Artwork : S.M. Wagh

Published by Sunil Sachdev and printed by Ravi Sachdev at Allied Publishers Private Limited, Printing Division, A-104 Mayapuri, Phase-II, New Delhi - 110 064

Invocatory Prayers

ॐ

Yogena cittasya padena vācāṁ
Malaṁ śarīrasyaca vaidyakena
Yopākarottaṁ pravaraṁ munīnāṁ
Patañjaliṁ prāñjalirānato'smi
Ābāhu puruṣākāraṁ
Śaṅkha cakrāsi dhāriṇaṁ
Sahasra śirasaṁ śvetaṁ
Praṇamāmi Patañjaliṁ

I bow before the noblest of sages Patañjali, who gave yoga for serenity and sanctity of mind, grammar for clarity and purity of speech and medicine for pure, perfect health.

I prostrate before Patañjali who is crowned with a thousand headed cobra, an incarnation of Ādiśeṣa (Anañta) whose upper body has a human form, holding the conch in one arm, disk in the second, a sword of wisdom to vanquish nescience in the third and blessing humanity from the fourth arm, while his lower body is like a coiled snake.

Yastyaktvā rūpamādyaṁ prabhavati jagato'nekadhānugrahāya
Prakṣīṇakleśarāśirviṣamaviṣadharo'nekavaktrāḥ subhogī
Sarvajñānaprasūtirbhujagaparikaraḥ prītaye yasya nityaṁ
Devohīṣaḥ savovyātsitavimalatanuryogado yogayuktaḥ

I prostrate before Lord Ādiśeṣa, who manifested himself on Earth as Patañjali to grace the human race in health and harmony,

I salute Lord Ādiśeṣa of the myriad serpent heads and mouths carrying noxious poisons, discarding which he came to Earth as a single headed Patañjali in order to eradicate ignorance and vanquish sorrow.

I pay my obeisance to him, repository of all knowledge, amidst his attendant retinue.

I pray to the Lord whose primordial form shines with peace and white effulgence, pristine in body, a master of yoga, who bestows on all his yogic light to enable mankind to rest in the house of the immortal Soul.

BY THE AUTHOR

This volume of *Aṣṭadaḷa Yogamālā* published by Allied Publishers, Delhi, is the third volume of the first part of the "Collected Works" of Yogācārya B.K.S. Iyengar. Each part comprises several volumes which are arranged according to the following scheme:

Articles

Interviews

Question and Answer Sessions

Techniques of *Āsanas, Prāṇāyāma, Dhyāna* and *Śavāsana*

Therapeutic Applications of Yoga

Garland of Aphorisms and Thoughts

General Index and Analytical Dictionary

Addendum

Also by the Same Author

Light on Yoga

Light on Prāṇāyāma

Concise Light on Yoga

Art of Yoga

Tree of Yoga

Light on the Yoga Sūtras of Patañjali

The Illustrated Light on Yoga

Yoga Ek Kalpataru (Marathi)

Ārogyayoga (Marathi)

Light on Aṣṭāṅga Yoga

Aṣṭadaḷa Yogamālā (Vols 1 & 2)

Yoga: The Path To Holistic Health

Yoga Sarvānaāṭhi (Marathi)

Also on *Iyengar Yoga*

Body the Shrine, Yoga Thy Light

70 Glorious Years

Iyengar His Life and Work

Yogapushpanjali

Yogadhārā

CONTENTS

Section IX – MULTIPLE ASPECTS OF YOGA

TABLES AND PLATES

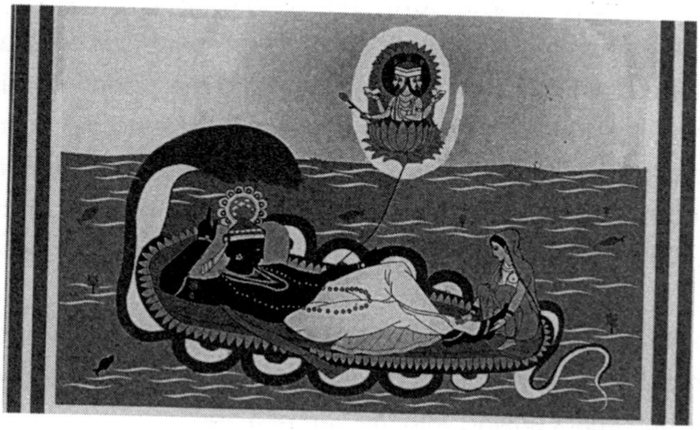

Ādiśeṣa

A note about the back cover:

The Universe evolves out of a primordial pre-elemental realm beyond limitations of time and space. Floating on this great "primordial ocean" is a coiled serpent – *Ādiśeṣa* – the couch of Lord Vishnu. Issuing from Lord Vishnu's navel – the root, the stem of a lotus extends with its flower floating above. Sitting on the calyx of the lotus is Brahma – the Creator. Vishnu indicates for Brahma to create. The creation acts as the seed, sprout and root of the Asvattha Tree (BG 15.1).

The Asvattha Tree is a giant banyan tree. Its roots extend deep and wide into the soil. Its trunk ascends, branching again and again carrying its leaves on the outer edge where they face the outer atmosphere, absorbing light, exchanging gasses and receiving the rain, directing its moistening fluid to bathe the entire organism. The banyan tree's uniqueness is that from the branches it grows shoots which return back to the soil as roots.

All that which exists in the macrocosmic universe exists within us on a microcosmic level. We are the Tree. Our brain is the root, the trunk is our trunk with its spinal chord, and the branches are the limbs; arms and legs. Like the tree, throughout our body run the nervous system which branch to form pathways for sending and receiving messages.

At our birth the head arrives first as the root. Then, in childhood we learn to stand. By disturbing this order, the root or the head is above with the rest of the body below.

Yoga practice (*āsana, prāṇāyāma* and *pratyāhāra),* gives us the tools for cleansing, toning and ordering the organism into a harmonious whole, so that it may flower and fruit. In the practice of inverted *āsana* the head is placed back in its original position with the brain or root down and the trunk and limbs above. The brain is bathed and fed from a reservoir of fresh oxygenated blood, like the roots of the mighty Banyan that is fed in the rich soil.

The health of each part is dependent upon the whole. Many *āsanas* are designed for this purpose. They keep the entire organism in a healthy state, in a wholistic way. With the placement of the muscles and joints, the various parts of the spinal column are aligned, the cerebro-spinal-fluid within flows up and down the column, filling and emptying the ventricles inside the brain so that the brain is benefited. When the amount and pressure of the cerebro-spinal-fluid is correct the brain floats within its own ocean, like Vishnu on his couch. With the correct placement and alignment of the various limbs and the torso, the entire organic body is benefited. Any organ can be targeted individually through the various actions which are deliberately augmented through complimentary and supplementary actions, or they can be wholly assisted to a state of harmonious interdependent functioning by the discretionary actions of the various *āsana*.

Yoga can be defined as **action orientated knowledge**. Through discerning placement and judicious adjustment, the use of correct pressure and direction, this knowledge flows to the practitioner like the nourishment arising with the sap of a tree.

As the practitioner understands the relationship between his subtle and "discrete" **action,** and placement of his "root, branch and leaf" in *āsana, prāṇāyāma* and *pratyāhāra*, he sends the **knowledge** that arises back as a "shoot" into the soil to be one with the root. This coming back in contact with the root brings a sea of changes. He aligns himself within as rhythmic re-**orientation** takes place in body, mind and self. From here on, his *sādhanā* unveils the covering of the inner-lamp and illuminates him from within.

On the back cover against the Banyan Tree, we have placed a vertical *Parivṛtta Ek Pāda Śīrṣāsana* along with a horizontal *Parivṛtta Janu Śīrṣāsana*. In both, there is a dynamic twisting action; which turns the core of the being; washing and cleansing the inner organic and nervous systems. Their vertical and horizontal aspects ensure the practitioner's intellect and emotions are balanced.

The tree is nourished,
its growth is healthy,
the tree flowers, and its fruit is abundant.

FOREWORD

I was hoping that this third volume of *Aṣṭadaḷa Yogamālā* would be released on the auspicious day of *Guru Pūrṇima* (2002). But, unknown situations caused the delay and yet I am delighted in my heart that I could complete the volume on this day. After going through the final reading, now I hope this volume will be released on *Vijaya Dashami.*

God is one, but we attribute him in many different ways. Similarly, the trunk of a tree is one but the branches are many. These sayings go well with yoga too.

In this volume, I offer a yogic cornucopia of subjects which will be of interest to the first timer as well as the discerning reader. I have shown how yoga casts its glorious light on subjects ranging from therapeutics and āyurveda to academics and sports, practice *(sādhanā)* and teaching as art, science and and way of life.

Here I have also discussed *sādhanā* not only from different dimensions, but also dedicated the sequential steps of grading the *sādhanā* as we improve in its practice, both as a teaching and a healing art. In this compilation, I have especially introduced the wisdom of yoga and its parallelisms with modern science as well as with *āyurveda.*

Lastly, I have discussed how yoga can be introduced in schools and colleges.

Yoga helps one to become a master of circumstances and I have given guidance with hints to those who choose yoga as a vocation.

Here, I wish to acknowledge once again the help and assistance of those without whom the undertaking of this project would not have been possible. Smt. Geeta S. Iyengar, for checking and helping with valueable suggestions for the subject. Mr. Faeq Biria and Patxi Lizardi for jointly co-ordinating the entire project along with Geeta. Mr J. Evans for editing the work into a cohesive and cogent language. I also cannot forget Stephanie Quirk for her technical assistance for layout and editing, Uma and Raya Dhavale for further assistance at the computer, Mr S.M. Wagh for the line drawings, Mr. Chandru Melwani of Soni Studios for reproduction of photos. Mr. Kokate for cover artwork. I am indebted to Mr. Surojit Banerjee for his final touch on the work, and last but not the least to Allied Publishers (New Delhi) for whom am grateful for publishing these volumes.

14. Oct. 2002

B K S IYENGAR

SECTION I

LIGHT ON PRACTICE OF YOGA

YOGASĀDHANĀ – A CULTURE OF CIVILISATION

The life of each individual is based on nature *(prakṛti)*, individual soul *(jīvātmā)* and Universal Soul *(Paramātmā)*. Nature extrudes *mahat* or cosmic intelligence. *Jīvātmā* is a part of *Paramātmā*, existing as *puruṣa*[1] or human soul. *Jīvātmā* has a vehicle in the form of *citta*, which is the off-shoot of cosmic intelligence. *Citta*, the subtlest form of *prakṛti* or nature, is constituted of *ahaṁkāra* ('I'ness or ego), *buddhi* and *manas*.

Though *jīvātmā* is pure consciousness, it has two facets. When it moves on the spiritual path, it is pure and divine. When it moves in mind – matter – energy, it becomes *buddhi-sattva* or mental consciousness. This *buddhi-sattva* often appears itself as pure *jīvātmā*, but in fact it is the instrument of the *jīvātmā*.

Yoga has been defined as *citta vṛtti nirodha*, which means to stop all internal and external forms of thinking which may sprout with or without volition. *Citta* stands for several things like life, inspiration, aspiration, drive, will power, intelligence, reason, consciousness and so forth. In yogic term, *citta* stands distinctly for three things. They are mind, intelligence and ego or the state which ascertains that "I know". Mind has no discriminative power, but has the power of gathering and feeling. Intelligence discriminates, reasons and comes to determinative knowledge. Intelligence is the nearest vehicle to the self. However, the I-ness interferes with intelligence and prides itself on being the true self. This is the creator of 'I' and 'Me' in man. One should know that the intelligence is the vehicle of the true self, whereas the I-ness is the impostor of the true self.

Man cannot be separated from his body as the trunk of a tree cannot be separated from the root. The physical body is a part of man. This body has three layers. They are known as causal body, subtle body and gross body. As the tree has branches, leaves, flowers and fruits this body of man functions in matter, mind, consciousness and energy as the anatomical intellectual and bliss bodies.

---

1 *Puruṣa, jīvātmā, ātman,* are used synonymously.

The causal body is the sheath of the soul. It is incorruptible and non-decaying. When man is not in this body, he loses his own *svarūpa* – true state – and dwells in the *citta*. This is the subtle body or the psycho-physiological sheath. The senses of perception and organs of action are the vehicles of the gross body and are dependent on the mind. Without the mind, the outer body cannot function. The gross and subtle bodies are interdependent upon one another. Man uses his senses to fulfill and enjoy the demands of the mind, as he is caught in the web of worldly desires. Like the spokes of the wheel, these enjoyments revolve between pleasure and pain. He becomes a victim of circumstances and environments, which creates a dual consciousness or dual personalities. This state in man is the seed of separation – *viyoga* – or pain and sorrow – *duḥkha*. It is interesting at this juncture to note that the art and science of yoga starts with the detailed explanation of the philosophy of sorrow or affliction.

Both afflictions of pain and sorrow and feelings of joy and pleasure, belong to the movements of the mind. Practice of yoga sublimates the mind through conscious effort to release the self from the web of pain and pleasure and leads one to experience that state which is beyond pain and pleasure. This state is the pristine pure state, *śuddha-svarūpa* or *jīvātmā-svarūpa*.

The consciousness *(citta)* has two facets, namely intellectual and emotional. The knowledge acquired through education is called *vidyā* or objective knowledge, and the intelligence developed through experience is called *jñāna* or subjective knowledge. The knowledge acquired through intellectual consciousness is developed by direct perception, false perception, imagination, sleep and memory, whereas the *jñāna* developed through emotional consciousness is understood through experiences in form of pleasure and pain, heat and cold, honour and dishonour, joy and sorrow, contentment and elation. The spokes of pleasure and pain move alternately and disturb the state of consciousness physically, emotionally and intellectually, creating imbalance or ill-health in man.

Yoga gives us the ways to develop harmony, balance and concord in physical health as well as emotional and intellectual health. Patañjali says that it is possible to achieve these either by practice and dispassion or by total surrender to the Supreme.

For an average man total surrender is not only difficult but an impossibility, which is why Patañjali insists on practice *(abhyāsa)* and dispassion *(vairāgya)*. These two are like wings for the *sādhaka* to fly from the world of matter to the world of the spirit. Practice means doing the *sādhanā* for a long duration without interruptions, but with dedication and devotion, while renunciation is intended for us to learn to minimise physical wants and emotional desires, so that sooner or later, the *sādhaka* develops desirelessness of the world and becomes attached to the Supreme – to God.

Through *abhyāsa*, the intellectual consciousness is stabilised and by *vairāgya*, the emotional consciousness is controlled. With a motive to develop harmony between the intellectual and emotional consciousness, man begins *yogasādhanā*. When harmony is achieved, then these two disciplines, *abhyāsa* and *vairāgya*, starting out as forced regimental discipline, become a natural process and the practitioner continues them without any motive or desire. From then on, his *sādhanā* becomes *vairāgyābhyāsa*.

In this state the practitioner develops stability in mind and steadfastness in his intelligence. He has no more disparities within himself or with his envelope – the body. His *sādhanā* becomes all in one and one in all. This is the true nature of one's self. This state of *sādhanā* can be called *prajñāna yoga*. This *prajñāna yoga* has two folds, *saṁprajñāta yoga* and *asaṁprajñāta yoga*. In *saṁprajñāta yoga* one is cut off from all external things and impressions but is alert internally. One is aware of one's *svarūpa*. In *asaṁprajñāta yoga* identity becomes cosmic as all the internal and external vibrations cease and the awareness of one's very self is lost.

Due to intensive *sādhanā* in previous lives, some are born with the conquest of elements *(prakṛtilaya)* while others are born with the deliverance of freedom from body *(videha mukta)*.

Jada Bharata was born as a *prakṛtilayan*.[1] Ramana Maharshi and Ramakrishna Paramahamsa were born as *videha mukta*.[2] *Videhi* is a *mukta* in this cycle of *kalpa*.[3] *Prakṛtilayan* is the perfect one in the previous life. He has a balanced mind and looks on things and events evenly without perturbation. He has a *samāhita-citta*. He has a calm and composed mind, a mind that is fit for *dhyāna* and advocates others to follow the same line of thought without giving importance to the other aspects of yoga. But Patañjali warns them to maintain the practice of all aspects of yoga so that they cultivate and maintain the essence of yoga in order to become perfect yogis.

For ordinary men like us, we have to start definitely from the principles of *yama, niyama, āsana, prāṇāyāma* and *pratyāhāra* as well as being friendly to all, compassionate towards those who are suffering, glad about those who are better placed than us and indifferent to good and evil, happiness and misery.[4] In addition to these the *sādhanā* should be coupled with faith, courage and energy, good retentive power, contemplation and wisdom.[5]

---

1 One who is merged in nature

2 The feel of non-physical existence or the non-feeling of physical existence.

3 4,320 million years of a mortal

4 *Y.S.*, I.33.

5 *Y.S.*, I.20.

Success in yoga depends upon our earnest practices. If our practices are casual, the effects are casual and if they are religious, the effect too is religious. It all depends upon the frame of mind and the amount of energy one aligns with faith, determination and discrimination. Both seriousness and sincerity are required.

What is faith? Faith is not just a belief. Faith is a trust, a confidence, veneration or respect. Faith at once creates zeal to act. It is a way, a key to *sādhanā;* whereas belief is an acceptance of views that one has heard. Acceptance being verbal, it may or may not ignite or incite zeal to act. So it does not become a key to *sādhanā*. Faith being a quality of trust and veneration, it demands not only confidence in the *sādhanā* but also reverence towards God. Patañjali calls God – *Īśvara* – the Supreme – the *Guru* of all *gurus*. He defines *Īśvara* as *Kleśa karma vipākāśayaiḥ aparāmṛṣṭaḥ puruṣa viśeṣa Īśvaraḥ.* (*Y.S.*, I.24). God is one who is untouched by cause and effect, action and reaction. He is free of affliction, action and fruition.

Due to our dual ways of thinking and acting, obstacles like physical, mental and spiritual ailments distract the mind, in one form or the other, from the one-pointed attention of self-realisation. They are to be checked, controlled and eradicated by the practice of yoga. Then that intelligence reaches discriminative knowledge and intuitive power dawns on the *sādhaka* for the light of clarity to shine. He perseveres in his path and develops that singleness of purpose whether he be in the waking, sleeping or the dreamy states. His intelligence becomes as clear as crystal. No tinge of doubt remains. The mind is freed from objects and becomes an autonomous entity in itself. It does not depend upon the organs of action or senses of perception. Time, place and space lose their identities. Habits are broken. The *sādhaka* reaches the highest state and tastes the true essence of yoga. You may call it *haṭha yoga*, *rāja yoga*, *rājadhirāja yoga* or *kṣetrajña yoga*. It all means the same.

For the practitioner of yoga, the body and mind are fallow lands lying untilled and not sown. He ploughs his body and mind with *yama* and *niyama*, removes the weeds by *āsana*, waters it with energy through *prāṇāyāma*, uses good thoughts and actions of *pratyāhāra* as fertiliser, sows the best of seeds – *dhāraṇā* – through the *bīja mantra Āuṁ*, tends it with *dhyāna* to reach the harvest of harmony and peace – *samādhi*.

Thus the art of yoga deals with the purification of body and mind. Yoga is *tapas* as it involves a blazing effort of discipline from the physical body, psycho-physiological body and self. Yoga is *svādhyāya* or study of the self from the skin to the self and from the self to the skin. Yoga is *Īśvara praṇidhāna* – a total surrender to the Supreme. Thus *tapas*, *svādhyāya* and *Īśvara praṇidhāna* are the golden keys that unlock the gates of the Self.

When the nation is careless and weak in defence, the aggressor attacks and occupies it. Similarly diseases are just awaiting outside our skin to enter the inner frontier of the body when its defensive energy is at a lower level, creating psychosomatic diseases and causing disharmony within and without. Daily practice of yoga not only destroys the obstacles, whether they are physical, moral, emotional, intellectual or spiritual, but also prevents the symptoms that come in the way of health. The practitioner of yoga – yoga *sādhaka* bridges the gap between the body, mind and self and becomes the master of these three. The knower, the knowable and the known become one. The journey of the seeker searching the seer comes to an end.

Thus by a constant culturing process from *yama* to *dhyāna*, he civilises himself and becomes an adept – a *kuśala*, a true owner of the sacred body. The light of wisdom dawns on him like a rain-cloud of justice – *dharmamegha*. As the *dharma* or duty of the clouds is to pour rain, the yogi's wisdom pours out knowledge which is ever pure, ever green and continues to live for posterity. He becomes *kṛtārthan*.

His way of living reflects on humanity like the reflection of the mirror and transforms it. Thus the culture of a yogi becomes the civilisation of the World.

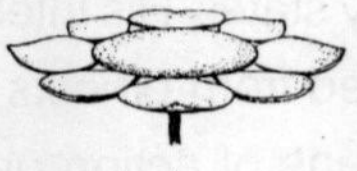

YOGADARŚANA

Darśana means seeing, looking, perceiving. *Darśana* also means showing or exhibiting. Yoga is called *darśana* as it gives eyes to see and behold thoroughly. The mirror reflects objects accurately. Similarly yoga not only reflects all thoughts and actions of the practitioner but also guides and corrects his vision so as to look into the inner self and gain sight of the soul. Yoga cleanses and illumines the mirror of consciousness by means of intelligence for the soul to be reflected directly and clearly.

Yoga is a practical method of art, science and philosophy embracing the life of man at all levels from the physical to the spiritual, thus making life useful, purposeful and noble. It enables each and every part of the human system to get attuned to its essence – the master within – i.e. the seer or the *Puruṣa.*

Patañjali, through his aphorisms *(sūtra),* shows ways of kindling the highest within the self whether one is initiated or uninitiated, intelligent or unintelligent, raising the *sādhaka* from the clutches of pain or sorrow. It helps the lazy body to become vibrant and active and transforms the mind towards balance and serenity. There are in all 196 *sūtra* divided into four *pāda* or chapters, namely *samādhi, sādhana, vibhūti* and *kaivalya.* Patañjali speaks on *dharma śāstra* in *Samādhi Pāda, karma śāstra* in *Sādhana Pāda, siddhi śāstra* in *Vibhūti Pāda* and *mokṣa śāstra* in *Kaivalya Pāda.*

In *Samādhi Pāda* Patañjali speaks for evolved souls, showing how they can reach the pinnacle of life. Such souls must be like Hanuman, Dhruva, Shuka, Prahlada, Shankara, Ramanuja, Madhva, Jnaneshvara, Matsyendra, Kabir, Ramdas, Ramakrishna, Ramana and so forth.

By beginning with *citta vṛtti nirodha,* he touches at once the subtlest sense of man – the *citta*

The *citta* is the seed from which *karma* (action), *karma phala* (fruit) and *janma* (birth) grow and diversify. Like an ocean, the *citta* is full of waves of thoughts.

The ocean is one but has many names such as Pacific, Indian, Atlantic, Arctic, Antarctic and so on. *Citta* too has many aspects. They are *vyutthāna citta, nirodha citta, śānta citta, ekāgra citta, nirmāṇa citta, chidra citta* and *divya citta.*

Touching the *divya citta* is the aim of yoga. Patañjali explains to both initiated and unitiated why yoga, and where yoga leads. He guides the initiated not to become complacent but to proceed further, and the unititiated to taste the untainted, clear and pure life.

Patañjali, as a great analyst of consciousness, shows the reasons for turmoil and disturbances in the improper and perverse actions and thoughts which result in endless pain. These endless pains are caused by direct indulgence, inducement and abetment, motivated by greed *(lobha)*, anger *(krodha)* and delusion *(moha)* which may be mild, moderate or intense in degrees.

Through introspection comes the end of pain and ignorance. The eight petals of yoga are the introspective measures so that the seeds of bondage are destroyed and eradicated in order to experience *kaivalya*. Hence, Patañjali says that yoga is meant to end all actions that create afflictions.

Patañjali explains the eight petals of yoga, namely *yama, niyama, āsana, prāṇāyāma, pratyāhāra, dhāraṇā, dhyāna* and *samādhi*. In the first chapter he begins with *sūkṣumendriya*, the subtle and the innermost *citta*, while in *Sādhana Pāda* he begins with *sthūlendriya* or gross *indriya*, showing ways and means to channel them towards the *antarendriya (buddhi, ahaṁkāra* and *citta*) so that the *sādhaka* reaches the aim of life, i.e. freedom from bondage. He explains the causes for pains and guides the *sādhaka* to control the organs of action and senses of perception through *yama* and *niyama*, to perfect the body by *āsana*, to steady the vital energy by *prāṇāyāma* and to stabilise the mind by *pratyāhāra*. He begins with the periphery by disciplining the gross *indriya* and then connects them to the subtle senses and takes them towards true *jñāna*.

Patañjali puts the eight petals of yoga in a capsule and calls them *kriyā yoga*, as *tapas, svādhyāya* and *Īśvara praṇidhāna*.

He speaks in clear terms explaining the qualities of God and asks the *sādhaka* to surrender to God completely and totally – *bhakti mārga* in *Samādhi Pāda*. As it is hard for the majority of people to surrender completely to God, he gives the yoga of eight petals so that they may surrender to God when maturity sets in.

He defines God as the Supreme Being *(puruṣa viśeṣa)*, who is totally and eternally free from afflictions and unaffected by actions and their fruits or by their residue. He mentions that God is the first and foremost *Guru*, the seed of all knowledge *(sarvajña bīja)*, and He is symbolized by *ĀUṀ* which has to be uttered with meaning and feeling.

See how Patañjali compares man to God in the *Sādhana Pāda*.

He says man is a product of the accumulated imprints of past lives, rooted in afflictions depending on class of birth, span of life and experiences, pleasant and painful states of life. From these impressions and experiences, thought waves sprout with painful or non-painful *vṛtti*, which again are dependent on afflictions, namely *avidyā, asmitā, rāga, dveṣa* and *abhiniveśa*. Nescience, ego, attachment, malice and sticking to life or fear of death churn the mind for a galaxy of thoughts to arise and make one act accordingly.

The mind *(manas)* is the connecting link between the outer and the inner body. It has the power to imagine, to think, to attend, to aim and to feel. It also involves the self with the tempting objects of the world. The mind is a very influencial factor in building up the imprints that are stored in the house of memory as latent impressions and desires *(saṁskāra* or *vāsanā)*.

This storehouse of memory generates either sensual pleasure or spiritual joy that is free from lust and infatuation.

Hence, Patañjali begins with *anuśāsanam* as *abhyāsa* – the practice – and *citta vṛtti nirodha* as *vairāgya* – the renunciation.

He explains implicitly the eight petals of yoga in *Samādhi Pāda* and explicitly in *Sādhana Pāda*. The mind – the outer layer of the consciousness – is first addressed so that the hoards of physical and mental ailments that accrue from afflictions and moods are quietened and one becomes free from bodily diseases, mental laziness, heedlessness, illusion, erroneous views, lack of perseverance, backsliding, sorrow, despair, unsteadiness in body and irregular flow of vital energy. He explains the new wisdom, free from taints, that comes to the *sādhaka* by interiorisation through the practice of eight petals of yoga.

All painful *vṛtti* are vanquished or brought to the minimum by the first five steps of yoga, namely, *yama, niyama, āsana, prāṇāyāma* and *pratyāhāra*, leading one to control the inner subtle *indriya* or senses so that *vṛtti* cannot crop up from *pratyāhāra* onwards and become *akliṣṭa vṛtti* or non-painful *vṛtti*.

Since the organs of action, senses of perception and mind, which are the gross senses of man, are used first for stilling the mind, it is called *bahiraṅga sādhanā*.

When *bahiraṅga sādhanā* of *sādhaka* is channelled, Patañjali asks the *sādhaka* to move further in order to know the depth of *bhakti, karma* and *jñāna* in *sādhanā*. He asks the *sādhaka* to discipline *buddhi, ahaṁkāra* and *citta* through *dhāraṇā, dhyāna* and *samādhi*. As the internal senses are brought under study, these three petals of yoga are called *antaraṅga sādhanā*.

In the first five petals of yoga, the elements of nature, (earth, water and fire), with their *tanmātra* (odour, taste and form), are controlled. Through *dhāraṇā* and *dhyāna* the subtle elements (air and ether), with their *tanmātra* (touch and sound), are stilled and silenced, so that the *sādhaka* enters the gate of the *puruṣa* through *samādhi.*

By this restraint of subtle senses *(buddhi, ahaṁkāra* and *citta),* Patañjali says the wealth of power appears as *siddhi.* He gives about thirty-four such powers ranging from knowing the past and future, reading the minds of others, becoming invisible at will, becoming strong like an elephant, graceful like a peacock, distinguishing concealed things, knowing about the solar system, lunar system, predicting world events, conquering hunger and thirst, walking on water, swamps and thorns, having divine visions and so on.

With all these so called supernatural or supernormal powers coming to the *sādhaka,* Patañjali cautions him so that he may not succumb to the temptations which lead to *chidra citta* or pores in the consciousness.

In order to keep the *sādhaka* in the esteemed state of untainted purity, Patañjali leads the *sādhaka* towards *Kaivalya Pāda*, by suggesting that the powers that one gains should be utilised with discriminative discretion so that the *sādhaka* does not become a victim of *bhoga.* By explaining the differences between *citta* - the consciousness - and *citi* - the eternal *puruṣa,* Patañjali encourages the *sādhaka* to become a *paravairāgi.*

Thus the summum bonum of yoga *(yoga phala)* is *ātma prasādanam,* the grace of the soul, whereby all actions are affliction-free and one lives in the pristine state of clarity and cleanliness moment to moment without getting involved in the spokes of the movements of time.

The kernel of yoga is that it takes one beyond time to live in the state of aloneness. The mirror of *citta* being cleaned, cleared and purified by the *yogasādhanā,* it reflects the pure soul. Hence, *citta* becomes *darpaṇa* (mirror) for the *ātman* to have its *darṣana* - the view. The viewer and view become one.

I would like to end with Vyāsa's quote - "Yoga is the teacher of yoga, yoga is to be understood through yoga, so live in yoga, to realise yoga, comprehend yoga through yoga. He who is free from distractions enjoys yoga through yoga."

Om Shantiḥ, Shantiḥ, Shantiḥ

FRESH MIND LEADS TOWARDS INTEGRATION*

Friends and fellow-seekers,

For the past thirty-five years I have been coming regularly to Europe and America, giving classes and demonstrations to bring the science of yoga to the people of the West. I regularly gave lectures and met students of yoga who wished to ask me questions and deepen their understanding of the subject. A number of my recent talks and question-and-answer sessions have now been brought together and rearranged in book form, and this book which you have in your hand – *Yoga Vṛkṣa, The Tree of Yoga* – can serve as a practical and philosophical companion to my earlier books, *Light on Yoga, Light on Prāṇāyāma* and *The Art of Yoga.* As you read it, you will discover the wealth and profundity of yoga which takes us from the surface of the skin to the depth of the soul.

I hope that this volume will be fruitful both for experienced practitioners of yoga and for those who are approaching the subject for the first time. It is my wish to share the joy of life through yoga with you all, and therefore I am glad to speak to you through this book. Yoga is bringing you and me together through these pages.

In the physical world one can climb a mountain from various directions. One way may be long but easy, another perhaps short but windy and difficult, still another straightforward but tedious. Yet by all these paths it is possible to reach the summit. It is similar in the search for spiritual knowledge. There are many methods, many avenues, many ways to experience the hidden core of our being, but we have to direct our minds which is caught up in the web of the pleasures of the world towards the very source of existence.

My subject is yoga. This path not only cultures the body and the senses, but refines the mind and civilises the intelligence to rest in the self. It is unfortunate that many people who have not penetrated the depth of yoga think of this spiritual path as being merely a physical discipline,

---

* From *Newsletter,* the B.K.S. Iyengar Yoga Association of Australasia Inc., vol. V, March 1989, on the occasion of the Australian edition of *Yoga Vṛkṣa, The Tree of Yoga.*

and consider it as a kind of gymnastics. But yoga is more than physical. It is cellular, mental, intellectual and spiritual – it involves man in his entire total being. It makes man an integrated person.

Think of the state of mind you were in before you began reading. The book was new and your mind too was fresh. You came with a fresh mind to look at this book. There were no ideas and no presumptions. If we can maintain that state in our daily lives, there comes integration. Fresh mind is untainted, untouched. Such a fresh mind can only get integrated. To be fully integrated means to integrate oneself totally from the body to the self and from the self to the body so that we live an integrated life with our neighbours and surroundings.

Integration is meditation and meditation is integration. Those who have no integration cannot speak of meditation, nor can those who have no experience of meditation say what integration is. The two are interconnected and interrelated. If you and I are integrated, the mind is silent in you and the mind is silent in me, yet we are alert and fully aware. If awareness is broken from time to time, it is known as distraction, and to bring the distracted mind again and again to a focal point is concentration. If this alert state of silence, which normally comes to us only in glimpses, continues for a very long time, then this concentration transforms into meditation.

When this uninterrupted awareness of integration of body, mind and self is retained, then there is no feeling of past or future. Time does not know past and future; time becomes eternal. That is integration, and in that state no differences or disparity can arise. I hope that if not today, then one day you may reach this state, the point of culmination. Remember, Self-realisation is culmination. Probably you might have heard something different – that the infinite cannot be seen or reached by the finite. But we have only finite means to know the infinite. When the finite merges in the infinite, everything become infinite. Here culminates the search of the Self.

Consider the sky. The sky is finite as well as infinite. None can touch it, yet we are in contact with it at every moment of our lives. Similarly, you and I have to use finite means – body, mind, intelligence and consciousness – to reach the soul which is the mother and father of all these evolutes. In this way, when we integrate ourselves to reach the infinite, we remain ever fresh, ever peaceful and intelligently aware.

God bless you all.

YOGA FOR PEACE OF MIND

Yoga, *samādhi* and *śānti* are synonymous terms which convey the same meaning. *Samādhi* is the experience of *śānti* or peace within oneself.

Samādhi means putting together, union, bringing into harmony, fixing the mind for attention on a thought, intense contemplation or meditation. *Samādhi* is an indivisible state of existence. It is to come face to face with soul.

Śānti means tranquillity, calmness, free from passion, an undisturbed state in the objects of pleasure or pain.

Yoga means to join, to bind and to unite the individual self with the Universal Self.

Before understanding the communion of the individual with the Universal Self one has to know how to bring union of one's body with mind and mind with the self. It is not easy to demarcate between body and mind and mind and self.

It is a known fact that there is no cohesion in man's body and nerves, nerves and organs, organs and senses, senses and mind, mind and intelligence, intelligence and will, will and consciousness, consciousness and conscience and conscience and self.

In order to bring all these evolutes of man in unison, sages codified the science of yoga. This vast scattered subject was systematised by sage Patañjali in his treatise with 196 terse *sūtra* about 500 to 200 BC and termed *aṣṭāṅga yoga,* comprising *yama, niyama, āsana, prāṇāyāma, pratyāhāra, dhāraṇā, dhyāna* and *samādhi.*

These aspects of yoga are like a gigantic mango tree which starts from the seed to the root, root to the trunk, trunk to the branches, branches sprouting into leaves, leaves aerating the entire tree supplying energy in the form of sap through the bark, and later blossom into flowers, culminating with tasty fruit.

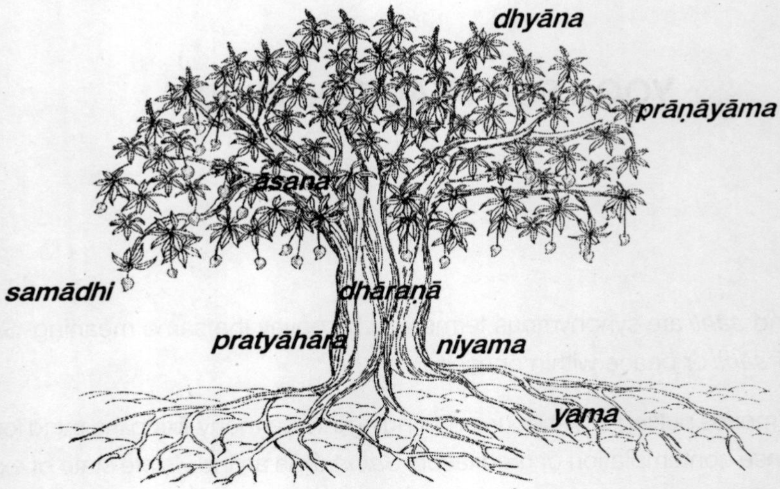

Plate n. 1 – Mango tree with the eight aspects of yoga

The eight disciplines of yoga are compared to the tree. The *yama* is the root; *niyama* is the trunk; *āsana* is the branches; *prāṇāyāma* is the leaves; *pratyāhāra* is the bark; sap the *dhāraṇā*, flower the *dhyāna* and fruit the *samādhi*. As the essence of the tree is concentrated in the fruit, the essence of yoga is in the experience of unalloyed bliss. This unalloyed bliss is *samādhi*, a spiritual bliss. As the fruit is the natural culmination of the tree, the art of yoga too terminates bringing the practitioner from darkness to light, from ignorance to knowledge, knowledge to wisdom and from wisdom to true happiness and unalloyed peace within himself.

THE EIGHT PETALS OF YOGA

Yama

Yama are *ahiṁsā*, *satya*, *asteya*, *brahmacarya* and *aparigraha*. These are considered universal ethics as they pertain to the whole of humanity all over the globe. They are logical virtues to be observed in life. *Yama* is the ethics that man has to follow while in contact with others. *Yama* teaches not to follow what is harmful to oneself as well as society. Such actions are known as actions of *vairāgya*.

Niyama

Niyama is the individual discipline which has to be observed within oneself. They are *śauca*, *santoṣa*, *tapas*, *svādhyāya* and *Īśvara praṇidhāna*. This is *abhyāsa* or practices to be observed daily.

Āsana

Āsana is for maintenance of health in the body and steadiness in mind. Health is not to be mistaken for mere existence. It is the balance of the body, mind and self. As far as the body is concerned, health is to bring the balance between all the three humours – *vāta*, *pitta* and *śleṣma*. These humours protect, sustain and support the body with the seven *dhātu* or ingredients, namely *rasa* (chyle), *rakta* (blood), *māṁsa* (flesh), *meda* (fat), *asthi* (bone), *majjā* (marrow) and *śukra* (semen). They not only keep the body immune from diseases but help to enjoy a positive, constructive and creative life.

The practice of *āsana* brings balance in the three humours and seven ingredients so that the three *mala* – faeces, urine and sweat – are thrown out of the body.

As far as the health of the mind is concerned, the practice of *āsana* keeps the balance in the three *guṇa*, namely *sattva*, *rajas* and *tamas*. These qualities illumine and activise the mind so that inertia does not take over.

Just as the goldsmith refines gold by heating and separating the ores, similarly the practice of *āsana* purges the senses of perception, cleanses the organs of action and strengthens the mind by dispelling its weaknesses. It frees the practitioner from the dualities of the body and mind, and mind and soul.

Prāṇāyāma

Prāṇa means energy. This energy may be physical, mental, intellectual, sexual, spiritual or cosmic energy. All vibrating energies are *prāṇa*. *Prāṇa* is the breath of all beings. The breath we draw in or out is the manifestation of the same *prāṇa*. The action and function of respiration is also *prāṇa*. *Āyāma* means extension, expansion, prolongation, regulation and restraint. Hence, *prāṇāyāma* means the prolongation and restraint of breath.

Prāṇāyāma has four actions. They are: 1) inhalation, 2) inhalation retention, 3) exhalation, and 4) exhalation retention. Inhalation is the intake of energy. Inhalation retention is the distribution of that drawn-in energy. Exhalation is the output of the used energy and exhalation retention is the state of pause for quietness in the body, nerves and mind. It is a resting period for the organs.

It is said in yoga texts that where there is mind there the breath is, and where there is breath there rests the mind. If the breath scatters, the mind wanders. If mind wanders, the breath scatters. So still the breath to still the mind. Mind is the king of the senses, breath is the king of mind. *Prāṇāyāma* makes the breathing rhythmic. The steady and rhythmic flow of energy in the form of breath depends upon the rhythm of *nāḍī* - the pulsation of blood vessels - and *nāda* - the sound and vibration of *nāḍī*.

This controlled and disciplined flow of breath helps the mind to concentrate with ease and *prāṇāyāma* acts as a unifying bridge between the mind and the self and helps the vital energy to flow uninterruptedly. It regulates man's habits, desires and actions and lead him towards the door of spiritual discipline.

Pratyāhāra

Pratyāhāra means keeping back or restraining the organs. After years of regular practice of *āsana* and *prāṇāyāma*, the mind and the senses are brought under control. When the senses are made to withdraw from the objects of desires, the mind is released from the pull of the senses. Hence, the senses cannot dominate over the mind. The mind which was held by the power of the senses finds release, turns inwards and the *sādhaka* is set free from the tyranny of the senses. This is *pratyāhāra*.

Dhāraṇā, dhyāna* and *samādhi

Dhāraṇā, dhyāna and *samādhi* are known by the technical term of *saṁyama*. *Saṁyama* means integration - integration of body, breath, mind, intelligence and self.

It is not easy to explain the last three aspects of yoga as separate entities. When concentration is prolonged in time, it becomes *dhyāna*. It is *samādhi* when absorption takes place. The object of attention, the instruments used for attention and the person who attends become one. In short, the knower, the knowing and the object of knowledge become one. *Dhāraṇā* means the act of holding, retaining or keeping the mind collected. So *dhāraṇā* is to bring the wandering mind into a single point of concentration or to be totally attentive in doing one's work with dedication and devotion. When one gets involved attentively, continually for a long period, it becomes *dhyāna* by itself. Body and mind, knowledge and experience get united. All actions from then on become effortless and pure. The only difference between *dhāraṇā* and *dhyāna* is that in *dhāraṇā* there is tension and stress. They are felt due to the action of bringing the scattered nerves and brain towards attention, whereas, in *dhyāna*, release, expansion, quietness and peace are experienced. The prolonged state of this quietness makes man free from attachments and indifferent towards the joy of pleasures or the sorrows of pain. Both are the same for him. The fruit of the discipline of *aṣṭāṅga yoga* is the experiencing of the state of oneness, *samādhi*.

Though man is born free, nature's heritage consists of three *guṇa*, *sattva*, *rajas* and *tamas*, which entwine him. He gets caught in the web of these *guṇa*. He is moulded and remoulded by his actions and reactions and his mind is endowed according to his own behaviour. Thus, he is caught up in deeds of his own making, the *preya* (pleasures) and *śreya* (auspicious and good).

The modes of mind, according to the predominance of *guṇa*, are categorised by Vyāsa into five states. They are *mūḍha*, *kṣipta*, *vikṣipta*, *ekāgra* and *niruddha*. *Mūḍhan* is he who is dull and stupid because of predominance of *tamōguṇa*. He begins with *yama* and *niyama*. *Kṣiptan* is he whose mind is scattered. Being in disarray, he hankers for objects but does not make efforts: he remains in a state of neglect. He is introduced to *yama*, *niyama* and *āsana*. *Vikṣiptan* is he who is agitated and distracted. He has the capacity to get what he desires, but his will is not marshalled or controlled. He is taught to practise *yama*, *niyama*, *āsana* and *prāṇāyāma*. As his mind oscillates between *tamas* and *rajas* or in *tamoraja* or *rajotama*, these aspects of yoga develop *rajoguna* in him to act. *Ekāgran* is he whose mental faculties are concentrated on a single object. He is very attentive and intensely active and knows exactly what he wants and rightly uses his powers to achieve his goal. This determined effort also makes him rigid, leading to selfishness. Hence, he is introduced, in addition to the above four aspects, to *pratyāhāra* (withdrawal of senses), *dhāraṇā* (concentration) and *dhyāna* (meditation). This makes him develop *sattvaguṇa*. Otherwise, *ekāgra* mind is of *rajosatva* or *satvaraja*, one slightly predominating over the other. *Niruddhan* is a highly *sāttvic* man. He practises all the eight petals of yoga, refines his intelligence and uses it meaningfully by synchronising ideas with facts and reason. His experiences and analysis tally with each other without room for doubts. This state is that of a healthy wise man. He is then a yogi and a saint.

The *Upaniṣads* and the *Bhagavad Gītā* proclaim that the mind, the cause of bondage or liberation, always plays a dual role. On the one hand it is caught up with the pleasures of the world and on the other it strives to gain freedom. Mind is bound with *avidyā*, *asmitā*, *rāga*, *dveṣa* and *abhiniveśa* (*Yoga Sūtra*, II.3).

Avidyā is the acceptance of non-eternal as eternal, impure as pure, non-Self as Self and living in material pleasures as if they were permanent pleasures. This causes egoism – *asmitā* – which in turn perverts the way of thinking. *Rāga* attracts more comforts and pleasures, and if they are not achieved, brings sorrow and hatred – *dveṣa* –towards his fellow beings. In spite of having all these afflictions and problems, there is a strong attachment to living – *abhiniveśa* – since there is a fear of death.

No doubt, today with his technological and scientific background, man has conquered ignorance, but he is caught in the pride of knowledge. This pride of knowledge brings competition between men and causes strains and stresses. In order to cope with competition, speed has crept into his thinking and action. These three, namely strain, stress and speed have made man a miserable creature on earth. His physical frame has started to wane, his nerves have got tight and tensed. He cannot release his tensions. So his thinking faculty has been affected and anxieties multiplied. Doubts and incapabilities set in. Attitudes of jealousy and malice have developed. He has become negative in his approach to life, evasive, reserved, indifferent, depressed, lazy, ill at ease and has created his own philosophy of illusion, seclusion and isolation. In order to find freedom from anxieties and restfulness, he has switched to artificial ways of living. He is addicted to tranquilisers, sleeping pills, alcohol and various other psychedelic drugs or sexual acts to find relief. These methods have allowed him to forget himself temporarily but the cause remains unsolved and troubles return unabated.

Most of us are aware that the reasons for our mental ill-health and imbalances are stresses, strains, incapacity to face day-to-day problems, depression, wrong concepts, false hypotheses, fanciful ideas, fears of insecurity, lack of desire, enthusiasm, will and drive, inaction, shunning society and so on. Patañjali, the codifier of yoga, had the foresight and vision to narrate the reasons which afflict man and disturb his peace and poise. They are: 1) *vyādhi,* 2) *styāna*, 3) *saṁśaya,* 4) *pramāda,* 5) *ālasya,* 6) *avirati,* 7) *bhrāntidarśana*, 8) *alabdhabhūmikatva*, 9) *anavasthitatva,* 10) *duḥkha,* 11) *daurmanasya,* 12) *aṅgamejayatva*, and lastly 13) *śvāsapraśvāsa.* All these can be further divided as dormant, attenuated, fluctuating or fully active.[1] From this division it is enough to say what extraordinary attention and action is required by man to keep his fortress free from the attacks of enemies as enumerated above in order to experience the unalloyed peace.

Yoga is the only science and art which eradicates all the above causes of affliction and disciplines the mind, emotions, intelligence, will and reason so that poise is gained in oneself leading to a renewed harmonious life without the prejudices of the past or future but with the present which is ever fresh. With this freshness we can do all our worldly duties, whilst maintaining mental peace in all situations.

Thoughts in our mind gush out like a turbulent river which can be tamed only with the construction of a dam. Similarly, the rising thoughts have to be controlled by developing a sound health in the body and nerves for the mind to think constructively, positively and usefully.

1 *Y.S.,* I.30. See the author's *Light on the Yoga Sūtras of Patañjali,* pp. 78-79, Harper Collins, London; see also in this volume, "Yoga For Stress-Free Life".

Just knowing about yoga is not going to give relief from sorrow, anxiety and depression. They may inspire, but daily practice of yoga alone will keep man to face the turmoils of life with steadiness and stability.

Along with the modern discoveries of medicine, mental and physical disorders have to be combated with one's own determined discipline, vigour and vitality, faith and earnestness.

I would like to bring to your notice that at a recently held conference on hypertension, the doctors were of the opinion that yoga and meditation offer no cure for such people. First of all, to differentiate yoga and meditation is wrong and, as far as my experience goes in the art of teaching, it is quite the opposite. My pupils, many of whom are physicians and surgeons, are benefited by yoga. Correct and persistent practice is essential in all these cases. Secondly no yogi with a thorough knowledge teaches *Sālamba Śīrṣāsana, Dhanurāsana* or *Mayūrāsana*[1] to such patients. In *Sālamba Śīrṣāsana* there is pressure on the throat and temples and respiration becomes heavy whereas in other two, the diaphragm is compressed which pushes up the blood-pressure. There are hundreds and hundreds of *āsana* which are used according to the condition, constitution and mental state of the person. A wrong diagnosis or wrong introduction of medicine does cause adverse results on the patient. So also in yoga there is a certain method to be adopted and it differs as the constitution differs.

Now let me say a few words about meditation. As man is a triune of intelligence, emotion and action, he is bestowed with head – seat of *jñāna* –, trunk – seat of emotion – and arms and legs – seat of action. Hence the great saints and yogis of yore discovered three paths *(mārgas)*, namely *jñāna, bhakti* and *karma*. In order to have perfect clarity in thinking and understanding, stability in mind and emotions and purity in action, *aṣṭāṅga yoga* was introduced as a fourth path.

Though *aṣṭāṅga yoga* is considered as a fourth path, it actually is a base for the three paths, namely, *jñāna, bhakti* and *karma*.

In yoga it is taught how to unite the body, the breath, the mind, intelligence and self, and all are made to balance evenly like the string holding the pearls of a necklace together. Then the practitioner is made to create a state of emptiness in his body, nerves, brain and mind through slow, soft exhalation without advising him to do deep inhalation. This creates in him a state of non-existence, bringing requisite serenity in the cells of the body. This in turn relaxes the facial muscles. When the facial muscles are relaxed, the senses of perception are released from tension. When the senses of perception are relaxed, the brain, which is constantly in contact with

---

[1] For a descrption of these *āsana* see *Light on Yoga*, Harper Collins, London.

these senses, becomes void. So no thinking process takes place. Intelligence, which is constantly in the head throughout the wakeful state is made to descend to its source, which is known as the sub-conscious seat.

In the *Chāndogya Upaniṣad* (VIII.3.3) it is said that, *Hṛdy ayaṁ iti hṛdayam* (The *ātman* dwells in the heart, hence it is called *hṛdayam* = heart). It is here that energy and intelligence take their origin. When one is active they move towards the brain and when one is at sleep they rest at their source. Realising this dual path of intelligence, we are taught to remain consciously in the source. Then our mind too is sublimated. This is stability of mind. When this is achieved, we are made to learn to stop the invading thoughts to enter either in mind or brain. Here we are made to experience a mindless state. When we develop these qualities, we do our work not only quickly but also well. We have a dynamic energy but will not allow it to dissipate unnecessarily. When man gains this condition of mind, how can he ever have hypertension! Instead of that our mind is cool and collected.

When such is the discipline and effect of yoga, I cannot comprehend the casual remarks of so-called scientific minds who think that they can criticise anything and everything which is not congenial to them. Have drugs found remedies for all ailments? If they fail in their treatment, they brand the disease an allergic disease. If yogis fail, they make a mountain of it. Many people die of heart attacks while in bed. Could anyone prohibit them to rest in bed? If a man walks or drives carelessly in the streets, he is bound to face an accident. So also if yoga is done thoughtlessly anything might happen. If it is done thoughtfully, no doubt it is a panacea for many ills. Yoga is an art, it is a science and it is a philosophy. As all other sciences and arts are respected, one should respect this also. If yoga was useless, it would not have withstood the onslaught of generations. It is still the most respected basic art for keeping the body, mind and soul in unison and peace. I sum up yoga saying that its essence is the dissolution of ego and development of humility and purity in thought, word and deed.

Before concluding, let me remind you that the person who practises yoga regularly will become a master of circumstance as well as the master of time. Yoga is the golden key that unlocks the door of peace, tranquillity and joy which have no limitations, frontiers or boundaries. He loves to live, lives to serve and serves the world with beauty and grandeur. This is the essence of life. Peace within and peace without. Peace in the individual, in family, in society and in the world at large.

Yoga leads towards *samādhi* and *samādhi* leads towards *śānti*.

RECOGNISE THE *VṚTTI*, KNOW THE *CITTA*, REACH THE SOUL

Today is Vyāsa Pūrṇimā day, which celebrates not only the emotional ties between a guru and śiṣya (teacher and pupil), but also the growth and expansion of intelligence that develops from this close relationship between the two.

You as pupils have come to me with some imbibed intelligence according to your capacities. Intellect is acquired through study and then gets further charged by putting the acquired study into practice, gaining the experience by which to reach matured wisdom.

Vyāsa Maharshi is considered as the incarnation of an exalted wisdom in whom the evolved intellect fully flourished into an ocean of knowledge. Vyāsa touched and tasted each and every faculty of knowledge.

Today is the day where we need to further sharpen our intelligence with wisdom. Though there are emotional ties between the teacher and the pupil, one has to keep these emotions aside in order to sharpen the intelligence.

Truth is harsh but stable. Similarly, the intelligence also is harsh and stable whereas emotion is not. In a way, you need to be firm within yourselves without excuses in order to have that wisdom. We have to excuse the mistakes of others, whereas as yoga *sādhaka* we have judiciously to face up to consequences without that word – excuse. We human beings normally remain harsh to others and soft to ourselves. We need to reverse this process in order to develop the characteristics of Vyāsa.

The meeting of *guru* and *śiṣya* today signifies the emotional base in the relationship. From tomorrow onwards, however, we have to forget these emotional knots but to walk on the razor edge of intelligence through *sādhanā*.

On this *pūrṇimā* day the moon shines gloriously and brilliantly. Let our intelligence, like the moon, shine brilliantly in our practices of yoga. The light of the moon is cool which soothes the heart. Let us together develop that coolness in the seat of our head and heart. Let us build up serenity in the heart and sharpness of awareness in the head. Let us keep our eyes wide open to see the full moon as we cannot see the sun with open eyes. From today onwards learn to keep the eyes open to see the inner dark world in your *sādhanā*. As the inner darkness begins gradually to fade, perhaps the Self may begin to shine on its own like the sun. See the moon (the waning and waxing of consciousness) first, then the sun (the *ātman*) will shine on its own. I have often said that the Self is sun and *citta* is moon. The moon has not got its own light, but borrows its light from the sun and illumines the night. In the same way, the brightness of the *ātman* illumines the *citta*.

Vyāsa for us is like the sun, who enlightens us in the knowledge of the Self. Let us all pray to him for his grace to dawn on us.

RECOGNISE THE *VṚTTI*

The word *cittavṛtti* is a compound word. *Citta* means consciousness and *vṛtti* means its waves in the form of fluctuations. If *citta* is subject, *vṛtti* becomes the object. Obviously we are caught up in the object and therefore we do not go near the subject. The first thing for us is to learn or know this difference between *citta* and *cittavṛtti* and to differentiate *citta* from *vṛtti*. *Citta* is the possessor and *vṛtti* is possessed. *Citta* is dressed in *vṛtti*. We need a sensitive intelligence to differentiate *vṛtti* from *citta*.

Often we think that tranquillity or peace *(śānti)* quietens the *vṛtti*. That is how people go to meditation. But peace or *śānti* is just a gross achievement. Normally, an average intellect recognises the disturbed mind and wants to calm down. As the person gets caught up in the mind, which is the outer layer of the consciousness, his mind makes him dance according to its whims and wishes. Hence, man hankers after *śānti* or for peace of mind. This *manaḥśānti* or peace of mind is neither the aim of yoga nor the end of meditation. Undoubtedly, *śānti* is a necessary element towards Self-realisation. No doubt it is required. It is acquired to a great extent by all of us in our practices of *yama, niyama, āsana, prāṇāyāma* and *pratyāhāra*. These practices do bring *manaḥśānti*. However, *śānti* is not the end but the essential step to move towards one-pointedness of the *citta*. When this essential step of tranquillity of mind is reached, there begins *dhāraṇā, dhyāna* and *samādhi*.

HOW TRANSFORMATION TAKES PLACE

Before attempting *citta vṛtti nirodha*, one has to have *śānti*, a pensive mind with which to identify the *vṛtti* of body and mind. We have *sthūla śarīra* – the gross body, *sūkṣma śarīra* – the subtle body, and *kāraṇa śarīra* – the causal body. In short this means that the body is *sthūla śarīra*, the mind, *sūkṣma śarīra*, and the Self, *kāraṇa śarīra*.

When you begin to practise yoga, the gross body and the outer mind have to be motivated to act first and then you have to bring the outer mind to come in contact with the inner mind. The body though gross in nature has its own way of behaviour. It has its moods, modes and fancies. The *vṛtti* of *citta* flow right up to the outer layer of body. Therefore body gets influenced by *vṛtti*. We all know that the mind gets affected by dualities such as heat and cold, honour and dishonour, hope and despair, success and failure and so on. At the same time we cannot deny the fact that these dualities of the mind affect the body too. The *vṛtti* of *citta* are categorised and crystallised into five forms. When a pebble or stone is thrown in the lake, we see the circles of waves forming around it. Each circle opens further to a new horizon and the biggest vanishes in the water. Similarly, the stone in the form of thought waves which could be *pramāṇa* (correct intelligence), *viparyaya* (perverse intelligence), *vikalpa* (imaginative intelligence), *nidrā* (sleep or restful intelligence) and *smṛti* (memory or remindful intelligence) is thrown in the lake of consciousness, *citta*. The circle of waves spreads upto the body and beyond leaving its imprint strongly on one's self.

The practice of *āsana* and *prāṇāyāma* based on the foundation of *yama* and *niyama* reverses the *vṛtti* so that the body and outer mind do not receive this onslaught of ripples. Here comes the judicious practice of *āsana* and *prāṇāyāma*. The *āsana* and *prāṇāyāma*, when practised attentively, accurately and meticulously, as I have explained very often, the physical body – *sthūla śarīra* – connects to the mental body – *sūkṣma śarīra* – and the mental body to the causal body – *kāraṇa śarīra*. The practice of *āsana* and *prāṇāyāma* is a religious practice. I mean the religion that is based on virtue and righteousness. Religion has no compartments. It is a science that is meant for walking on a right and honest path and at the same time remaining within contact of the core of being. Earlier I said that *citta* is the subject and *vṛtti* is the object. Similarly the mind is the subject and the body is the object. And above all, the Self is the subject and the body, mind, intelligence and *citta* are the objects. As *vṛtti nirodha* has to take place, the *śarīra nirodha* also has to happen in the same way. While practising *āsana* and *prāṇāyāma* the body is moulded, shaped and disciplined in order to reach the inner mind. The practice in this sense has to be deep and penetrative.

No doubt, the body is the temple of the soul. Still, know that the body is *tāmasic*. *Tamas* is darkness. If the shrine itself is dark, how can you see the God dwelling inside? Let the shrine be lighted for it to radiate the light of knowledge *(jñānadīpti)*.

On new moon day, the moon is not seen in the sky, because the side of the moon facing the Earth remains opposite to the sun. The light is not reflected and that is why it is dark. Similarly, when all the evolutes of *prakṛti*, namely *śarīra* (body), *karmendriya* (organs of action), *jñānendriya* (senses of perception), *manas* (mind), *buddhi* (intelligence) and *ahaṁkāra* (I-ness) are occluded, there is darkness. They are illumined when the light of the Self is lit.

What is that dark era? It is ill health or disease that affects us. Hence, all the evolutes of nature from body to intelligence have to be trained, toned and tuned, to get rid of mental discomfort and physical disturbances so that one comes in close contact with the *ātman*. In order to experience this state, we have to reverse the movements of *vṛtti* from external worldly thoughts towards internal spiritual thoughts.

Let us see how the *vṛtti* fluctuate on the surface level. When you begin your practice, fluctuation occurs like, "Should I do or should I not do? What should I do? From where to begin? Oh!, I think I can do *Utthita Trikoṇāsana*. No, let me do some other *āsana* easier than *Trikoṇāsana*." This way of thinking and tossing the mind, are these not fluctuations? To choose the *āsana* without having any logical base or discipline of mind is also a fluctuation. So know these as *vṛtti*.

You may do *Utthita Trikoṇāsana*. The body performs. But you do not penetrate your intelligence and awareness into your inner body. As a result, you remain completely disoriented. The legs remain in one direction, the trunk is pulled in another direction, the head is thrown forward or backward. Where is the inner network? The arms, legs, trunk, head as well as the skin, muscles, bones, joints, including the organic body, remain disjointed without any inter-connection. Not only do you deviate from one *āsana* to another but you deviate even in that chosen *āsana*. Keep in mind that this does not work at all to lead you towards the final aim of emancipation. Practice of *āsana* and *prāṇāyāma* in the right sequence stabilises the scattered mind which in turn helps the body to remain firm and stable.

While practising, you do not feel what is wrong and what is right. You do not observe what is perceivable which could be corrected. For example, in *Utthita Trikoṇāsana*, you do not apply your logical deliberation to look and feel whether the distance between legs is perfect or notice what happens when the distance is more or less. Often you do not remember the instructions given by the teachers. The organs of perception fail the imprints of memory. If an *āsana* is done absent-mindedly, where is the project of single mindedness? All these are the disturbing *vṛtti* in practice. In our every day's work, if there is no attention and the mind remains undetermined, disoriented and scattered, how can such a mind suddenly be brought under control through meditation? Before jumping into *dhyāna*, you first need to discipline, plan and organise the mind. This is what the *āsana* and *prāṇāyāma* teach.

Suppose you plan to do standing *āsana* and begin *Utthita Trikoṇāsana* without attempting *Taḍāsana*, the disorientation begins. Again, when you are asked to check your feet, toes, ankles, legs, arms, wrists, fingers and trunk, you may think you have aligned, but you do not verify whether these actions done are really aligned. Is it not a misconception of mind? You imagine that you have done it. Here, the imagination is self cheating. If somebody gives a false promise, you know that you have been cheated. Similarly in *sādhanā*, heedlessness and carelessness is like cheating yourself. Hence, inter-action is needed within oneself in body, mind, intelligence and consciousness. I studied on myself in this way and practised with prudence *(nīti)* with a distinct method *(rīti)*. Through these means, I repeatedly recognised my own *vṛtti* and examined by study to reach a steady state in body, mind and self.

In *Sālamba Śīrṣāsana*, if I forget the presence of my legs, there is a sleepy state of mind. Then I do not experience my legs. If I take for granted that my legs are straight, it is just a cherished dream and not the actual or factual happening. People cherish the dream as if they have bought and won a lottery ticket.

While in an *āsana*, watch your body, organs of action, senses of perception, mind, intelligence and consciousness and the most intricate one, the actor, dramatist in you – the impostor or the duplicator of the Self, the ego. Let them not project themselves as Self. Especially watch the 'I', which says, "I am doing. I have done, I am perfect. I have not committed a mistake and I have conquered the *āsana*. Hence, I do not need any correction." This type of dialogue is not from *buddhi* but from the ego. The ego shuts the door of *buddhi* and says, "I am perfect and I am serene". This is the threshold of failure which may in course of time make one a *yogabhrasta*.[1]

Learn to transform the mind, intelligence and 'I' to go from outside in. Your practice has to change for the better in the physical body, nervous system, behavioural pattern, character, psychological interaction and sublimation of 'I'. Therefore, Patañjali has introduced *yama* as the first aspect. Through *yama (nīti)*[2] and *niyama (rīti)*,[3] he asks you to check your behaviour and action. Through *āsana* and *prāṇāyāma*, he wants your body, mind, intelligence and I-consciousness to be transformed towards deeper and higher knowledge. As discipline is the first fundamental required quality for the transformation, Patañjali introduced the first steps as *yama, niyama, āsana* and *prāṇāyāma*.

Unfortunately, today the "fast food trend" has entered even in the spiritual field. Every one wants everything fast and expects the results faster. Painkiller is a fast reliever from pain. A caesarean is quick relief for pregnant mothers. Fast food is a convenience for householders. Similarly, meditation is considered as a fast food in yoga – "Meditate and get freedom". As the fast food, painkillers and unwanted caesareans all are harmful and futile in the long run, so also this fast meditation is bound to be harmful and futile.

---

[1] One who has fallen from the state or position of yoga.

[2] *Nīti* – A right, moral and wise conduct.

[3] *Rīti* – A way, course, custom, a method of practice.

As *guru* transmits his light of knowledge to *śiṣya* or sun enlightens the moon, similarly each aspect of yoga transmits and enlightens the next aspect. In yoga, *yama* casts light on and strengthens *niyama*. *Yama* and *niyama* for *āsana* and *prāṇāyāma* practice and so on. In fact the *śānti* or placidity of mind is gathered from each aspect of yoga like the bee gathering honey from each flower. This peace or placidity is the touchstone for transformation. The practitioner has to watch the role of *vṛtti* in the three layers, body, mind and Self – *sthūla, sūkṣma* and *kāraṇa śarīra*. The waves of *vṛtti* remain gross at gross body level, subtle at that of the subtle body and causal in root form at the causal body. Through practice of *āsana* and *prāṇāyāma*, one learns to recognise their existence at all levels. They cannot be swept away as easily as you sweep your room. They need to be transformed through practice and renunciation *(abhyāsa* and *vairāgya)*.

From now on, watch these *vṛtti* while practising. See how they change their mood and modes. See how the *vṛtti* get restrained. The clouds covering the moon make the moon invisible. *Vṛtti* covering *citta* make the *citta* invisible. The wind moves the clouds aside. Let your *prāṇāśakti* move and melt the *vṛtti* for you to see the *citta*. *Citta* is like a dark cloud on the Self. Let *citta* be brightened and illumined with clarity so that the Self shines like the sun.

The message for today is that while practising remove the *vṛtti* that cover your body, mind, intelligence and 'I' so that peace and placidity set in and make you become a new person, a new being and a yogin.

KĀYABRAHMA TO *ĀTMABRAHMA*

Taittirīya Upaniṣad[1] says, *Annam brahma, prāṇam brahma, vijñānam brahma,* – the *ātmā* is *brahma*. Similarly, for us *āsana* is *brahma, prāṇāyāma* is *brahma, dhyāna is brahma* and know that the body is also *brahma,* which is nourished, nurtured and kept alive by food – *(kāya brahma, kāya* is body).

There is a very educative story in *Bhṛgu vallī* of *Taittirīya Upaniṣad.*[2] *Ṛṣi* Varuṇa had a son called Bhṛgu. He was known as Bhṛgu Vāruṇi. Bhṛgu was studying *Veda* from his father Varuṇa. As he was progressing in his studies, he developed much interest in *Brahmavidyā.* He approached his father with humbleness and asked him to teach and enlighten him so that he might know *brahma. Varuṇa* spoke thus to his son, "Know well that food, energy, eyes, ears, mind and speech are *brahma".* What did he mean by this? He meant that *annam* – food, *prāṇa* – energy, *cakṣu* – eyes, *śrotṛ* – ears, *manas* – mind and *vācā* – the organ of speech, are the gateways, the instruments to know *brahma.*

Then the son asks his father how to know this. Varuṇa *ṛṣi* asks him to do *tapas* and makes him understand step by step, stage by stage, what *brahma* is. Knowing very well that spiritual knowledge does not come without *tapas,* Bhṛgu does *tapas.* First he realises, *annam brahmeti* – food is *brahman.* The very seed of our birth is in food. The parental body which is nourished and nurtured on food forms *sapta dhātu.*[3] The sperm and ovum are built up on food. Human beings remain alive because of food and after death they merge back into the food-chain. Therefore, Bhṛgu realises at the first stage, *annam brahmeti vyajanāt* – know that food is *brahma.* When he approaches his father Varuṇa, he is told, "Go again. Do *tapas".* He says, *"tapo brahmeti"* – *tapas* itself is *brahma.* "Do *tapas* and know *brahma".*

---

1 *Taittirīya Upaniṣad,* III *(Bhṛgu Vallī).*

2 *Taittirīya Upaniṣad* has three chapters, *Śikṣā vallī, Brahmānanda vallī* and *Bhṛgu vallī.*

3 *Rasa* (chyle), *rakta* (blood), *māṁsa* (flesh), *medha* (fat), *asthi* (bone), *majja* (marrow) and *śukra* (semen) or *śoṇita* (ovum) are the *sapta dhātu.*

And in this way Varuṇa *ṛṣi* asks Bhṛgu to do *tapas* and through *tapas* he asks him to realise *brahma* by peeling off each sheath.

Brahma is a word derived from the verbal root *'bṛih'* which means to grow, to expand. It indicates a strong and vast expanse. The root question of Bhṛgu here is what the substratum is and what is the ultimate and supreme which is both all and above all. The answer is *brahma*. *Brahma* is in us and we are in *brahma*.

Varuṇa indicates how food, energy, the *ātman*, everything is *brahma* and *tapas* is also *brahma*.

If *tapas* is *brahma*, can't we say *āsana* is *brahma*, *prāṇāyāma* is *brahma?* Of course one has to practise in that manner.

So let us transform the *śarira brahma*, the temple of the Soul into a real shrine in which the Self may shine. That is why so many *āsana* were given, for the simple reason that some weaknesses unknowingly may set into our system. It may be a physical ailment, an organic ailment, nervous ailment, biological ailment, mental ailment, intellectual ailment or whatever. The innumerable *āsana* are meant to keep the shrine clean and sacred. If *āsana* is *brahma*, *prāṇāyāma* is *brahma*. We need to see whether our practice of *āsana* and *prāṇāyāma* proves this saying of *Upaniṣad* that everything is *brahma*. The *sādhaka* has to elevate his *tapas* to the highest stage to realise that his *tapas* (instrument) is *brahma* and his goal is also *brahma*.

We need to search the *brahma* in our practice of *āsana* at each area within our bodies, since *brahma* is all pervasive and interwoven length-wise, cross-wise, width-wise, all-dimension-wise (ota-prota).

If I point out just a remote area like inner and outer armpits, one may laugh at me but you may not know of even lift or stretch in the armpits. For me *brahma* is there and *brahma* is in an *āsana* too. This observation and re-orientation is *tapas*.

I give one example of right learning which you can all begin to understand. You have all done *Vīrabhadrāsana* II. Right? And when you do *Vīrabhadrāsana* II you want to extend your armpits while stretching both hands. When the teacher says to go to *Utthita Pārśvakoṇāsana* from *Vīrabhadrāsana* II, you forget the attention on the armpits. Watch your inattentive mind at that moment to understand how *āsana* teach you to sharpen your intelligence. You lose your attention to extension on the side you are doing. You do not know how the mind which existed in the armpits of *Vīrabhadrāsana* II disappeared when you went to *Utthita Pārśvakoṇāsana*. Mind is also *brahma*. One should not shrink it. Can anybody say that he retained the armpit as it was

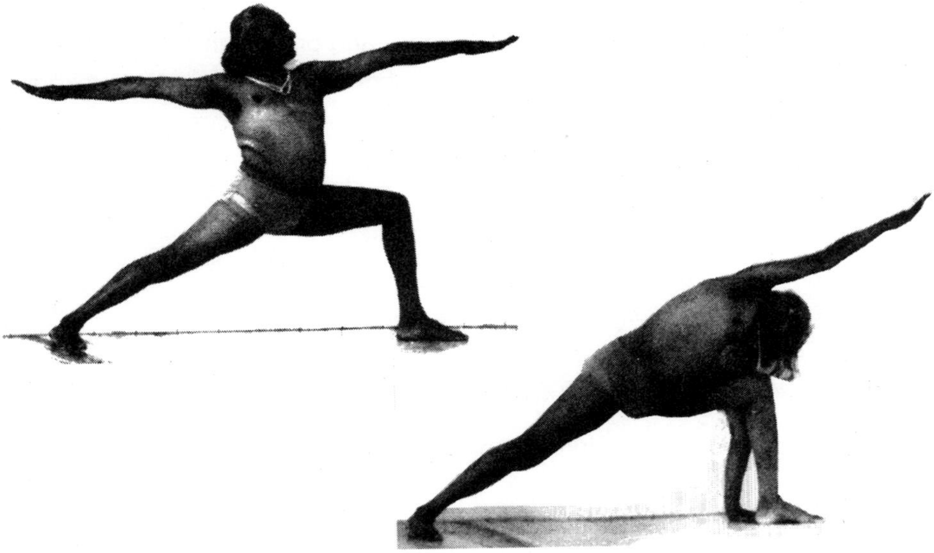

Plate n. 2 – *Vīrabhadrāsana* II and *Utthita Pārśvakoṇāsana*

in *Vīrabhadrāsana* II? Can anyone lift a finger saying, "Yes I do keep it?" Find out. The moment you go to *Utthita Pārśvakoṇāsana* you shrink the armpit, you shrink the body, you shrink the mind, you shrink the self. And if you forget this way, how can you know the self? Just one example is sufficient to know the waning and waxing of your mind and consciousness. Even in *Utthita Pārśvakoṇāsana*, when your teacher tells you to stretch your armpit, you do not stretch both banks of the armpit evenly and totally. Bhṛgu obeyed the orders of his *guru* Varuṇa. But you do not. Only a compartmental stretch of the armpit is done by all of you, but not the full armpit stretch. Probably you do not understand at all, or you are not aware of the existence of the armpits. You may have been doing this for years but the mind does not come there and reach to expand and stretch. It means the grace has not still fallen on your efforts. So when you see even one point with that intensity and honesty which I gave you just now as an example, and you start projecting that point you will know that you also will be graced by God because God as all pervasive witness ever-watches to see if people are well understanding their *annamaya śarira brahma*, so He can say, "Let Me go and guide them to understand the *ātma brahma*.[1] God is light, God is knowledge.

[1] *Bhṛgu vallī: anando brahmeti vyajānāt* (III.6.1).

In each *āsana* there is a hidden knowledge which one does not explore at all. One needs to do *tapas* for it. The others who do not know the value of *āsana* at all, call it body culture. They do not know the positioning of the body properly and pride themselves as Self-realised persons. Not that they are ignorant, but they are absent-minded. So you have to take away the absent-mindedness from your practice. Absent-mindedness is night, whereas present-mindedness is day. You will enjoy *āsana* when you have developed this present-mindedness.

It is said in the *Bhagavad Gītā:*

Yā niśā sarvabhūtānāṁ
tasyāṁ jāgarti saṁyamī /
Yasyām jāgrati bhūtāni
sā niśā paśyato muneḥ // (II.69).

Day for a sage or a *muni* is night for normal human beings and what is day for human beings is night for the sage.

Day to the *muni* is when he lives in the *Ātman*. For others it is night, since they live and dangle from the vehicles of the *Ātman*. If you practise with full awareness and presence of mind, the Self, like the daylight, shines brightly. If your practice is with absent-mindedness and carelessness, then you are dependent on the vehicles of the *ātman* and this is darkness in your *sādhanā*. The practice has to be such that the vehicles of the soul gravitate towards the soul. *Āsana* teaches you to be in that daylight – to be with the soul.

The mind keeps you in the dark. The body is already in the dark. Pleasures lead you towards darkness. Once in a while pains awaken and sensitise you but you do not pay attention. You want to be in the web of pleasures, thinking that it is heaven. You develop aversion to pain but you do not know that the pain is the eye-opener. It says, "My dear friend, pleasure is the ground for pain. Avoid pleasures, I will be no more". But you do not listen to it.

The way I have explained is just one aspect of an *āsana*. If you act from the bottom of the feet to the tip of the middle finger and from head to foot in each *āsana*, then you experience:

pūrṇamadaḥ pūrṇamidaṁ pūrṇāt pūrṇamudacyate
pūrṇasya pūrṇamādāya pūrṇam eva avaśiṣyate.[1]

You are full here, you are full there and from fullness you live in fullness. There is no emptiness here or there. Learn this language. There is no emptiness. There is *śānti*, not in terms of emptiness but in terms of fullness.

---

[1] Whole is that, whole too is this; from whole, whole comes; take whole from whole, yet whole remains. *(Īśopaniṣad,* the opening invocation).

Kāyā is *brahma, manas* is *brahma.* The word *brahma* itself indicates fullness, completeness and vastness.

If *āsana* has to be complete, you cannot forget any part. You cannot remain absent anywhere. The body and mind both have to be free from pleasure and pain to experience fullness in the practice of an *āsana.* The completeness brings contentment. Contentment leads towards quietude.

Today everybody says, "Close your eyes and do the *āsana.*" Find out yourselves whether that leads to fullness or emptiness. See the meaning of *pūrṇa* in *pūrṇam adaṁ* and *pūrṇam idaṁ.* What a difference it makes for us who are the practitioners with eyes open to interpenetrate and bring completeness and fullness in *āsana.* But things are twisted conveniently. You see only convenience and contentment, and not beyond. But is it a real contentment? You do not test whether it is real or unreal, full or partial, basic or superficial. So with convenient contentment, which is momentary, you are happy.

The mind is a big cheater. It is said that mind is a friend and foe. Often it proves to be a foe. You need to befriend it by the disciplines of yoga. Caught in the spokes of organs of action and senses of perception, mind flies like a kite with the thread of attachment in the sky of pleasure, not knowing that pain and pleasure lay side by side. It is very difficult to liberate the mind from this attachment to pleasure and aversion to pain. It keeps on oscillating and fluctuating between them.

The practice of yoga undoubtedly calms the fluctuations of mind. Know very well that you have tremendous latent energy resources which can be awakened and channelled by the practice of *āsana, prāṇāyāma, pratyāhāra, dhāraṇā* and *dhyāna.* I am not omitting *yama, niyama* or *samādhi.* These five aspects can be carried on successfully only on the firm foundation of *yama* and *niyama.* And when these five practical aspects are carried out completely (and not compartmentally), *samādhi* is the result. All the *sādhanā* has to be converted and terminated in *samādhi.*

But, you need to carry the *yoga-bīja* in your *citta-bhūmi.* The seed of yoga has to be sown in the field of consciousness which is covered by the stones and rocks in the form of body, senses, mind, intelligence and ego. All these make the land barren. One needs love, devotion, dedication, attachment to yoga and to sacrifice all that is unyogic and unethical, merely giving worldly pleasures.

Let me explain *pūrṇatva* in *prāṇāyāma.* You may do simply a deep, soft, slow inhalation *(pūraka),* which takes you gradually from inner core·to the vast space. The *prāṇa-brahma* expands to reach vastness. Energy and consciousness unite to know their own incarnation of vastness – the *bṛhad*[1] form. When there is fullness and completeness, you reach a natural retention – *pūraka-kumbhaka,* which makes you experience the fulfilment in fullness – a state of *pūrṇatva.* Again when you exhale *(recaka),* it is the returning process of the *prāṇa-brahma* after having reached the state of fullness with satisfaction and contentment. It is not an emptiness but a process of reaching the inner core or the inner being. By this completeness in *recaka,* there is natural pause – *recaka-kumbhaka,* which comes on its own as a full stop. In this process, the *pūraka* is complete, *recaka* is complete, and both types of *kumbhaka* are complete. Nothing is lessened, nothing is compartmental *pūrṇaṁ adam, pūrṇaṁ idam* –inhalation is complete, the inhalation *kumbhaka* is also complete. Similarly, the exhalation is complete, so exhalation *kumbhaka* is also complete. *Pūrṇāt pūrṇaṁ udacyate* – the complete meets the complete and *pūrṇasya pūrṇam ādaya pūrṇam eva avaśiṣyate* – the completeness contributes completeness and in all states, only completeness remains.

When your awareness has reached everywhere, there comes a full stop. This is completeness. At this stage grace has dawned spontaneously through ripeness in practice and wisdom. From now on, you do not forget yoga and yoga does not forget you. You are yoga and yoga is you. You and yoga are now inseparable.

You just listened to the *bhajan.* The composer of the *bhajan,* Sahajobai, was willing to forget God but not ready to forget her *guru,* Charaṇḍas. The text of the *bhajan* was,

Rāma tajū pai guru na visāru I
Guru ko sama hari ko na niharu II
Charaṇḍāsa para tana mana vāru I
Guru na taju hari ko taja ḍāru II

meaning, I may abandon (forget) and sacrifice Rāma but never do I forget my *guru* – Charaṇḍās. I may meditate on *guru* rather than Hari (Lord Krishna). Oh! Charaṇḍās, my *guru.* I surrender myself totally (my body and mind) to you. I may sacrifice Hari (God) but not the *guru.*

The *bhajan* reminds me of my statement that I will not leave the practice of what I have learned, even if God tells me to leave. Sometime ago I said something which appeared in the papers and magazines, 'If God comes and tells me to stop my *āsana* practice, which is now

---

1 *Bṛhad* – vastness, expansion.

enough, I would say, "I had better think of my *āsana* practice and not of You."' The critics took advantage to criticise my statement, remarking my pride. But think of what the feeling of the saint was to her master Charaṇdās. She says, "I don't care for Rāma or Krishna but I will think of you, my *guru*." So for me, my *guru*, T. Krishnamacharya, opened my heart to my inner *guru* who guided me to this subject, so I cannot leave that even if God does not want to bless me. I say, "Never mind, the *guru* inside me has blessed me so I carry on." That's why I have not oscillated in my subject since the day I started. I have met and taught great intellectual wizards of the world. I got them to adopt yoga. I influenced them through yoga but they could not influence me. I have maintained my practice and I am refining it every day. I have stuck to yoga and made the intellectuals feel what yoga does for them and they continued their practices as yoga brought transformation in them.

This shows that the inner Grace was abundant in my practice. That's why I said that this *deha* (body) has changed into *brahma* by my yogic practices. For me, the very *sādhanā* is *brahma*. Therefore I want you and your body to change into that state of sacred *Brahma* through *tapas* of *yogasādhanā*.

God's blessings be upon you all.

THE GEM OF LIFE IS IN YOUR HANDS*

My heart is touched by your respect for me, which I gather from the vibrations of your loud applause. Even the sound was divine.

Friends, we are stuck with our limitations and hence, we have not found the depth of wealth this ocean of yoga has to offer. When children taste the water of the sea they say, "It is salt and nothing else." Whereas the scientists say, "The wealth of the world is hidden in the ocean." Similarly, the wealth of yoga is hidden.

The followers of yoga like you and me have to dip into it and bring out the jewel of yoga to the surface. Then not only do you taste the flavour and essence of yoga, but share the same with others so that they too taste yoga, not as salt water of the ocean, but as the hidden jewel of the mind.

You all go to the temple or church as the devotees of God. You pray and worship. But tell me, how many of you who have gone to a temple or church, have really concentrated on God or the cross more than five or ten seconds, though you may be there for hours? Even when we visit the holiest temples or the holiest churches, are we not tempted to turn our eyes in different directions and lend our ears to somebody talking? Is it not true that our attention and meditation on God is lost, whether it is in the temple or in the church? Similarly, in yoga we ramble and we lose that attention which is needed to trace the eternal *tattva* (truth), that is filled from within and without. In yoga we call this *puruṣa tattva* or the *ātma tattva*. We often think of all other things of the world; but we think of the *ātmā* only in a flash and forget about it immediately. Patañjali gave this art and philosophy of yoga so that the rambling and unsteadiness of our mind may be minimised or come to an end.

When Patañjali speaks about various impediments that come in the way of realising the soul, he guides us with compassion by ways and means to eradicate them, so that we cultivate

---

* *Guruji's* message, 14th Dec, 1999, RIMYI, Pune.

strength and vigour to face the Self with courage. Even highly sensitive intellectuals with their intellectual intoxication get frightened when they come face to face with the Self, because they do not train the mind for stability. Patañjali indicates the unsteadiness of the intelligence and calls this unsettled state *anavasthā*. When stability gets disturbed, fear of facing the immortal self sets in, but the intellectual pride or ego momentarily covers this fear. Even intellectuals may face this fear but appear on the surface to be stable personalities though remain unstable and empty within. Only through the stable growth of the intelligence, is the emptiness within eradicated.

A mirror covered with dust does not reflect properly. Similarly the *ātmā* or the Self, when tainted with *vṛtti* (thought waves), gets veiled, preventing the Self from revealing its own state. As a result of the closeness of the Self the thought waves get involved with the fluctuations of the consciousness which in turn build up imprints as *saṁskāra* (latent imprint) for future life.

When the mirror is left uncleaned over a long time, it may not reflect clearly at all. Though one takes more time to wipe it, some particles may stick and tarnish the mirror, refracting the image. Similarly, when the Self identifies with the continual imprints of the objects seen, it develops an impenetrable veil *(āvaraṇa)* that may take lifetimes to move. Therefore, in order to see that the Self is not covered by the dust of thought waves or mental rambling, Patañjali speaks of *yoga anuṣṭhānam* – the stable, ascetic and devotional practice of yoga. Yoga needs *anuṣṭhānam*, which shows the ways and means, through proper guidance, to recover and rediscover what we have lost in our mundane thoughts.

The ramblings of the *citta* go on moment to moment. We do not know in what thought wave we were a few seconds before and how one thought wave jumps to another, without any link. This is how disturbances in our thought waves continuously take place. In order to control these unlinked thought waves, Patañjali gave a *mantra* in the very first *sūtra* of *Samādhi Pāda: Atha yogānuśāsanam,* meaning "Follow the discipline which comprises eight petals".

In the fourth *sūtra* of the same *pāda*, Patañjali explicitly explains, *vṛtti sārūpyam itaratra,* which means the ramblings that take place in the consciousness entrammel the Self . These ramblings have a tremendous power over consciousness causing both the consciousness and the self to be in a state of unsettledness *(anavasthā)*. This is what I would like to bring to your attention, how fickleness continues to taunt the consciousness, distracting it from going towards the Self. Hence, Patañjali's teaching in the aphorism *yogaḥ citta vṛtti nirodhaḥ* (I.2) is to bring discipline and restraint to the waves of consciousness through yoga.

When the divagations of consciousness come to an end, the *puruṣa* keeps away from those thought waves, breaks the contact with the *vṛtti* and rests in its *avasthā* state. Patañjali thus concludes, *tadā draṣṭuḥ svarūpe avasthānam* (I.3), meaning "The Self, thereafter, dwells in its own pure and true splendour". If this pure *avasthā* was stable and steady in us throughout, Patañjali would not have used *tadā draṣṭuḥ svarūpe avasthānam.* This *sūtra* clearly mentions that due to the *vṛtti,* we are not able to trace the steady state of the Self and doubt the Self's splendour. We do not understand this missing link and hence we are all in a state of *anavasthā.*

In the third chapter Patañjali grooms and combs the same central idea or theme of the above *sūtra* as, *etena bhūtendriyeṣu dharma lakṣaṇa avasthā pariṇāmāḥ vyākhyātāḥ* (III.13). The rambling of the mind is its *dharma* and *śāsana* is *lakṣaṇa dharma. Śāsana* is to govern or discipline. This *lakṣaṇa dharma* is to bring out, govern or monitor the right attitude in the thought waves with a qualitative intelligence. You irrigate the field to cultivate good crops. Similarly you have to irrigate the good, pure and auspicious thought waves. This is known as *lakṣaṇa.* The quality which you have to build up in them has to soak totally into the *puruṣa* so that they are quietened. This is the intelligent act of making the seer abide in his own pristine pure state. This is actually what we have to attempt, to reach this optimum level of non-oscillation so that no *anavasthā* comes in between our practices from the start to the end. This being the gamut of yoga, we have to take this *śāsana* to our heart in our *sādhanā.*

As I said earlier Patañjali gives *mantra* in the first *sūtra. Mantra* is composed of two words – *manana* and *trai. Mananāt trāyate iti mantraḥ,* – *Manana* is the process of having thoughtful and careful deliberation, reflection and meditation with full of reverence. *Trai* is to protect, cherish, preserve or defend. The thought which protects or defends is *mantra.* Every mantra has *tantra. Tantra* is the main characteristic feature of the technique or the methodology. The practice of yoga explained by this *mantra* and *tantra* in the first *sūtra* lessens the load on the consciousness.

Take *Utthita Trikoṇāsana.*[1] When a teacher tells us to turn the right foot with right leg out and without disturbing the left leg to turn the left foot in,as a novice, one turns the right foot out and left foot in through one's own law of instinct. This instinctive movement is *dharma pariṇāma* of the flow of instinct.

If I ask you whether you have experienced the change of vibrating sound in the form of waves between the right leg and the left leg, you may not be able to answer as you have not studied or thought about it.

Listening to the waves of vibrations and adjusting them evenly by study is a descriptive qualitative change. As you do not study this way, the *āsana* is not a *mantra* for you. You do not reflect *(manana)* and feel *(bhāvanā);* whereas for me it is a *mantra,* because I study the quality of vibration. I observe how it vibrates and feel the condition of the vibration.

---

[1] See plate n. 25

When I turn my right foot with the entire leg out, I watch the movement of energy and its vibration. Similarly, I study the type of energy wave moving in my left leg. Observing whether it is rhythmic or not, passive or active, aggressive or non-aggressive, I reconstruct the left leg in the *āsana (lakṣaṇa pariṛāma)* for the vibrating sound to move evenly on both sides with steadiness and stability by right re-adjustment (*avasthā pariṇāma*).

In this way, I deconstruct and reconstruct the instinctive orientation towards a right and rhythmic re-orientation. Then it becomes an *āsana* in the real sense.

Compare for yourself when you turn your right leg out, whether it is stable or unstable. Similarly, study the left leg and know its state. In the same way compare to know the differences between the right leg and foot, the left leg and foot, between the legs and the trunk, and so on. Note that the variations in the body, like the *vṛtti* of the mind, do not imprint on your mind or intelligence. Though there are differences in the placement of the muscles and flow of energy, you feel as though you have stabilised the *āsana.*

The teacher makes the pupil pronounce the words of *mantra* exactly as heard to get the best effect, as wrong pronunciation may be harmful or ineffective. Similarly, the body has its own sound waves, just as the mind has. Hence, use the right type of force while performing the *āsana.* It should be like uttering the *mantra* in the exact manner. In doing *Utthita Trikoṇāsana,*[1] the sound waves in the body are not grasped by you, and hence there is no *manana* or reflection of the *āsana* in you. Without *manana* there is no *bhāvanā* – felt feelings. As the reflection is not there, the feeling is not going to be exact. You have to grasp in *Utthita Trikoṇāsana* the power of *prāṇa śakti* and *jñāna śakti* moving evenly in your right or left leg. If the *prāṇa* in the left leg is strong, it holds the *āsana,* while the stretched right leg being passive shakes. Watching this difference, study how to get an even vibration, harmony and symphony between the left and right leg by reconstruction and re-adjustment. From this you get a thorough co-ordinated understanding between the right leg and the left leg. Then it becomes the right *Utthita Trikoṇāsana.*

If your left leg is aggressively powerful, then that leg is in the state of *hiṁsā* (violence). You have introduced *hiṁsā* in that leg, whereas on the right leg, as it remains light and passive, shakiness remains. Unknowingly you introduce *hiṁsā* in the right leg through non-attention. That is why you have to reflect and study *(manana)* on the placement of energy in the right and left leg. You have to listen to the various movements and *prāṇic* waves taking place in the right and left leg simultaneously. Then try to work out with discriminative intelligence how to bring evenness in the flow of energy through a methodology *(tantra),* which consists of doctrine, scientific theory,

---

[1] See plate n. 25

rule and regulation. So the *tantra* stands for the method, since it has to protect us and not destroy us. Therefore, *mantra* and *tantra* go together as *mantra.* While doing any *āsana* or *prāṇāyāma* through *pūraka, recaka, kumbhaka,* understand that there should be no difference in the vibration. Vibration is nothing but sound. *Nāda* is sound and *nāda* also means vibration. There is *nāda* in body, muscle, joints, bones, nerves, organs and brain too. In *Utthita Trikoṇāsana* the waves – *nāda* – or the power of sound on the right leg and on the left leg have to remain identical.

Take *Utthita Pārśvakoṇāsana.*[1] It is a different *āsana* and therefore the vibration differs, but you have to adjust the rhythm of vibration in concord. As the sound waves in each *āsana* differ, so observe and adjust the vibration. The waves in *Tāḍāsana*[2] are like a rock. It cannot revolve, whereas in *Sālamba Śīrṣāsana*,[3] the structural body remains firm, but the energy circularly rolls within the body between the arms, thighs, calves and knees. We have to go on observing and learning about the vibration of *Tāḍāsana*, the vibration of *Sālamba Śīrṣāsana* and so on with a fresh mind. This way of study is essential for the flame of the mind to attend to the flow of the sound waves in each *āsana,* according to the format of an *āsana.*

In this way, you begin to understand, realise and think what type of changes have to take place and what type of adjustments are needed in order to do the right *āsana.* Learn to experience the symphony and the melody, as well as the tone of each *āsana.* This becomes the *bhāvanā* or correct feeling. That is why I say that *āsana* are my prayer and *āsana* are my *mantra.* Study while you are staying in the *āsana*, in which way you have to move, and how much you have to move without disturbing the other parts of the body. Suppose in this *āsana*, you turn your head, the vibrations in the legs change. Have you noticed these changes that take place? If you do not observe and re-adjust, then you develop instability *(anavasthā)* in that *āsana.* You should maintain that smooth wave of *prāṇa śakti* and *jñāna śakti* in the body so that you do not waver at all. This is known as *avasthā* or stability of body, mind and self as a single capsule in that *āsana.*

To ramble is the natural character *(dharma)* of the mind. Change the mind from the rambling state by discipline *(lakṣaṇa dharma).* From this stage move to achieve a total and complete stability *(avasthā dharma)* through *mantra* and *tantra.*

Yogasādhanā needs a tremendous inward penetrative and introverted state of mind. You have to be very, very sensitive to the inside body. Look at a leaf. See its end and its middle. When there is a gentle breeze, the middle of the leaf may shake or not, but the end of the leaf vibrates because that part is not only thin but very sharp and sensitive. Your intelligence should

---

[1] See plate n. 26.
[2] See plate n. 27.
[3] See plate n. 28.

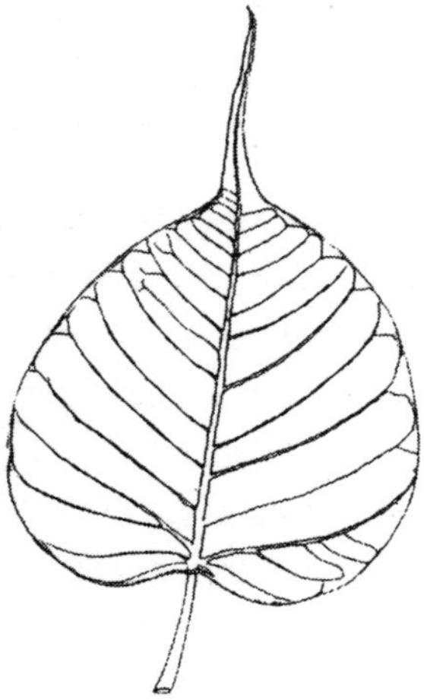

Plate n. 3 – A leaf

be sharp like the thin edge of the leaf. If your intelligence is as sensitive as the thin end of the leaf, I am sure you will understand the presentation of the *āsana* far better than now. The skin at the corners of our torso, legs or arms is like the thin edges of the leaf. Skin has the power to contract *(sunkucita)* or expand *(vikāsata).* If the skin has no power to contract or expand, neither can the muscle. Medical science only speaks of the muscle contraction and expansion. Nobody thinks that the skin has the power to accommodate the muscles. If skin was incapable of expansion and contraction, it would have torn easily, ruptured easily, and the blood would have oozed out. Skin creates the space for the inner body. Skin is infra-structurally ether. This ethereal body, the skin, has a tremendous touch-sensitivity *(sparśa).*

The *āsana* teaches us the subtle *(sūkṣma)* element of the ether through skin. Each and every part of our body has a certain amount of ether, which expands and contracts. For example, when you do *Utthita Trikoṇāsana*[1] on the right side, the ether expands on this leg while it contracts on the left. That is why you move the right leg easily for adjustment. In the left leg the earth element is strong and hence you cannot adjust and move your left leg with ease. So learn to change the earth element in the left leg into the ether element to adjust. In the right leg you change the ether element into the earth element to gain stability.

Similarly, in *Utthita Trikoṇāsana*, you have to adjust the right hand as well as the left hand, so that the self says, "I am not here, you are dragging me, I am contracted here." This way the self brings your attention to move the arms evenly and vertically up and down as separate entities. This way study in each *āsana* how to make the self to feel and dwell in the body.

In *Utthita Trikoṇāsana* the air element shakes in the right leg as the earth element in that leg is unstable. In the left leg the earth and ether element bring the firmness. Co-ordinate these two elements of earth and ether so that the skin gets space in both legs. From this you have to

[1] See plate n. 25.

learn to use the element of air and earth on the right leg with the help of the element of fire as an agent to develop rhythm and concord. If you study this way in each *āsana* you will be surprised to know that you exist everywhere in the entire body, transforming each cell into a self.

In the first chapter, *sūtra* 41, Patañjali states that, *grahītṛ, grahaṇa, grāhya,* (subject, the instrument of knowing and object), unite. While practising *āsana* there is a flash from the elements of nature that has to be caught by the flasher (self). The elemental body as an object flashes the corrections and disappears, but the mind as an instrument has to be sensitive to catch these flashes coming from the body. Use the *grahaṇa śakti*, the power of intelligence for the *grahītṛ*, the self, to engulf the *grāhya*, the body while practising *āsana*. In this state of practice, there is no object, no subject and no instrument. They all disappear and everything appears as subject. That is how the *āsana* has to be practised with a mature state of intelligence and sensitive understanding. Patañjali calls this intelligence *ṛtaṁbharā prajñā*. I am sure that a day will come for you all to experience this *ṛtaṁbharā prajñā* (truth bearing state) as you go on practising with reflective observation and absorption.

In the Nobel prize winning book, *Man – The Unknown,* the author wanted the physiological and physical body to be made to speak. The knowable is more unknown than the unknown – the self. It is difficult to know what it is possible to know. Or I say, "We say we know, but we do not know."

Patañjali presents to us that we can change and transform the physical, the physiological, the emotional and the intellectual sheaths, and in the end submerge all in the sheath of the self. The self has to engulf from the bottom skin of the foot to the crown of the head. It is said that the self is subtler than an atom and larger than the Himalayas. This is what we can learn from our practices. We can make our *ātmā* to become a *mahātmā*, the large, the vast.

Today meditation has become so popular that classes are opened on every street by anyone at all. We have reduced spiritual knowledge to a commodity. For me life itself is a meditation. Life is nothing but a reflection of one's own self. We have to live moment to moment on each of our physical, mental and intellectual movements. But do we pay attention, or observe all these movements? If we observe life like a stream which is one from the beginning to the end, we learn that meditation is a stream of life from birth to death, a steady flow of energy and intelligence maintaining continuity without any breaks in between.

Meditation is not escapism. It is a positive force where you like to study and cleanse your own behavioural pattern with the zest for worthy living and noble growth and for salvation: meditation is life that is free from prejudice and intellectual pride. Patañjali brought in meditation as the seventh petal of yoga as it is difficult for individuals to reach that state without sensitive, subtle and matured truth-bearing wisdom *(ṛtaṁbharā prajñā). Dhyāna yoga* was part of Patañjali's *aṣṭāṅga yoga* taking the *sādhaka* from *vikalpa* to *savikalpa, nirvikalpa, savicāra, nirvicāra, sānanda, nirānanda* and *sāsmita prajña,* and then on to reach the subtlest of the subtle states – *nirāsmita prajñā.*

With these words I hope that from now on you make an attempt not to perceive on the physical level but to start from the intellectual and spiritual level. Reverse your mind. Instead of going from the periphery, start from the core. Bring the core to reside in each cell.

If you practise yoga this way, the Gem of life, the *puruṣa,* is in your hands.

*ANUKRAMA SĀDHANĀ ŚRENI**
(Successive, Sequential Ascension in *Sādhanā*)

Sādhanā is never done in a haphazard manner. *Sādhanā* is essentially a planned programme in order to reach the goal. There are definite links in *sādhanā*. These links conduct us to the ultimate aims of our pursuits. The aims may vary according to the frame of each individual's thinking capacity and mental stature; still the links are not broken. My *sādhanā* had to be of various moulds as I had to start from scratch on account of my unhealthy, unfit body and my raw mind. No doubt, I took yoga for health in the early stage of my life. When yoga is done for health, it is often branded as physical yoga. Similarly, when people see varieties of *āsana* from simple to complicated ones, they call it physical yoga. So the critics branded my practice as physical yoga. But remember well that nobody will continue *sādhanā* his life long as physical yoga.

For no reason people divide yoga by terms such as physical, mental or spiritual yoga. But all these divisions are humbug. There is no part in our body which is not touched by the mind, intelligence or the self.

Though I started *yogasādhanā* for health, I began tapping the hidden psyche in every part, every organ and every cell of the body after gaining health. The psyche is hidden in tissues, tendons, ligaments, flesh and skin. Soma and psyche go together. Wherever there is soma, there is psyche and vice versa. It is intellectual arrogance that divides psyche and soma considering soma as inferior and psyche as superior.

Again it is a wrong notion of the people who say that the practice of *āsana* is related to body and the practice of *dhyāna* is related to mind. Can anybody do meditation without the body?

In the name of spirituality, let us not judge divisively that one path is higher than other paths. For me this is humbug. I am using this word purposely and deliberately.

---

* Talk given on 14th December, 2001, Pune.

MOULDING OF THE BODY FOR A RIGHT PERSPECTIVE OF THE *ĀSANA*

Yoga is not just a theoretical subject. It is a very practical one. Yoga is essentially connected to *sādhanā*. Without *sādhanā* yoga cannot be experienced. *Sādhanā* has no other colour except practice with reverence. However, by imitating my way or method you cannot reach the end. The method shows the means which are known as moulds in *sādhanā*. Moulding is just a means, and it is a means to find out where it leads the *sādhaka*. My method or my way of practice is moulded in such a way that you can definitely mount on it to reach the goal; but finally it is you who have to touch the goal.

My *sādhanā* has made me touch that point where you as my students consider that the hierarchy of *sādhanā* reaches its zenith. My effort to reach the depth of each *āsana* or *prāṇāyāma* has given you courage to make an effort to evolve through this hierarchy. But what is this hierarchy? You will never know unless I open my mouth and tell you. You have all done *Tāḍāsana* for days, months and years. You may imitate the *āsana* as I do. But this imitation is external. What I do from inside is unknown to you. Therefore, let me explain to you a bit.

Many of you have been doing yoga for ages. If I put you a question regarding the gauge of the successive changes *(anukrama)*, or the successive imprints that have been gathered by your psyche or intellect, you may find it hard to answer.

In *Tāḍāsana*,[1] for instance, do we feel the psyche? Do you know where the mind is aware of sensation? Often, the psyche remains moving in one leg, whereas in the other leg the psyche recedes, or it wanes like the moon.

Have you ever observed or felt while doing *Tāḍāsana* that one arch of the foot extends and the other contracts? Do you ever feel that the outer foot of one leg in *Tāḍāsana* is in firm contact with the floor whereas the other one wobbles? You can guess now how much your intelligence has to peep inwards to penetrate, to study and understand *Tāḍāsana*. In this way, you need to reach the other areas of body and mind in *Tāḍāsana*. Often, you are present at one area and absent at another. You do not find the body and mind coming into the sphere of attention and awareness in a total sense. But when your psyche touches soma everywhere, your intelligence too, penetrates everywhere. This is integrating the whole hierarchy of *Tāḍāsana*. Even if one considers this as just a physical movement, see how much the mind, intelligence and self have to be involved to get the right *Tāḍāsana*.

---

1 See plate n. 27.

Watch yourselves doing *Tāḍāsana* tomorrow, look at your metatarsals. If the head of one metatarsal is in line to the big toe, the other one will be slightly sliding towards the outer foot. You do not know on which part of the feet you are standing, where your intelligence is and where it is not. You do not observe the length, width, or breadth of the heels and soles and which part is in contact on the floor and which is not.

Similarly, when you are doing *Utthita Trikoṇāsana* on the right side, you lose the quality or the hierarchy of the *sādhanā anukrama* of *Tāḍāsana*. When I say do *Utthita Trikoṇāsana* on the right side with legs apart, you remain stable on both the legs. The moment I say move the right leg to the side, the left becomes light and flies in the air. You lose the sensation of its firmness. The moment you turn the leg to go to *Utthita Trikoṇāsana*, you do not know that not only is the rear leg in the air, but the left knee moves higher than the right knee and, at the same

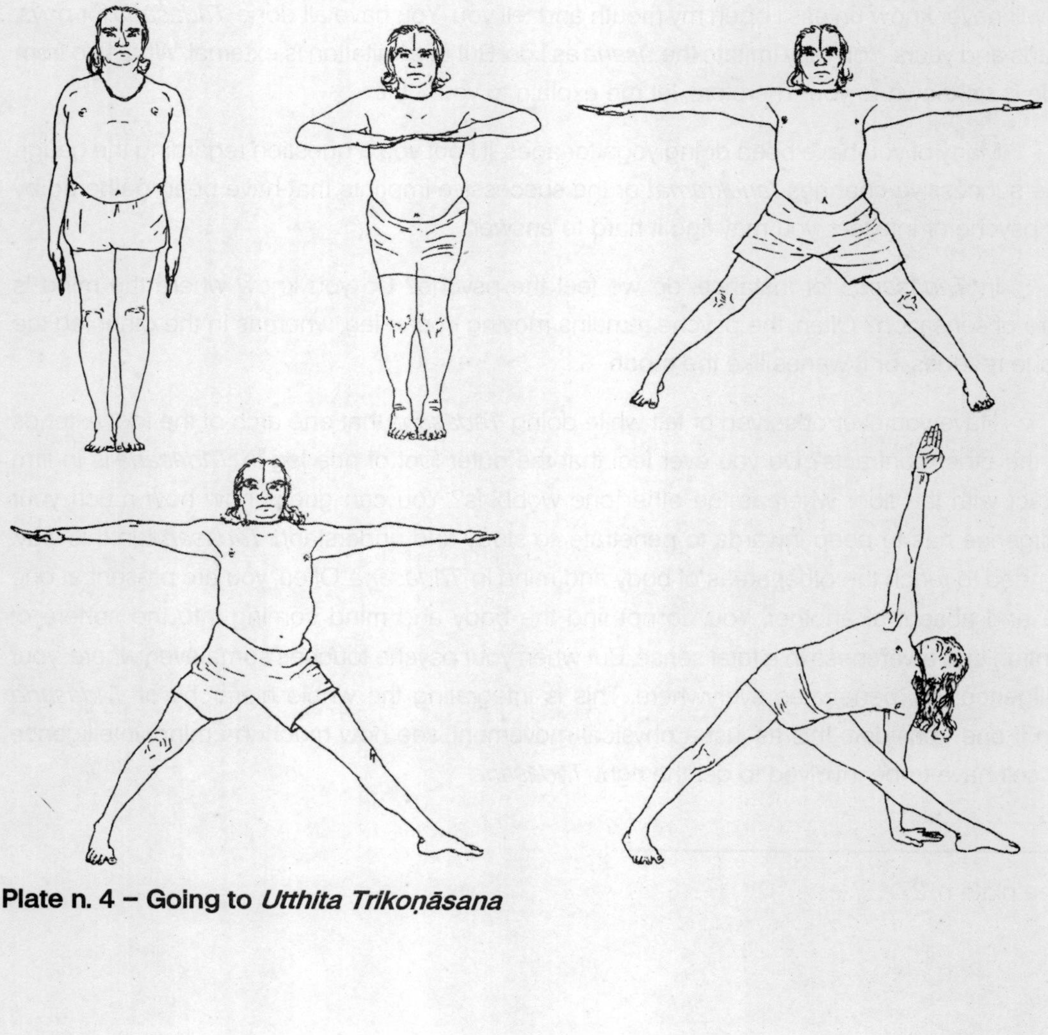

Plate n. 4 – Going to *Utthita Trikoṇāsana*

time, you only feel the right leg on the floor. If I ask you about the condition of the left leg, you become blank. If you draw a line and bring successive pressure and energy in both the legs and arms, then *Utthita Trikoṇāsana* becomes a meditative *āsana*. You can even make further progress by looking at the right foot and follow the line from the big toe up to the groin. You start adjusting the distorted movements and bring the groin in line to the big toe. By adjusting this way you realise that the energy which moves like a brook begins to flow evenly in the banks of the legs, giving a feeling of contentment and satisfaction.

Now, let me also tell you how one has to learn to observe. Many people do the *āsana* but do not understand how to observe. Often the body does the *āsana* but the mind goes somewhere else. After a few years of practice, if the mind attentively comes to be in *āsana*, then you see some parts are shrunk or narrowed. This means that you see only a part and not the whole. Here you need to learn to train your mind. For example, while you are doing on the right side, learn to look at the right leg with your eyes as the right leg is visible and perceivable. As the left leg cannot be perceived by the eyes, it has to be conceived by the mind for rhythmic adjustment. This way the *sādhaka* has to use his senses and mind in each *āsana* perceptively as well as conceptively.

While doing on the right side, it is a perceivable adjustment and on the left, it is a conceivable adjustment. On the right side, the senses of perception help the mind to work for correctness, while on the left side the mind directly conceives and guides the senses of perception and action to adjust to a required condition by spreading the intelligence, *prāṇic* energy and the self evenly in all parts of the left leg. Similarly, when you do *Utthita Trikoṇāsana* on the left side, the perceivable adjustments will be on the left side and the conceivable adjustments on the right side. In the same way in each *āsana*, the front of the body is perceivable whereas the back of the body is conceivable. In lateral twists, the lateral sides of body become perceivable while the front and back become conceivable parts.

ARCHITECTURAL ELEMENTS IN THE ARCHETYPAL ICON[1] OF *ĀSANA*

The *āsana* that you see on the walls of the main hall of the Institute are not the pride of Iyengar or the decoration on the wall. These pictures are meant to be looked at and observed by you. They are meant to make you understand their depth. For me, when I practise these, they are divine. For a devoted practitioner like me, it is worship.

---

1 The Oxford English Dictionary (3rd edition), says, "In platonic philosophy, archetypal is applied to the idea or form as present in the divine mind prior to creation, and still cognisable by the intellect independent of the *ectypal* object." Icon is an image, figure or representation.

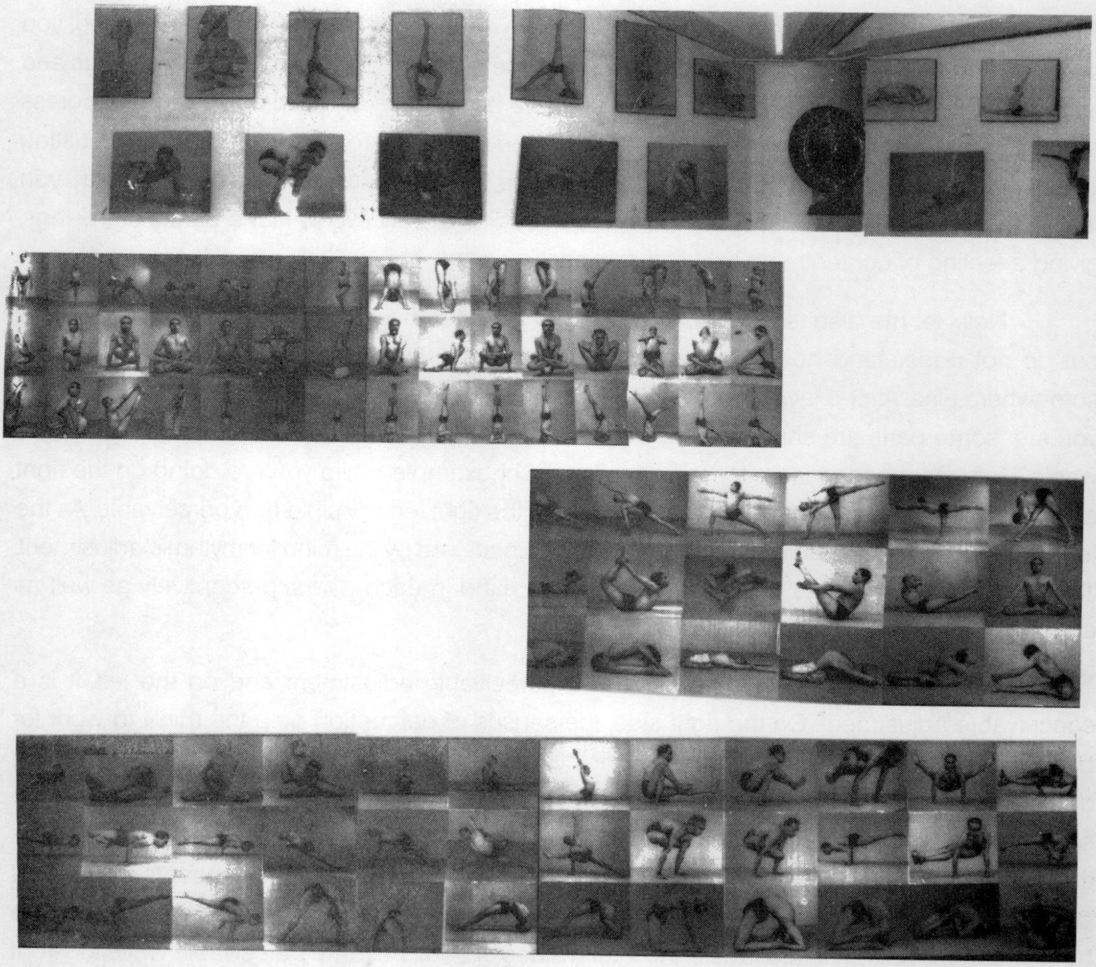

Plate n. 5 – Photos in the Main Hall of the Ramāmaṇi Iyengar Memorial Yoga Institute

They are archetypal icons using architectural elements within the frame of the human body. The architect designs the house and the sculptor shapes the sculpture employing external means and materials. The practitioner of yoga uses his own elemental body, vital energy, mind, intelligence, consciousness and the conscience in order to shape and design the body with each *āsana* and make it lively with divinity. He moulds his body through his intelligent discretion and creates various icons in different architectural shapes to get the archetypal beauty such as triangular shapes (i.e., *Utthita Trikoṇāsana* and *Parivṛtta Trikoṇāsana*), angular shapes (i.e., *Gerandāsana, Uttāna Pādāsana, Kala Bhairavasana* and *Vasiṣṭhāsana*), square, rectangular shapes (i.e., *Utthita Pārśvakoṇāsana*), dome shapes (i.e., *Eka Pāda Viparīta Daṇḍāsana*), weaving in *Paripūrṇa Matsyendrāsana* and *Pārśva Kukkuṭāsana,* and so on. (see Plate n. 7)

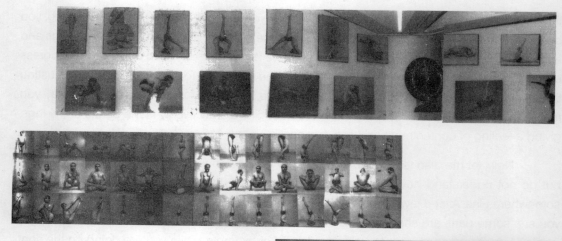

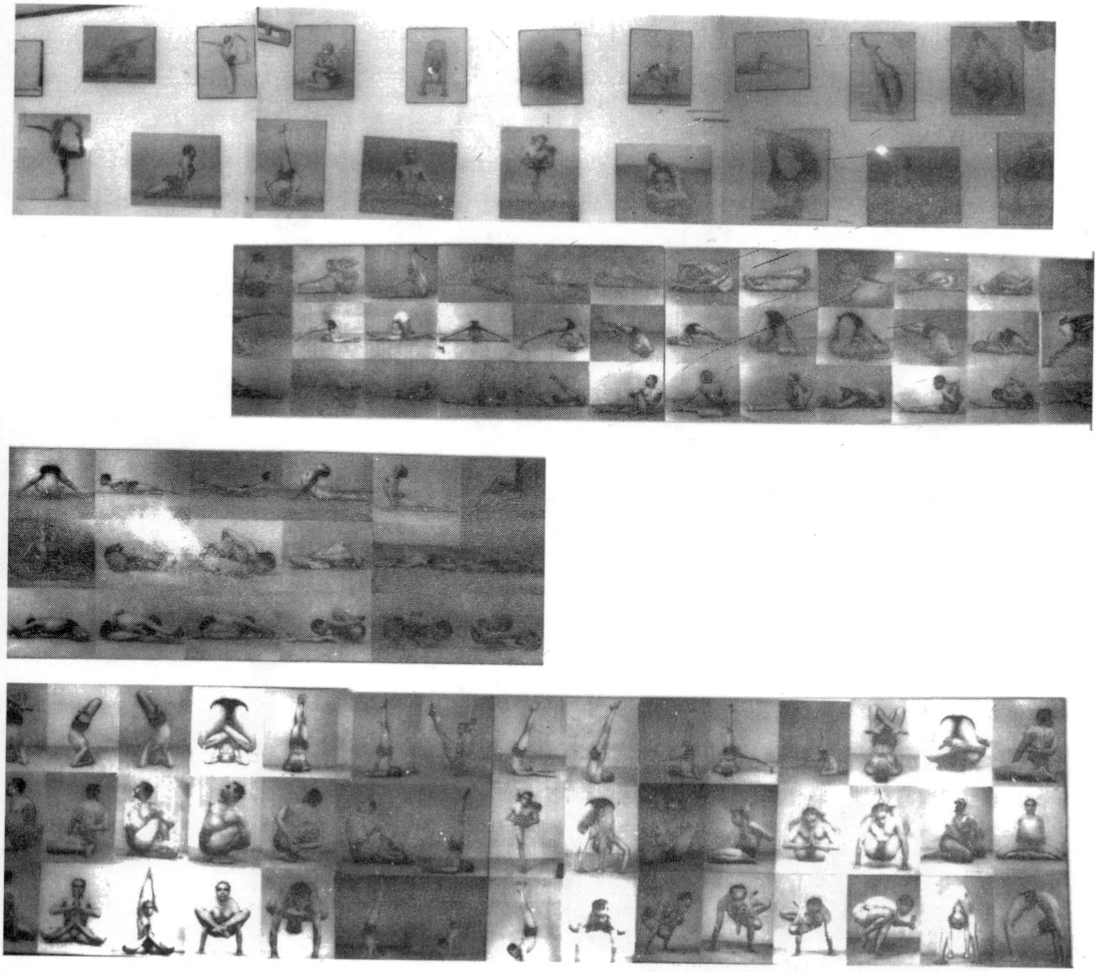

Plate n. 5 – RIMYI photos cont.

If evolution in our *sādhanā* has to take place, then we have to work along the following line. You have done *Sālamba Śīrṣāsana.* How many of you know where the dome shape, the triangular shape and round shape come in *Sālamba Śīrṣāsana?* If there is no dome shape of the crown of the head while placing the centre of the head and triangular shape between lower and upper arms, *Sālamba Śīrṣāsana* is bound to go wrong. When you are doing *Sālamba Śīrṣāsana,* watch and observe your arms, whether there is a triangular shape or not and on the back of the upper arm if there is a dome or not? As the dome has a centre, the upper back arm should have a dome shape in *Sālamba Śīrṣāsana.* If it leans like the leaning tower of Pisa, it is not *Sālamba Śīrṣāsana.* Hence, watch the upper arms and form a dome in the upper back arms by bringing the flesh and the skin exactly on to the middle portion. Similarly, work and adjust the joints and

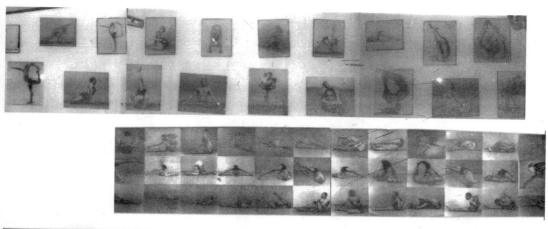

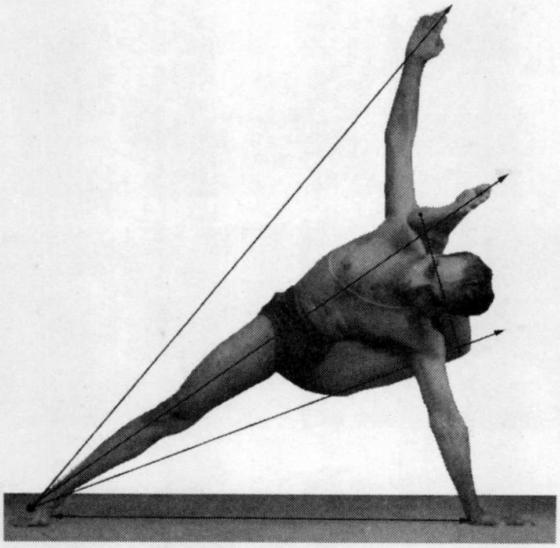

Kāla Bhairavāsana

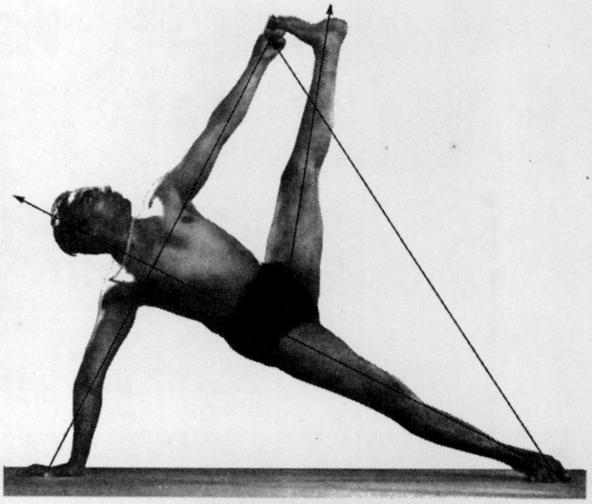

Vasiṣṭhāsana

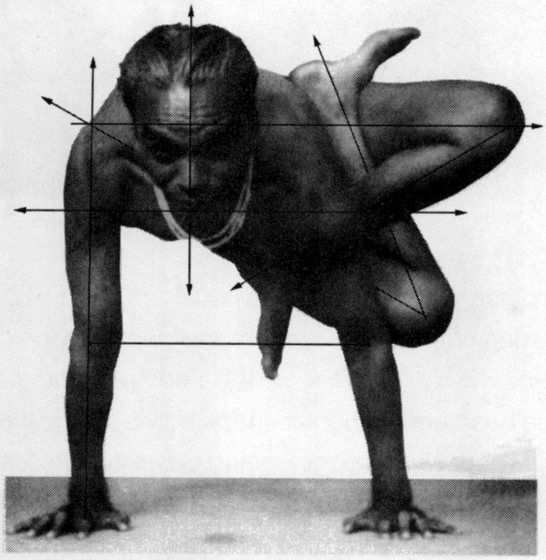

Pārśva Kukkutāsana

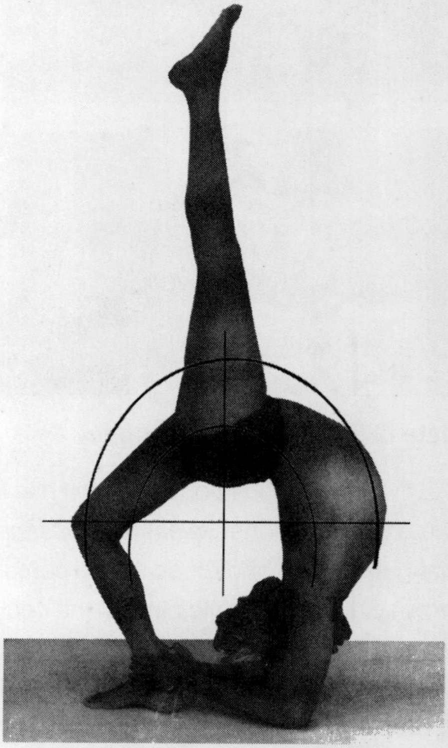

Eka Pāda Viparīta Daṇḍāsana II

Plate n. 6 – The architectural shapes in *āsana*

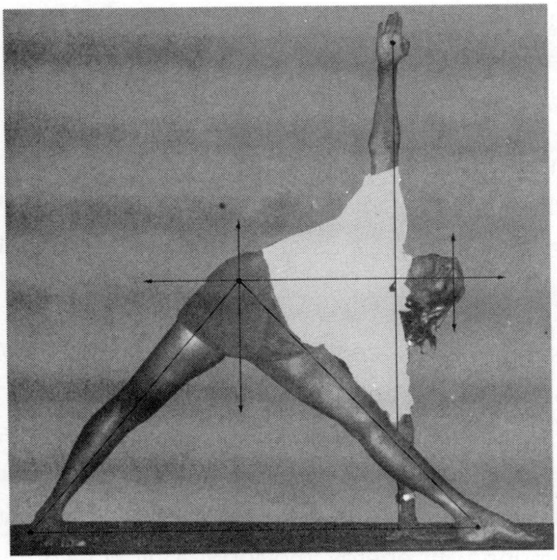

Utthita Trikoṇāsana

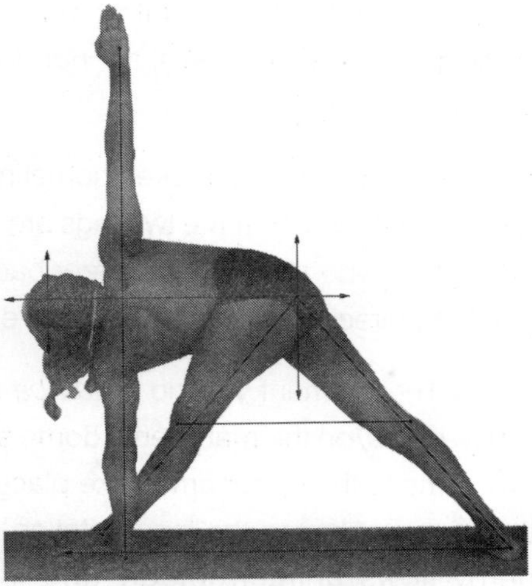

Parivṛtta Trikoṇāsana

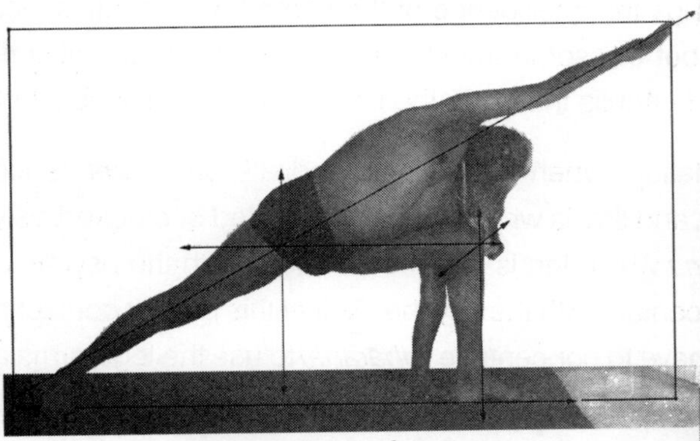

Utthita Pārśvakoṇāsana

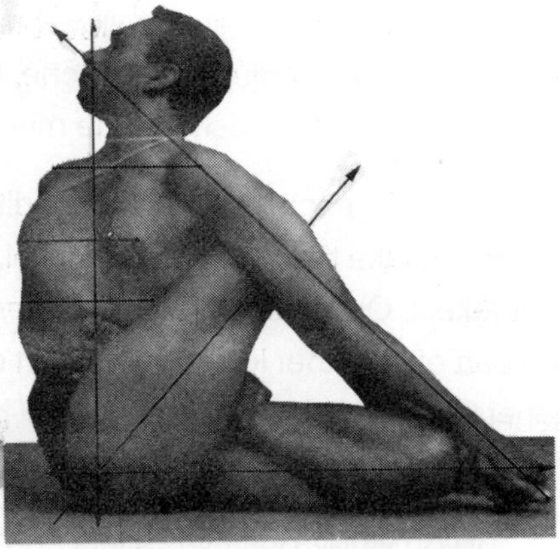

Paripūrṇa Matsyendrāsana

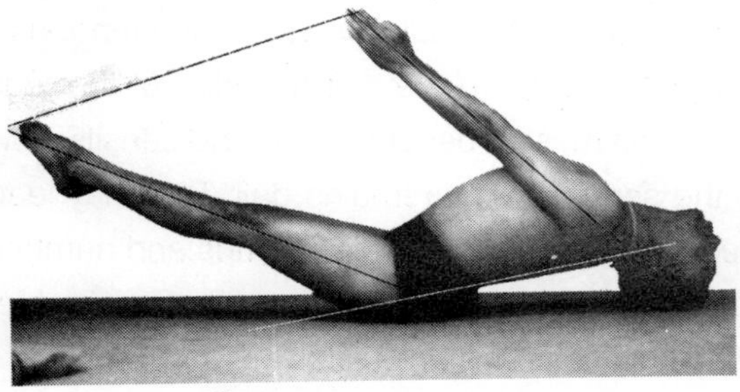

Ūttana Pādāsana

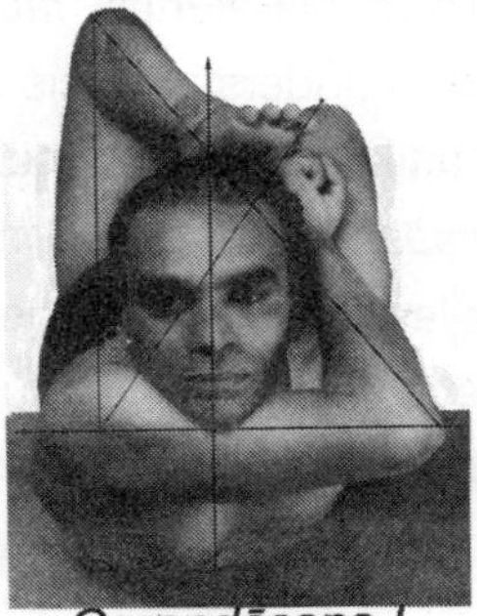

Geraṇḍāsana I

Plate n. 6 – The architectural shapes in *āsana* cont.

the muscles of the legs to turn round circularly like pillars. These movements of posing and reposing, or the adjustments, are not possible unless the psyche intensively penetrates all the areas of the body.

You might have looked sometimes in the mirror while you were in *Sālamba Śīrṣāsana.* Have you seen whether the two legs are straight or which one is straight and which one is tilted? You might not be able to get the feedback due to want of intellectual sensitivity or you might not be able to direct the flow of the *prāṇic* energy in the required areas.

The moment you do *Sālamba Śīrṣāsana,* with the centre crown of the head *(Ūrdhva-madhya Śīrṣa)* on the mat, then a dome shape in the upper arms and a triangular shape from the lower arms to the upper arms take place and as a result the legs turn and come closer to each other. If you enhance the inner rotation of flesh and skin in the legs, the compactness comes, energy flows uninterruptedly and intelligence gets alerted immediately. Here comes communication from the intelligence to commune with energy, moving it to flow with rhythm everywhere. This type of energy-flow brings the intelligence of the soma for right adjustments. Here, one does not adjust the psyche, but the soma transforms into psyche and adjustment takes place instantaneously. As the mind engulfs the body, the body is no more felt as a body.

For me, each *āsana* is a meditation. When I practise, I meditate on *āsana* as icons whereas you take them on a fitness level, and that is why your body gets tilted or crooked, as you do not reflect. Observe while in the *āsana* which leg is in perfect contact with the psyche and which part of the other leg is not at all in contact with the psyche. To feel this perfect contact and to generate awareness in the mind, you have to concentrate *(dhāraṇā)* to use the legs, arms and spinal column as a forceps or pincer action[1] to tap the dormant psyche to surface.

If you study, observe, reflect and do right adjustment in each *āsana*, then you realise the feel of the words of Patañjali, *tataḥ dvandvāḥ anabhighātaḥ*[2] (*Y.S.,* II.48). It takes a long time for you to begin to understand this *sūtra* and translate it into the cellular system, the tendons, the fibres, the cartilage and the muscles. For example, compare the calf muscles of the legs in *Sālamba Śīrṣāsana.* In one leg the inner edge of calf muscle becomes thin and sensitive, while in the other leg intelligence does not grasp the sensitivity but remains dull. This may lead to imbalance even in the spinal muscles and duality sets in causing pain, cramps and numbness. And what about the nerves if such imbalances affect them? Apart from these physical problems, which are at somatic level, the psyche gets affected. The above defect shows that your mind has

---

1 The "pincer" action, is where the upper thigh, at the level of the femur heads, are rotated from outside in as well as moved directly in towards the centre.

2 From then on, the *sādhaka* is undisturbed by dualities.

not reached the calves. It is a fact that you cannot perceive them nor conceive them either. When the inner edges of both the calves are extended to make them thin and sensitive, it is not that they have become shapely, but rather that mind has pervaded that area. The mind is no more in a dual state.

These details are required in each and every *āsana*. They are not merely techniques to deal with parts of the body. These elaborate technical explanations with details are meant so we can visualise and experience the architectural elements in the archetypal icon of an *āsana*.

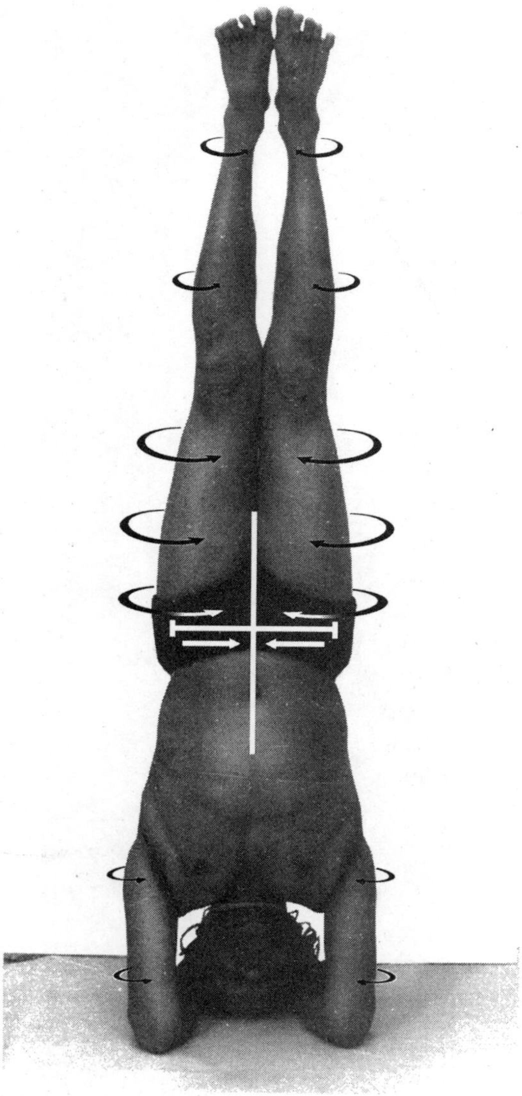

Plate n. 7 – Pincer action in *Sālamba Śīrṣāsana*

SĀDHANĀ KRAMA AND *SĀDHANA-TRAYA*

In the practice of an *āsana*, apart from these elements, which connect the soma to psyche and psyche to soma, the connecting of the mind to intelligence, intelligence to consciousness and consciousness to conscience in the sequential order is essential. Then only the *āsana* performed would be like the archetypal icon. This is the *sādhanā krama* or the sequential ascension in *sādhanā*.

The body is the outer cover of the mind. The mind is the outer cover of the consciousness and the consciousness is the outer cover of the soul. Therefore the *sādhaka* requires *kāyaśuddhi* (purification of body), *manōśuddhi* (purification of mind) and *cittaśuddhi* (purification of consciousness). Patañjali explains this *sādhanā krama* – the sequential order of approach in a capsule called *kriyā yoga*, which consists of *sādhana-traya*, the three-fold practice. *Tapas, svādhyāya* and *Īśvara praṇidhāna*[1] are the *sādhana-traya* which correspond to *kāyaśuddhi, manōśuddhi* and *cittaśuddhi.* He elaborates *tapas, svādhyāya* and *Īśvara praṇidhāna* in the eight aspects of yoga namely, *yama, niyama, āsana, prāṇāyāma, pratyāhāra, dhāraṇā dhyāna, samādhi.*[2]

The practice of each aspect or each petal has the same sequential order. Each aspect is first followed by the physical body at the gross level to bring *kāyaśuddhi.* Then the body is connected to the mind. The defects and the tricks of the mind are detected. The mind is cleansed by eradicating these defects in each aspect and finally the body and mind are connected to consciousness. The consciousness is purified by taking off the unwanted, defective and painful *vṛtti.*

Again in each aspect, there is *tapas,* there is *svādhyāya* and there is *Īśvara praṇidhāna.* This is not only interesting for you to know but also thought provoking. For instance, *yama* has five petals namely, non-violence, truthfulness, non-stealing, celibacy and non-covetousness. Now all these five moral aspects are practised on the level of *tapas,* level of *svādhyāya* and *Īśvara praṇidhāna.* The body, mind and consciousness, all three need to undergo the transformation and purification in a gradual but sequential manner to digest and assimilate these principles into the deeper system of *citta.* You, as a *sādhaka,* can now imagine how the five principles of *niyama* have

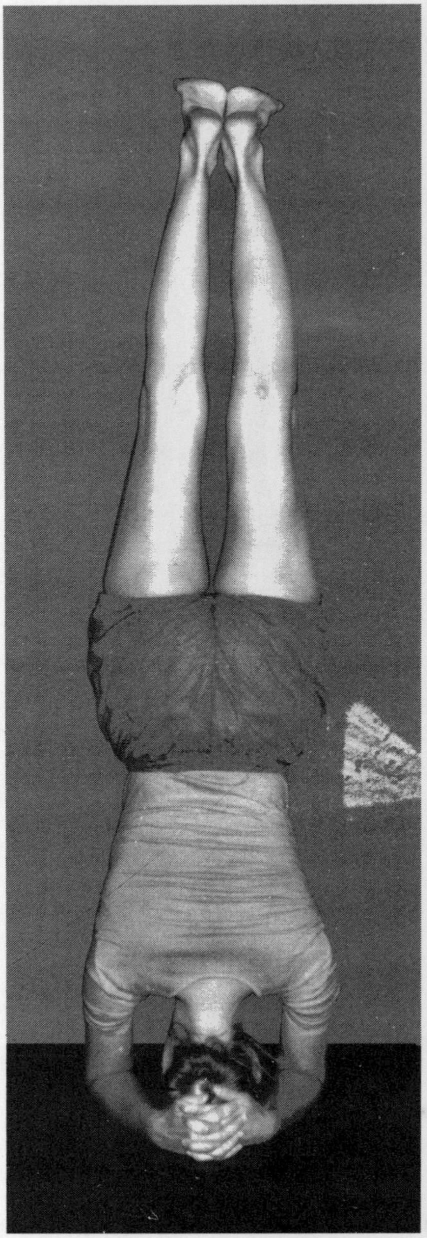

Plate n. 8 - Calf muscles in *Sālamba Śīrṣāsana*

[1] See *Aṣṭadaḷa Yogamālā,* vol. 2, pp. 42-44, and the author's *Light on the Yoga Sūtras of Patañjali,* pp. 102-104.
[2] See *Aṣṭadaḷa Yogamālā,* vol. 2, section I, and the author's *Light on the Yoga Sūtras of Patañjali,* pp. 26-31 and 134-135.

to be practised and absorbed in the human system. Similarly, there are varieties of *āsana* and *prāṇāyāma*. The *āsana* are considered to be innumerable. If all these thousands of petals of yoga have to be adopted in *sādhanā* and assimilated, then the sequential order remains the same as *tapas, svādhyāya* and *Īśvara praṇidhāna*.

Patañjali shows ways of using these thousands of petals of yoga through *tapas* by *yama, niyama, āsana* and *prāṇāyāma*, through *svādhyāya*, by *pratyāhāra* and *dhāraṇā*, and through *Īśvara praṇidhāna* by applying the knowledge of *dhyāna* and *samādhi*. Hence, *tapas, svādhyāya, Īśvara praṇidhāna* become *sādhanā-traya* as *kriyā yoga*. They become the three limbs of practice, the three aspects of practice. These three correspond to work, word and wisdom. *Tapas, svādhyāya* and *Īśvara praṇidhāna*, all three cleanse, clean, purify and sanctify the God-given *trikaraṇa* (*kāya* – body, *manasā* – mind, and *vācā* – speech).

TRIKARAṆA ŚUDDHI

God has given us *trikaraṇa*. *Karaṇa* means instrument. The body, speech and mind are the instruments of the human being. We call them, *kāyā, vācā*[1] and *manasā*. Patañjali first speaks of *tapas* for *kāyaśuddhi*. He wants the body to remain completely pure. Then *svādhyāya* for *manōśuddhi*. *Svādhyāya* is to acquire knowledge and use it as a means to purify the mind, intelligence and consciousness. *Īśvara praṇidhāna* is for *vācāśuddhi*. *Japa* in the form of *Īśvara praṇidhāna* is said to purify the *vācā* or speech. *Vāk* is the organ of speech as one of the organs of action. *Vācā* is the very action of speaking or speech. Speech – *vācā* – is often caught in the web of lust, anger, greed, infatuation, pride and envy, which are known as *ṣaḍripu* – the six enemies of human mind. Speech is affected and influenced by *ṣaḍripu* and emotions. That is why *Īśvara praṇidhāna* is introduced. *Japa* is a part of *Īśvara praṇidhāna*. By doing *japa*, the tongue is brought under control. *Japa* frees the *sādhaka* from bad usage of words. You can bring the mind under control but not speech. As the mind is purified, speech is cleansed. Speech is the outlet of the mind. If the mind is introduced to *japa* with the feeling of devotion to *Īśvara*, speech is controlled and restrained. Hence, this comes under *Īśvara praṇidhāna*. Further with *Īśvara praṇidhāna*, the *asmitā* – the very existence of "I, mine and me" which causes mental turmoils, is purified and sanctified.

Again, each of three instruments *(trikaraṇa)* is purified in sequential order by *tapas, svādhyāya* and *Īśvara praṇidhāna*. For instance, let us take *japa*. *Japa* is the repetition of the sacred *mantra* or the name of God with feeling and understanding of its meaning. Repetition of

---

[1] See *Aṣṭadaḷa Yogamālā*, vol 2, table n. 9, p.238.

the *mantra* is a physical action done by the tongue as the body of speech. This is *tapas*. The mind and intelligence have to be involved in understanding the meaning, which comes under *svādhyāya*. To get the feel of the word and its meaning, one has to soak body, mind and speech in *Īśvara praṇidhāna*.

This is why Patañjali puts *aṣṭāṅga yoga* in a capsule as *kriyā yoga*.

By *tapas* one conquers *tamōguṇa*, by *svādhyāya rajōguṇa* and by *Īśvara praṇidhāna sattvaguṇa* so that one later becomes a *guṇātītan*. Hence, the yogic science of *tapas, svādhāya* and *Īśvara praṇidhāna* is meant to sanctify the body, mind and speech for the consciousness to shine in purity. That is why I often say that yoga fits even an atheist on account of its quality of cleansing body, purifying mind and sanctifying consciousness.

A HINT TO DO *ĀSANA-SĀDHANĀ*

The *sādhaka* has to do *āsana-sādhanā* and watch what is coming and what is not coming; what is happening and what is not happening. I have already described, while in *āsana*, how to bring psyche to penetrate soma. The *sādhaka* needs to watch out for these lapses. At the beginning stage of *sādhanā* everyone acts at physical level, very mechanically. I too performed mechanically in the beginning. As it did not satisfy me, I did not give up the practice, but tried to find out the lapses and gaps which process fascinated me to continue the *sādhanā*.

We must learn to see and feel, perceive and conceive. The *kāyā* (body) does *āsana*, but *manas* (mind) has to penetrate. The *vācā* (speech) has to find an inlet while doing *āsana-sādhanā*. This speech is the inner dialogue with ourselves, with our body and with our mind. While doing *āsana*, we must look at each mistake that we come across so that it becomes a turning point for us to study, rethink and proceed further. When I say, "*Āsana* is my prayer and body is my temple", it is not a casual or sweeping statement. It is a genuine experience and true devotion. My devotion to practise *āsana* was not blind. It was an eye-opener for me.

Patañjali mentions the five mental modifications, namely *pramāṇa* – valid knowledge, *viparyaya* – perverse knowledge, *vikalpa* – indecisive and imaginative knowledge, *nidrā* – sleep, and *smṛti* – memory, which you all know.[1] I am not going into details here. Let us take the help of *pramāṇa*. Patañjali does not ask us to restrain the *vṛtti* straightaway. He asks that we sort out

---

[1] *Y.S.*, I.5-6. See the author's *Light on the Yoga Sūtras of Patañjali*, pp. 50-52.

through the *sādhanā* the disturbing and non-disturbing or the afflicting and non-afflicting *vṛtti*. Let us see a part of it in the context of *āsana-sādhanā*.

Patañjali says in *sūtra* I.7 that valid knowledge has to be checked with three resources namely, *pratyakṣa* – direct perception, *anumāna* – imaginative[1] way of thinking with a logical base, and *āgama* – scriptural text or authentic authoritative experience.

In my early days of *āsana* practice, I had no means for direct perception *(pratyakṣa)* nor logical imagination *(anumāna)*, because I had not seen anyone doing those *āsana* which I was doing. My teacher never showed me the *āsana*. He would say, "Do *Kandāsana*,[2] turn the knee and ankles."[3] I had to apply imaginative inference. I also approached the qualified masters of those days *(āgama)*. As I could not get a logical reply to my questions, I depended upon this above *sūtra* and read it in a reverse order, that is *āgama, anumāna* and *pratyakṣa*. By reversing the *sūtra* I.7 of Patañjali, I learnt the importance of the *sādhanā*. I took each *āsana*, whether it is *Utthita Trikoṇāsana*, *Tāḍāsana* or *Vṛśchikāsana*[4] as a spiritual scripture *(āgama)*. For me each *āsana* became a literary book. Knowing that each *āsana* is an archetypal icon of the body, I worked to get that fineness in each one. For this I used the middle guideline of Patañjali, to apply my own logical imagination *(anumāna)*. Then I practised using the pros and cons in different ways. Suddenly I experienced naturalness, concord, grip and rhythm with various parts of the body, and lightness in mind. This feel of concord in body and lightness in mind led me to valid knowledge *(pramāṇa)*. This valid knowledge led me towards intuitive perception *(pratyakṣa-pramāṇa)*.

This way I began experimenting and aiming at each *āsana* for a further firmness which I built up in each of them as an icon and thereby experienced the *āsana*. The *āsana* no more remained only as prayers, but the prayers led me towards *antaryāmin* (the Lord within).

TRISĀDHAKĀ **(three types of practitioners)**

Having spoken on *sādhana-traya, trikaraṇa śuddhi* and three *pramāṇa vṛtti*, let us move on to three types of *sādhaka* that Patañjali explains. For example, whatever *Utthita Trikoṇāsana*[5] you did today as a beginner, you cannot do the same way after ten or twenty years. Look at *sūtra* I.22:

[1] *Anumāna* is the process of deliberation based on inference. Inference has a logical base. We infer that if there is smoke, there is fire. Now, the fire is not seen but its existence is inferred from our experience. We don't see the fire but we can imagine the fire because we have seen the fire earlier. If we lack the imagination, we cannot infer.

[2] See *Aṣṭadaḷa Yogamālā*, Vol 2, plate n. 16.

[3] See *Aṣṭadala Yogamālā*, vol. 1, pp. 25-26.

[4] See *Light on Yoga*, Harper Collins, London.

[5] See plate n. 25.

mṛdu madhya adhimātratvāt tatopī viśeṣaḥ, in which Patañjali explains the types of *sādhaka* as feeble, average or of intense degree. Commentators demarcated the *sādhaka* as if they can be categorised permanently to those levels. When I started yoga I was feeble but later moved on to become a *tīvrasaṁvegin* (see I.21). Similarly, when you started yoga, were you an *adhimātra* or *mṛdu sādhaka?* Do you practise now as a feeble practitioner? Do you want to remain a feeble *sādhaka* throughout your *sādhanā?* Patañjali wants the yoga *sādhaka* to move to higher stages. This is hierarchy in *sādhanā*. He wants us to move from this feeble quality of practice towards average practice with intellectual attention. This is the *madhyama* stage.

It is said that the union of the individual soul with the Universal Soul is yoga; *saṁyogayoga ityukto jīvātma paramātmanaḥ.*[1] As a feeble practitioner in *sādhanā*, the *sādhaka* is made to understand the structural body. When the structural body gets mobility, would one like to stay there alone or like to go a little further? Naturally you prefer to learn something more. The moment that arises in a feeble *(mṛdu) sādhaka,* he likes to be upgraded to *madhyama sādhaka*. This aspiration in your practices means moulding oneself to build higher aims in the *sādhanā*. And what is this higher aim? It is to bring union *(saṁyoga)* by associating the flesh and the skin or the motor nerves with the sensory nerves and vice versa. The moment you think and start practising, you connect the *karmendriya* with the *jñānendriya (indriya saṁyoga)*. Here you become a *madhyama sādhaka*. In *sādhanā* you need to become a sensible person. I am indicating here how your sensitivity has to increase to reach from skin to soul and from soul to skin.

The mind and intelligence are connected to the entire skin of the body. As the skin envelops the inner contents of the body, it cannot be said that it has no intelligence here or has intelligence there. A *sādhaka* cannot be of a thick skin. So in feeble *sādhanā* you use the muscles and joints while in *madhyama sādhanā* you begin to feel the imprint on the skin, the actions of the fibres or spindles of the motor nerves. By this contact *(saṁyoga),* the skin conveys whether the stretch in an *āsana* is harsh or fine. The skin tells one whether the actions are refined or not. The skin as sensory nerve conveys the subtle touch of the motor nerves from within.

Skin being the cover of the flesh, you and I have to practise *āsana* or *prāṇāyāma* to learn to move the inner body in such a way that the various layers of the skin are touched not aggressively or forcefully but gently, as the sensory nerves of the skin are non-aggressive.

In our *mṛdu sādhanā* there is *hiṁsa* and *ahiṁsa,* though we may not know this. When the motor nerves are overused, it is violent – *hiṁsak* – yogic practice. The skin being non-violent – *ahiṁsak* – by nature, overstretch does not give the feel of the stretch on the skin, hence you do

---

[1] *Ahirbudhnya Saṁhitā*, 32.15

not get the imprints of the inner action on the skin. In *madhyama sādhanā,* while using the muscles, you are made to watch carefully whether the skin gives room for the expansion of the muscles or not. If you put a folded letter into a small envelope, the envelope tears, does it not? Though the skin is the envelope of the inner body, it has the capacity not to tear at all, but an ordinary envelope tears. In *sādhanā* the skin does not tear, but the inner tendons, ligaments or muscles can tear. We commonly hear people complaining, "I tore my hamstring, or this or that muscle." Why did the muscle tear? Because the skin did not give room for its expansion. In *madhyama sādhanā* you study how the skin is made to co-operate and co-ordinate to give room for the stretch of the muscles. In this *madhyama sādhanā,* practice of *āsana* is changed from the physical level to the psycho-physical and psycho-physiological levels. You understand the union *(saṁyoga)* of *jñānanāḍī* (channels for senses of perception) with the *karmanāḍī* (channels for organs of action).[1] From here on you realise that the knowledge of yoga begins in *āsana-sādhanā.*

From understanding and experiencing the co-ordination of *jñāna nāḍī,* the *madhyama sādhaka* begins to transform himself towards the *adhimātra* stage.

In this stage he traces the defects in his *sādhanā* and corrects them. When he does *Sālamba Śīrṣāsana*[2] he will notice that one side of his skull feels the texture of the mat and the other side of the skull does not get the feel of the touch of the mat. While in the *āsana* one leg may be thick and the thigh stable, the other leg may be fumbling and wobbling. Correcting these imperfections in practice is to invoke the intelligence to seep in. Then it becomes *adhimātra sādhanā.*

According to Patañjali feeble practice is meant to get rid of bodily pains *(kleśa vṛtti nivṛtti).* In *madhyama sādhanā* or average practice, one learns to still the movements of the mind *(manōvṛtti nirodha).* In the *mṛdu* state *kāyā* is adjusted and in the *madhyama sādhanā* the mind is restrained. Then one becomes an *adhimātra sādhaka.* Here the *adhimātra sādhanā* is meant to correct the defects *(doṣa)* in one's presentation through the discriminative intellectual power in order to achieve the archetypal icon of the *āsana* in the body. *Adhimātra* teaches where the seed of defects *(doṣa-bīja)* is in the *sādhanā* and it is guided by *buddhi* to eradicate them so as to reach the iconic *āsana.*

---

1 See *Aṣṭadaḷa Yogamālā,* vol. 1, p. 148.

2 See plate n. 28.

First *tāmasic guṇa* of the *śarīra* (body) is removed in *mṛdu sādhanā*, inertic nature of the mind is minimised in *madhyama*, and in *adhimātra sāttvic* nature is developed by making the body and the mind work together and finding the missing links through *prāṇic* and intellectual penetration to make the self live instantaneously by engulfing the body and mind.

For example you all have done full arm balance - *Adho Mukha Vṛkṣāsana* - and elbow balance - *Pīncha Mayūrāsana*. When you do these *āsana* and touch the wall with your heels, you will be surprised to know, you will never touch the same part of the heels on the wall. You may be balancing but the sensations of the skin tell you that the motor nerves are elastic on one leg and on the other side they are contracted. See in *Paśchimottānāsana*, the same part of the heel or the hinges which are close to the ground will be a little higher on one leg than the other. Why does one calf muscle on the inner side stretch towards the heel while on the other the energy does not move and intelligence gets blocked and shortens the stretch or makes the energy move towards the knees? In one leg the shin bone is alert while in the other leg it sleeps. This is known as defective practice - *sadoṣa-abhyāsa*. If we observe these defects and remove with *anumāna* (imagination with logical application) through pros and cons, this becomes the *āgama* or the scripture of the *āsana*. This comes in the *adhimātra sādhanā*.

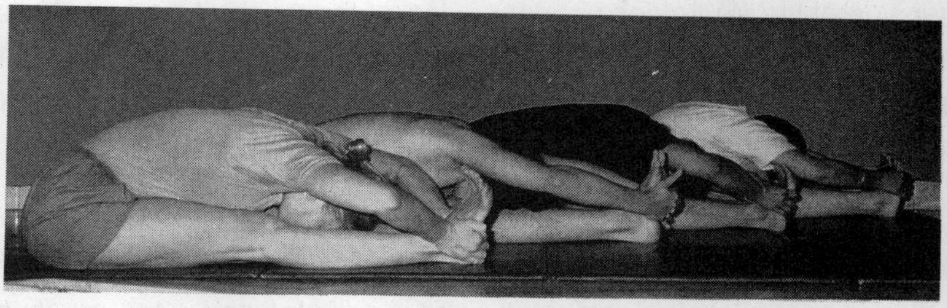

Plate n. 9 – Heel hinges in *Paśchimottānāsana*

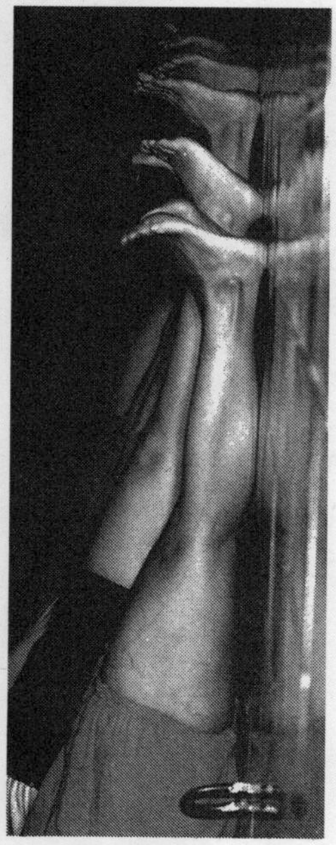

Plate n. 10 – Heel hinges in *Adho Mukha Vṛkṣāsana*

Thus these *tri-sādhaka* are closely connected with *tapas, svādhyāya* and *Īśvara praṇidhāna* according to our intellectual calibre. From here begins *tīvra saṁvegānām āsannaḥ* (*Y.S.,* I.21). At this stage everything is instant and fast for the *sādhaka.* In the 49th *sūtra* of the third chapter[1] Patañjali says that *kāyā* (body) moves as fast as the intelligence. This means that defect is eradicated, *doṣa* is dissolved and perfection in *āsana* has set in where the imprint of the body energy is one with the intellectual energy. This is the transformation – *pariṇāma* – of soma into an intellectual sheath. The union of these two energies – *prāṇic* and *bauddhik,* vital and intellectual energies – moves the self to cover the whole body as Self. The disparity or the division between body, intelligence and self terminates and unity is felt. Here you realise the meaning of *tataḥ dvandvāḥ anabhighātaḥ* (II.48). The duality between the skin and the flesh, the duality between the flesh and the bone, the duality between the cartilages, the duality between body and mind, intelligence and self culminates. Till then you have not mastered *āsana.*

This way *āsana* and *prāṇāyāma* teach us to bring all these loose ends together so that all deformities and disturbances in body, disturbances in intelligence and pride *(ahaṁkāra)* cease to exist. In this state one touches the end of yoga. This is *āsana jaya.*

---

[1] *tataḥ manojavitvaṁ vikaraṇabhāvaḥ pradhānajayaḥ ca*

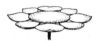

TEACHING YOGA: VIGOUR OR RIGOUR*

For me this is a very happy moment. I know this place very well, as my first public appearance in Manchester took place in this very hall, and it gave a very strong impetus to the audience who watched me on that day. Though I had come earlier to Manchester, probably in 1968; it was later when I gave a demonstration here, which had a tremendous impact on the public and attracted people towards yoga. Naturally, I am grateful to Manchester University, who gave me the opportunity to present the yogic art, and we are here again to celebrate the Silver Jubilee function of the institute at the same place, which is touching, particularly to me. The seed I put in this hall then has now grown into a healthy tree. I am grateful to all of you, and to those who started then, though I do not know whether all have kept to their practices or not. As I see lots of my old students here, it means to me that they have maintained their practice, creating enthusiasm around them for others to take to this practice.

In today's world we have lost the sense of good health. We have lost the sense of human communication. We have become individualistic to a very great extent. Probably, the practice of yoga may transform individuals not to be individualistic, but to think of society and the community at large. You as yoga students have imbibed the effect of yoga, and you may share this with others so that they may experience that same joy.

Today is not a lecture-day. I am nearing 80 and I think it is the right time for me to say good-bye. And when I see so many students, it is the students who should now take the lead to present this art according to the modern way of living and thinking. When an old man like me speaks on yoga, naturally some youngsters may think, "Oh! He's an old man, what does he know about the present way of life?" Therefore, I want the youngsters to come up. It is the youngsters and the middle aged people who can talk to their colleagues of the same age group. Why do I refer to the youngsters? This morning I read in the paper that in 1995 about 5 billion dollars of trafficking in the United States took place through the drug trade. You can imagine what an amount of money was spent just to have a little triggering of the peripheral nervous system and

---

* Address at the Silver Jubilee of M.D.I.I.Y. (U.K.) on the 11th of November 1997.

then to suffer for the whole of life. That's why I say if I talk about this, then many youngsters may take it with a pinch of salt. But youngsters who have experienced the same triggering, the same exhilaration through yogic discipline, may be able to guide those who have spoilt their future life by becoming victims of drug addiction.

No doubt, yoga demands discipline and the young do not like to be disciplined. They want to be free birds, having no control over themselves. They want everything to happen like fast food. Fast food has no nourishment at all and hence diseases are increasing. New names are given for various diseases because of this introduction of fast food. Food affects the mind. Wrong food, wrong mind! That's why we have become individualistic and are interested in making money by hook or by crook, just to enjoy life. We have not realised that life is meant for something more than just momentary sensual pleasures.

The *ṛṣis* of yore gave four aims in life for human beings. Those aims are *dharma, artha, kama and mokṣa.* The first one is *dharma. Dharma* means a sense of duty which expresses the virtuous qualities of life, but now it is wrongly represented as religion. *Dharma* does not mean religion but 'right way of living.' Then comes the financial aspect, the *artha,* which means economy to lead a contended self-esteemed life. Then comes lust, *kāma.* The last one, *mokṣa*, is liberation. Why did even such great yogis, who had practised and mastered yoga keep these two main pleasures of the world - the *artha*, finance which brings joy to a person, and the *kāma,* lust, sensual joy, within the borders of right living - *dharma*, and liberation - *mokṣa*, i.e., to be free from this worldly net? They have not said, "Renounce." Unfortunately, today what you hear from the neo-yogis is the word 'Renounce'. But the geniuses have not said, - "Renounce." On the contrary they have told us to enjoy the worldly joys with discipline, limiting them within the banks of right living - *dharma*, on one side and the liberation from that sensual net - *mokṣa,* on the other side. In case one falls into that net of *artha* and *kāma* and gets caught in them, the wise people then knew that yoga was the only answer. That's why yoga was very popular in the early days. It was so popular that the definitions were increasingly lost and only the effects were remembered. The effects of breathing, the effects of postures, the effects of meditation and so on became the focus of attention.

When I started practising yoga there were not as many books as there are available today. These days even a novice brings out a book, within six months of practice, on the subject of yoga. The books which were available in those days had brief explanations and very little to convey. You may find those books even today. If you read the techniques explained in those books, and compare the techniques to the given illustrations, you find no coordination at all between the techniques and the presentations. That was the time when I felt that everyone was writing so much about the effects of *āsana* but the technique of doing them was scanty and brief.

So I used to read about the effects, and through the effects I built the technique. There is no technique in the yogic texts on *āsana* or *prāṇāyāma*. But from the effects they give, I had to work to find out the means to get those effects and that's why people call my method of presentation "Iyengar Yoga." I traced. I picked up the explanation, the effects of the *āsana*, the effects of the *prāṇāyāma*, and worked on them to get the effects that had been written about. That is how I found out the balance between the old texts which give the effects of the *āsana*, and the present day technique of mine so that the effect and the technique could meet and go hand in hand.

Many people are in doubt, "Why are so many postures needed?" Our body is made up of thousands of muscles, hundreds of joints and trillions and trillions of cells. The brain has maximum cells. Now, imagine how the yogis of yore thought of *Śīrṣāsana* and the rest of the inverted *āsana* as important in value.[1] Though they did not go to the depth of explanation; they could think of how to supply the blood to those areas where millions and millions of cells are situated in an important organ like the brain. Today the doctors may say, - "Oh! Head balance is injurious." But the people who practised found out the way that one should do it, so that there was no micro-hemorrhage while practising head balance and on the contrary, it gave serenity and tranquillity in the lobes of the brain.

The reason why so many *āsana* were given to human beings is that they could play a game of 'kite' with their bodies. You know very well when children play with kites, they grip the thread very tight and they try to play where the wind is strong. The kite is made to move in the direction of the wind. When the kite comes down or dips, they shorten the thread to get a grip on the kite. They pull it down in order to readjust and move it once again in the direction of the wind blowing in the sky.

The yogis too gave diverse *āsana* so that we, the yoga practitioner's can use the body like a kite.

The intelligence within us is a thread. The body with various limbs, the muscles, the bones, joints and the nerves, is nothing but different kinds of cells, like the multi-coloured kites. Each cell has significant life. All these cells are kept under the control of the thread of the intelligence; so the kite does not get dropped or caught anywhere. Again all these various limbs of the body like kites are connected through the thread of intelligence to the central lobe of the brain, just like the thread of the kite to the original reel.

This is the cause behind introducing the innumerable *āsana* which, unfortunately, people of today call "physical yoga," without proper knowledge, logic or reasoning.

---

[1] These *āsana* can be seen in *Aṣṭadaḷa Yogamālā,* vol 2, plate n. 5.

It is a statement that comes out of a poor intelligence and which does not understand the inner depth, the interior feelings, which are only realised through the practice of yoga.

Since I am addressing the students whom I am seeing for the first time, I must clarify the meaning of the *sūtra* - *sthira sukham āsanam.* (II.46) The definition given by Patañjali is misunderstood and misinterpreted by many. Go to any yogi, he will say, - "Sit in any *āsana* in which you are steady and comfortable."

The modern generation is so much attached to the word "comfort" that they hate the word "discomfort." Therefore, they are very happy if they are given freedom to be in any comfortable *āsana*. But they should remember that as the kite can get lost in the sky if the thread is cut, similarly, they can get lost in the practice if comfort disconnects them from within.

They forget the next aphorism which speaks about *prayatna śaithilya* - the ceasing of efforts. Efforts end only when nothing remains to adjust and readjust. When the kite has gone high in the sky the string holder just holds the thread in his hand since he has not to pull or loosen the string repeatedly. Similarly, when repeated mechanical effort is transformed into a natural course, division disappears.

So this present day misinterpretation of practice of *āsana* has brought a bad name to the subject as though it were merely a conative action, without realising the cognitive functions of the mind, intelligence and consciousness.

Āsana is a position where you have to adjust and re-adjust, using your bodily attitude and mental attitude, to balance in such a way that the challenges and the counter-challenges of the mind act and react to find an exact and correct position by re-aligning so that the attention of intelligence and the awareness of the consciousness are kept flowing evenly, and at the same time feeling the touch of the life force in every part and parcel of the cells.

It should not be just a rough touch. There are millions of leaves in a tree. Similarly, there are millions of sensations, millions of leaf-like cells in the skin which receive feedback through the tendons and the spindles of the muscles at work during the *āsana*. They send messages from the cells on the skin for the intelligence to re-think and re-act so that the right position is obtained. This is how one has to do and define the *āsana*. This is the real definition of an *āsana*; the actual meaning of *sūtra*. The *āsana* has got two sides: One known as *samāna āsana* or *sama vṛtti āsana*, and the other is known as *viṣama āsana* or *viśama vṛtti āsana*.

Samāna means equal. As I told you just now that our body has hundreds of muscles, hundreds of joints, trillions and trillions of cells, you have to know how you have to balance the body, using the elements which are existing in our system – the earth, water, fire, air and ether, and their counter-parts, smell, taste, shape, touch and sound. I feel that the five elements (*pancabhūta*) are physical properties, their infra-structural atomic qualities or substances (*panca tanmātra*) are chemical properties. These physical and chemical properties have to be measured and set properly, mixed and blended in each and every āsana for right nourishment of body, mind and self. This requires a lot of discriminative discretion and tremendous intelligence. When all these are attended to while doing an *āsana* then it is known as *samānāsana*. But moving the limbs and the anatomical structure of the body without giving time for feedback leads only towards *viṣamāsana*. Here, there is absolutely no thinking process involved at all. It becomes a conative action and lots of people do this conative action and say that they have done *āsana*. This way of practice is called physical yoga. Bringing the outer mind to touch the inner mind in your practices or internalising the outer mind to penetrate deep inside in order to trace the invisible parts and make them appear as visible parts in each and every *āsana* is the *samānāsana*. *Samāna* means equilibrium, equanimity in each and every part of the body. For instance, while stretching the arms in any *āsana*, if the biceps of one are shorter or longer than the other then you should know that it is *viṣamāsana*, and not a *samānāsana*.

Suppose you are balancing in *Bakāsana*,[1] and your one shin is closer to the armpit and the other is slightly farther away from the armpit, then that *āsana* becomes *viṣamāsana*. In order to balance this *āsana* evenly, one needs a keen observation and application of the scale of justice from the centre. You have to learn to apply the mind evenly on the right side as well as on the left side and then with attention, bring the mind to the centre to balance evenly. You have to study carefully and then use that intellectual justice of the right and the left sides to adjust and play together. This kind of balancing is the process of internalising your external mind by using the body as a unifying agent.

When we do the *āsana*, we use what you call the four lobes of the brain: the right, the left, the front and back. At that time, we greatly need to use all the four parts of the brain - the analytic frontal brain and the synthetic back brain. Medical science speaks of the front brain as biological brain; and back brain as old brain. While practising the *āsana*, we need to trace how the back brain and the front brain react in keeping the discriminative faculty and serenity intact. When analytic and synthetic parts of the brain synchronise together, real sensitivity develops and leads us to experience a state of silence and stability.

For example, when you do backbends, you use the frontal brain and when you do forward bends, you use the back brain. When you do *Setu Bandha Sarvāṅgāsana* with props,

---

[1] See *Light on Yoga*, Harper Collins, London.

you keep both the parts of the brain silent.[1] This way one has to search how the reaction of each *āsana* works not only at a physical level but also at chemical, bio-chemical and meta-physical levels. Then you understand how meditation is involved in the practice of *āsana,* when you are observing the changes and transformation that take place.

Without knowledge you cannot contemplate. This knowledge is to make the analytic and the synthetic brain act so that when these two faculties come together, contemplation sets in unbidden. You need not say, "I want to do meditation". It becomes automatic and happens naturally.

In *prāṇāyāma*, if you observe carefully the in-breath, you experience that it is not done by the head at all. If the in-breath is done by the head, you feel the eyes burning, the ears blocking, the head becoming tense. If you observe yourself carefully you notice that you cannot inhale from the head. You inhale only from the divine source which is hidden within you, i.e., the intelligence of the heart. If the *āsana* make you work from the intelligence of the head, *prāṇāyāma* makes you work from the intelligence of the heart. No strain is felt on the analytical or the synthetic brain in *prāṇāyāma*. There is only the movement of the "I". The words "Know Thyself," or "Know who I am," are tapped and used in inhalation. *Prāṇāyāma* teaches you to go into the source of life - the core at the very start of inhalation. The start of in-breath will take you to know "Thyself." That is *jñāna* - knowledge. Here, the mind or the brain does not inhale but the one that is the cause of life alone starts inhalation and continues to draw in throughout.

Now, after inhalation, you say that you are holding or retaining the breath. Instead of asking you how long you hold the breath, I question how long you hold that "Self," which has been tapped in inhalation. The "I" which has surfaced in the inhalation, can you maintain that without disturbing? When you inhale, at the starting point alone, you observe the awakening of the subjective intelligence. As you proceed, the subjective intelligence gets converted into objective intelligence. If this happens you have lost the source intelligence. So you have to go on watching whether you maintain the pure intelligence of "I" (subjective intelligence) throughout.

Observe very carefully while you are exhaling. Your exhalation is done from the lobes of the brain and not at all from the seat of the heart. While explaining about *āsana* I used the word internalising. In the process of exhalation, you learn how these two lobes of the brain internalise to reach the spot which is "I" in each individual. If this background of *āsana* and *prāṇāyāma* is understood, I am sure, all of you who practise and follow this guide line will experience the real

---

1 See *Aṣṭadaḷa Yogamālā,* vol 2, plate n. 11.

existence of 'I' or 'Me' or 'You', the very source, at least to some extent. You will experience the divinity existing in you. If you can tap this latent divinity with more attention, with more awareness, then there is certainly a hope for your transformation. Perhaps, the glow that shines in your practices may make others come to you. And you may be able to transform them by your teachings. Though you have all practised, I advise you to think from now on how to internalise the consciousness by using the body as a kite, and the ways to trace this divinity which is also the source of that holder of the thread of a kite. If you all practise with this kind of understanding and awareness, I guarantee that you need not search for spiritual light or life. You are already in spiritual life and see no difference between you and spiritual life.

This is what I wanted to convey to you today, though it is an informal gathering and I have not come here to give lectures. From now on see that there is a feedback in practising *āsana* and *prāṇāyāma* between the body and the mind; between the head and the heart, heart and head, and between the intelligence and consciousness with the inner being. For the time being I may be in my head-intelligence and you may be in the heart-intelligence. I want your heart to receive what I said from my head. Because today though I have said something from my head, I have already experienced it from my heart. Today, the professors come, lecture and go away without bothering to find out whether the students have understood what has been said. But the professor believes his job has been done, while teachers of yoga teach with patience till the students are made to experience and get the feel of what has been taught.

Since you and I have practised yoga, you and I should come closer to each other. You might have practised for 25 years, I have practised for 60 years. Probably, if you are very sensitive your experiences may be far superior to mine. Or my experiences of 60 years may throw some more light on yours, in case you have not reached my state. So I feel that if you have any doubts in your own practices or if you have had any confusion, well, I can talk about it, so that you and I come closer to each other and discuss to find the means. Otherwise the subject talked about is over and we just go out to have a cup of coffee, and then claim that the gathering was good.

After this meeting the staff members of the university held a tea party for us all. Let us have intellectual coffee or tea before we can have that coffee or tea (laughs). This is the only chance. Remember that I have come all the way, though the Committee members knew that I was not keen to come. They insisted that I come. I said, "I should withdraw from the world," and I have been saying it for years, but still circumstances force me to come. People know that I am a very hard task master. This propaganda has spread like wildfire and it cannot be stopped. The stories pile up. The gossip goes on. Those who spread such gossip do not differentiate between the words of my teaching and the words from the dictionary that they all choose to write about me.

From the very first day of my teaching, I have faced attacks on my practice and as usual on my teaching. From the beginning the writings about me, calling me "a physical yogi who kicks and uses abusive language", "a violent teacher," and so on, never left me in peace though my practice was continuing. With all these onslaughts I continued and faced all the challenges and you see still I have survived. I am still here. I have swallowed all opposition, but I know exactly what I am doing. Those who criticised me went on and on. My conscience trusted my wisdom. Those who saw my teaching and my practice saw everything only externally. As one tastes sea water and says, "Salty," but does not see the hidden jewels of the sea, similarly, those who criticised me did not try to find the 'in-depth' of yoga. They did not distinguish their rigour from my vigour. I was, and I am a vigourous teacher, and not a rigourous teacher. My vigourousness is meant to create vigour in you people, so that you are also lit by that flame which is latent in you, which otherwise might never catch light. I came and used the torch in such a way that the hidden fire in you may burst into flame. That's why I was very strict, taking you deeper and deeper to understand the *āsana*, though I was using only the words known in those days. I could not speak in depth on philosophy, since it was beyond the average intellectual standard. So I was interpreting philosophy in the language of the common man. For this I was criticised by academics and intellectuals all over the world. It is not that I am speaking of the early magazines, but even in the magazine "Yoga and Health" that started in London, you found more articles of attack on me than on yoga. Though I was restfully practising, due to the criticism I was restless because others were putting so much pressure on me that was irritating my inner being. I was alone, I had to fight single-handedly, without using wrong or abusive language. I have not criticised anyone. Look in other people's magazine articles and compare them with mine. Have I spoken anywhere against any yogis in the world? I took all the attacks as a guide. Fortunately since a few years ago, not only here but also in my own country, people have respected my work. This shows that they have changed their ways of thinking regarding my practice and I am happy that the fruit of my work has changed and is changing their thoughts on my yogic discipline.

Rigour is a conative action, whereas vigour is an intellectual action. Unfortunately even in those days, they did not know my vigourous way of teaching. They called it violent teaching. Vigour is connected to the mind, and not to the body. A few days back, I was reading a book called "Power Yoga". Nobody is criticising "Power yoga," calling it physical yoga as I was criticised in those days. Only, if Mr. Iyengar does it, then it is physical yoga, if others do it, then it is power yoga. Is it fair? Find out in any book, any review, on this subject. And see what they have done. They have presented only what you see in the book *Light on Yoga*. But what is the difference? The performers of "Power Yoga" have shown that they are people with muscle-power whereas I have shown the same thing with elegance, and not with muscles. This is known as discriminative power. I used discriminative power and did not do it as physical yoga though others interpreted it as such.

I see that each and every part of my joints and my skin flashes with the elegance of light. But nobody saw it or said that there is something special and specific in my practice. They branded it as physical yoga. Today, the "Power Yoga" includes the muscular actions, jumping, flexing of the muscles, developing them like wrestlers - a kind of gymnastics and acrobatics. And that is considered as wonderful yoga. What will this lead to? People say, "Oh! Mr. Iyengar's yoga is too deep, too complicated; whereas 'Power Yoga' is a strong action and therefore we are doing it". It means they are doing the conative action. If you come back to the conative action, is it going to help? Is that the way to learn yoga? Is that the way to write on the subject by reducing and degrading such a noble subject to conative action, just for the sake of name, fame and money when every practitioner wants to know something of the inner body, the inner mind, the inner intelligence, the inner judgement, which yoga can so generously offer?

So please give it a thought. You are all students of yoga. Direct your thought and find out while you are practising what type of mind you have? What type of intelligence do you have? After practice, what type of intelligence do you have? Why did this change take place so soon? Then you realise what the external mind is and what is the internal mind, how the internal mind functions in yoga and how the external mind functions in the external activities of life. This will help you to understand the value of yoga. I still say that though you have not experienced that depth, do not stop your practice. Who knows at what time grace comes. It does not come on your demand or on your command, but it comes with religiousness and divinity in your practice. Grace comes when the divinity – the Universal Self – sees the ripeness of religiousness in your practice. So continue practice as a religious student of yoga, not as an extrovert student but as an introvert student of yoga. May God bless you.

PROGRESSION IN LEARNING THE ART OF TEACHING

The *Yoga Sūtra* of Patañjali explains four types of aspirants namely, *mṛdu* (mild), *madhyama* (average), *adhimātra* (keen) and *tīvra* (intensely intent). Similarly, *Śiva Samhitā* defines four stages of *prāṇāyāma* according to the grade of the aspirants. These stages are *ārambha* (commencement), *ghaṭa* (intent endeavour), *paricaya* (intimate knowledge) and *niṣpatti* (consummation). I would like to connect and compare the four types of this classification from the *Yoga Sūtra* and the *Haṭhayoga Pradīpika,* which also holds good for the four kinds of teachers. Hence, students as well as teachers depend on these four types of classification and as well for the learning process. The teacher is called *adhyāpaka*, the students are called *adhyāyī* and the very learning or studying process is called *adhyayana*.

The teachers could be of four types according to their capacity and calibre, such as mild, average, keen or intensely intent. When knowledge or understanding is limited and unsure, obviously the teacher will be mild. Similarly the students, as beginners, will be mild. The standard of teachers may differ according to their grades. For instance, the teacher at the *ārambha* stage may commence with the explanation of connative actions in *āsana* which involve more of the movements of the muscles and joints. The teacher at the *ghaṭa* stage may proceed a little further in order to explain the cognitive actions in *āsana* where the students begin to understand some inner actions and self-adjustments. The teacher at the *paricaya* stage may introduce the students to his own intelligence and awareness so that they begin to feel the inner communication. The teacher at the *niṣpatti* stage may bring the graceful extension and expansion of consciousness for the students by leading them towards their *citta*. However, I would like to add one more stage and that is the graceful expansion of the Self – *citta prasādanam* and *ātma prasādanam.*

The above description is not only for those who have potential to take to the art of teaching, but also those teacher trainers who have to build up the needed characteristics of teaching. There is less depth in understanding and direction in the earlier or primary levels, but the senior teachers should help to guide and lift them, so that the juniors begin to understand the points which are essential to reach the higher level. It is possible that one may demonstrate well but lack in expression in the art of teaching. Therefore, the teachers need to develop an eagle eye. They need to learn how to see all the gross as well as subtle movements, modulations, modifications and vibrations. They need to observe and penetrate with the torch of consciousness from toe tip to the crown of the head and from the crown of the head to toe tip, as well as from skin to soul and from soul to skin.

If the *Tāḍāsana*[1] of the introductory level teacher and of the senior level is identical, how can one distinguish between them? The instructions should show the ascendance in the understanding and an increasing depth of subtlety.

A certain margin is given for Introductory *(mṛdu)* level instruction because it is a developing process. One does not expect this from a senior level teacher. One expects a better and brighter explanation from the senior level teachers or students. That is why stages of growth are given from the mild level to the intensely intense, as well as from commencement to consummation. In this way teachers have to develop from one level and move further into the advanced stages of growth.

OBSERVE, RE-DO AND RE-LEARN

Senior teachers have to watch and see that the base level of instruction is maintained and build upon that to higher levels as confidence grows. Their instructions should bring right adjustments in the body without distorting its anatomical structure. Correcting the *āsana* without distorting the anatomical structure is important in higher levels as attention is focused on alignment; first on the alignment of the physical parts and later on the alignment of the outer or seen physical body with the mental and intellectual bodies.

In the beginning one has to put in effort to observe and re-learn. One has to observe everything about the students who come to the teacher. When one repeatedly observes and repeats to re-learn, only then will one's teaching become effective.

The teachers may gain knowledge by reading, but they have to study, reflect, adjust and readjust all that they have read in their own *sādhanā.* They have to get the feeling of it and experience it themselves before they guide students how to learn from their shortcomings on their own body.

Today teachers want to give crash courses to students who want to become teachers but the teachers forget that the wealth of experiential knowledge that comes through observation and re-practice cannot be given in a short time. If the teachers themselves have taken a long

1 See plate n. 27.

time to understand, how can they train the student-teacher in a short time? The teachers have to make the would-be teacher aware of this fact also. Unfortunately, the acquisition of knowledge seems to be directed to making money *(dhanārjana)* whereas *sādhanā* is intended to earn knowledge *(jñānārjana).*

GET TOGETHER

Teachers should get together and study each other's *āsana* and the position of the body in *āsana.* This gives a great chance to observe each other's body structure, the differences in the positioning and adjustments. The teachers understand each other's problems. This leads them to develop the art of observation and correction and guides them how to help each other in the art of teaching.

Here, I choose *Tāḍāsana.* Observe the thickness, thinness, shortness and fineness in the muscles, the symmetry or asymmetry of their placement, then the texture; smoothness and roughness of the tissue, where the bulging is, where there is hollowness and erosion. Look at the colour and lustre of the skin and eyes.

Watch the bony skeletal structure, the placement and shape of the head of the bones and the symmetry of the joints. Compare the length of the arms and the side torso. Study the central axis of the body, from the eyebrow centre, tip of the nose, centre of sternum, navel, pelvis, inner thighs, inner knee joints and ankle, see that all these are maintained in one straight unbroken line. Are the ears, jaw lines, armpits, elbow crease, pelvic heads, hip joints, patella and ankles arranged along perfectly parallel horizontal planes up and down the vertical axis? The eyes of the teachers need to get accustomed to watch all these in order to develop and improve the sense of alignment. This also makes them catch defects quickly.

The comparison between two persons also gives some depth to understand what the right means are. The teachers begin to understand what is right and what is wrong. Watch whether they stand on the centre of the heel, do they open the back legs evenly, do they lift the side walls of the chest evenly, equally rolling the shoulder bones back. All these are the visible points to be observed in the structural body. From this study of the structural body one begins to see the underlying body of organs and nerves. As one penetrates to the deeper level in one's own body in *āsana* and *prāṇāyāma* then one develops the ability to see the deeper layers in the student's *āsana.*

One can also add to one's knowledge by watching when someone walks. Often one shoulder blade moves and one does not move. One shoulder goes up and the other does not. Observe and understand and work to find out why one moves up or down, while others move differently. Then, as a teacher, one has to imitate and work on one's own body to see which muscles are held unknowingly tight and which muscles are released. This way one becomes one's unknown teacher. As a teacher, one has to catch the good as well as the bad points of each student and work on one's own body to get a mental imprint and improve the art of teaching.

Observe the person who flexes one elbow and not the other elbow. He may bend one better, while the other does not go back. If you observe you will know which muscles are working and which are not. This is how you pick up clues.

Look and build up. When I tell you to open your eyes like the lidless fish, I mean that this will make you keep your intellectual eye ever alert.

One can learn to correct by looking at the way people stand. *Tāḍāsana* is very important for developing the right quality of presentation in the various *āsana*. One has to maintain without deviating the muscles, or without distorting the shape of the muscle from the oriented shape of attentive *Tāḍāsana*, and see that it does not get a disoriented shape in the other *āsana*. This is how I began to learn to look, observe and learn.

This is what learning at the senior level means. Learning here is actually acting, doing, studying, investigating and analysing in order to know the direction of one part of the *āsana* in relation to another counterpart. Teaching is also a self-studying process. Feel from which part elegance flows and which part feels the strain. If one does not pay attention to these things, then what difference is there between an introductory level certificate holder and a senior intermediate level certificate holder? One should not ask for up-grading because he or she has been teaching for a number of years. If the presentation and instructions of the *āsana* by senior, intermediate and introductory level teachers are the same or the understanding is identical, then how does one assess the different levels? In higher grades, there must be better observation, quality and depth in the presentation and maturity in explanation.

INTERACTION

The teacher, while practising, has to interact with himself. He has to interact with his body, with each muscle, each bone, each joint, each tissue, his own senses, mind, intelligence and consciousness. Linking of one muscle with the other is a necessity in order to develop quality in practice. Go on observing from one area to another and study which parts show deficiencies deformities and imbalances in the muscles and joints, which part responds and which does not. If any part gets distorted and crooked, how can there be elegance?

The interaction is not only of the various muscles, ligaments and fibres of the body, but also of the mind that has to be co-ordinated. The sharp mind has to learn to see and observe observe and to feel the felt movements of the body and how it has to be readjusted to break its disoriented position and move towards the orientation of the structural position. Even if the *āsana* is complicated such as *Viśvāmitrāsana,*[1] it should not be disoriented, distorted or contorted. The advanced teacher should think of how to bring the higher quality of smoothness in the *āsana.* This is what one expects higher grade teachers to excel in.

A senior level teacher needs to have the understanding of the elegance and rhythm of the introductory and intermediate level *āsana.* Elegance is that when each and every part of a muscle directed by mind, intelligence and consciousness interacts and co-ordinates to maintain freedom through the placement of the banks of each muscle evenly. The shape, tone, length, smoothness, fineness, with the creation of space in between the muscles, tissues and ligaments have to be maintained in each *āsana.*

From the intermediate and senior level onwards one must imbibe the sensitivity and depth in the practice and make fine adjustments to tune the entire *āsana* as a single unit. Like a well tuned violin that produces an accurate sound, the senior teachers have to produce a right resonance and serenity in the vibration of each and every aspect of the *āsana.*

SĀLAMBA ŚĪRṢĀSANA

Sālamba Śīrṣāsana is taught by the teacher at junior and senior levels to the beginners as well as advanced students. When the junior and senior level teachers are doing *Sālamba Śīrṣāsana* there must be a pronounced change in the positioning of the *āsana,* so that they can impart that to their students. They should roll the back of the legs, stretch the side of the legs, rinse the front of the legs, and open out the lateral parts of the chest. While doing *Sālamba Śīrṣāsana,*[2] the side trunk may be shrinking but at the Introductory level of teaching it will not be explained. The teachers should know that while teaching the students at the introductory level, the instructions should be more on stretching the legs, thighs, tightening of the knees and lifting of shoulders.

When the student progresses, explanations for corrections should take place that keep the front of the chest, the back of the chest and the sides of the chest maintaining the same length and height.

---

1 See *Light on Yoga,* Harper Collins, London..
2 See plate n. 28.

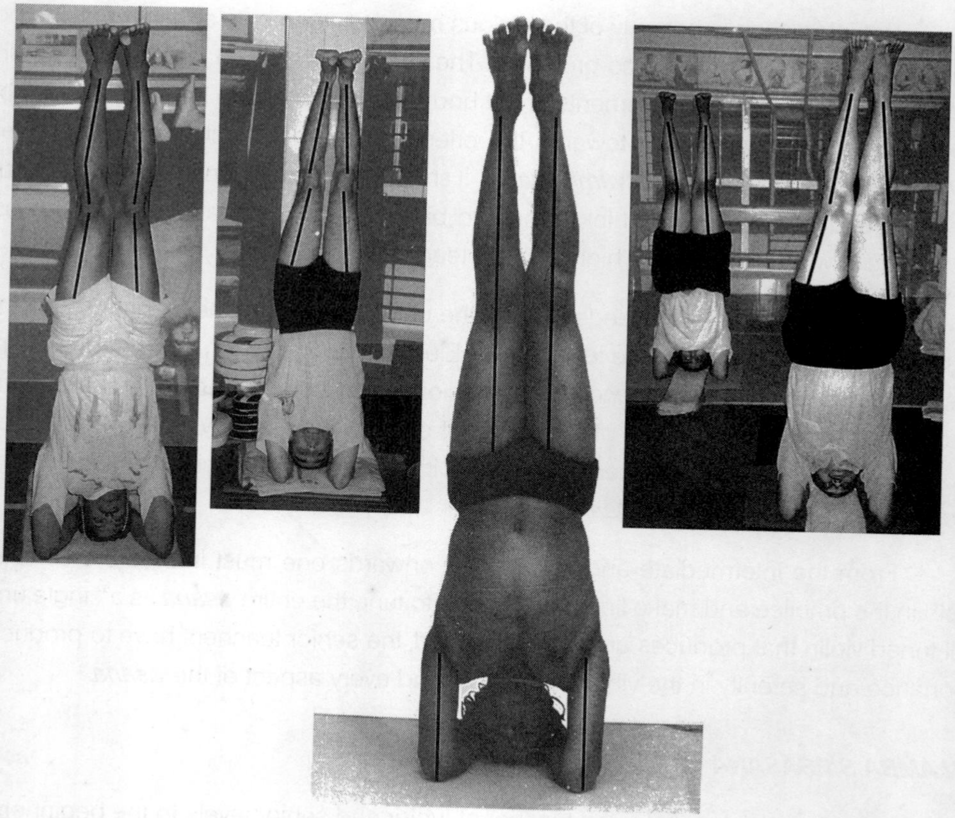

Plate n. 11 – Showing differences in *Sālamba Śīrṣāsana*

In *Sālamba Śīrṣāsana* draw parallel lines on the outer corners of the body. If you find that the shins turn inwards and the thighs do not, rather they turn out, or the skin and muscle turn at different angles to each other it is a disintegrated *āsana*. These are the things that have to be taught by the senior teacher so that uniform presentation comes to one and all. Then the mind and intelligence of the junior teachers begin to penetrate and pierce the inner body. That peeping inside is not only the process of observation but also interaction within. Observation is an ongoing aspect of yoga for all the teachers as well as students.

The moment re-orientation takes place in an *āsana*, the mind becomes fluid and with ease fits in those places where one has to be quick to catch on. Then one can integrate the parallel lines between the right outer side and the inner side, at par with the middle line of the trunk, the arms and legs as well as the back of the trunk. This readjustment of getting an even feeling on both the sides begins from discrimination. The elegance then starts setting in.

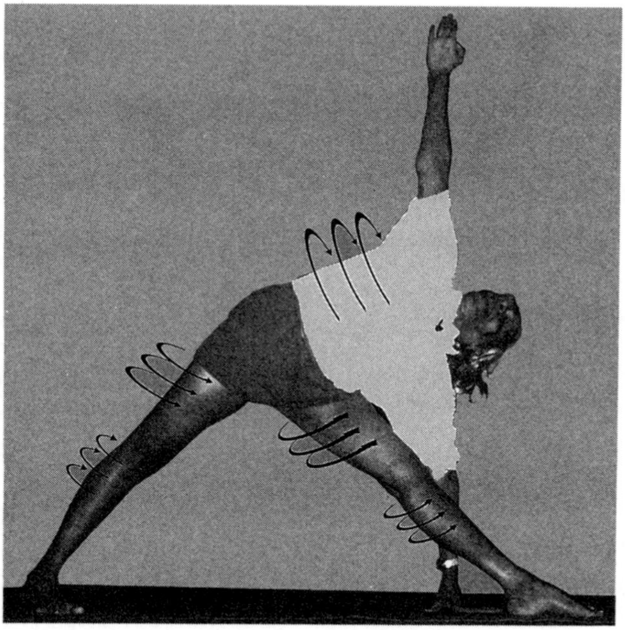

Plate n. 12 – Parallel aspects of the legs in *Utthita Trikoṇāsana*

The median plane in the body is very important for studying the form of the *āsana*. See also *Utthita Trikoṇāsana*. It is the fibres of both the legs that have to be parallel to trace the median plane of the legs and positioning of the pelvic girdle which helps to perceive the median plane. In *Sālamba Śīrṣāsana*,[1] the balance of the pelvis must be equidistant from the pubis. For this, one must attend to the rotation of the pelvic heads in towards the pubic bone.

The teachers have to notice the median plane of every part of the body and learn to stay in that plane. Also watch the inner pubic plate. Is the inner plate of the pubis perpendicular to the floor? Are the bottom and top parallel?

While practising ask yourself, "Am I far away from the centre, which way are the outer legs facing? Which pelvic head is far away from the centre, and which is closer to the centre? Here one has to introduce a pincer action in the legs to get into the median line. This action of rolling the frontal thighs in and making the femur heads come in line with the pelvis is a closing in or pincer action. If one makes these adjustments towards precision, then one becomes a sufficiently advanced teacher to teach advanced students.

---

[1] See plate n. 7, in the article *Anukrama Sādhanā Śreṇi*

Watch the breath. Does each breath disturb and make the body wobble? Or is the breath stabilising the body? This is how religiousness in *sādhanā* is cultivated and the mind learns to peep in. You have to develop this character of the penetrative mind, which is the beginning of observation.

It is important to note, through *svādhyāya* or self-study in *āsana,* when and where the outer body has to move in and when and where the inner body must move out.

ARDHA MATSYENDRĀSANA

Now, let me take *Ardha Matsyendrāsana.* This *āsana* is a great gift for one to study. This is the *āsana* in which many actions and movements are involved right from the beginning. As a teacher and practitioner, one has to develop the eyes to see how not to break the flow of intelligence.

When one prepares to sit for the *āsana,* one sits on the middle of the foot (a) without turning. But as soon as one begins to place the arm, one does not maintain the same position or character of the leg that has been maintained before turning. As a teacher one may point out that the placement of the legs in *Ardha Matsyendrāsana* are good and correct, but one has to pay attention to maintain that sitting position without disturbance when one brings the arm over the other leg (b). Watch the structure and shape of the leg and foot on which one sits (right leg in the picture). It looks as if it is in *Śavāsana,* though bent and divided evenly at the knee (c). Next, look at the shape of the lifted left leg. It should be in a triangle. Similarly, watch the arm crossed over the leg to see whether it maintains the triangular shape (b). Feel the chain of changes that take place while adjusting the legs and arms to triangularity.

Does one notice the upper arm shortening when bent in order to place the forearm in this *āsana?* If the length of the forearm from the elbow is about sixteen inches, it should remain the same but it does not. Ask yourself why.

Perceive and follow the sense of direction in *Ardha Matsyendrāsana,* while catching the wrists on the back of the trunk a bridge-like grip has to be formed (d). This helps to move both the sides of the spinal vertebrae in a correct direction. This co-ordination of one part of the body with other parts should bring a sense of oneness and a feel of ease all over the body. When clasping the wrist in the *āsana,* watch the tilt of both wrists. They should not run zig-zag but run at the same angle (e&f).[1] This is the the *prāṇa* flowing without ripples. Balance various muscles of the *āsana* so that they do not break that flow, though the arms link together, one to the other,, the wrists maintain the same plane and do not disturb the rhythmic flow of *prāṇa.*

[1] In plate n. 13 the figure (e) shows the hand position "zig-zag" with the wrists facing different directions. In (f) the wrists are facing the same direction

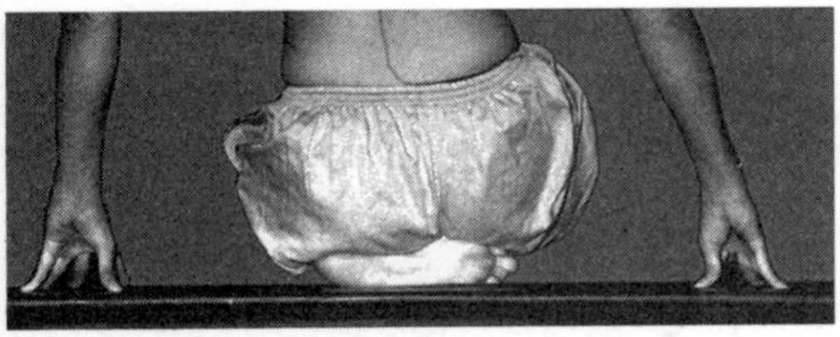
(a)

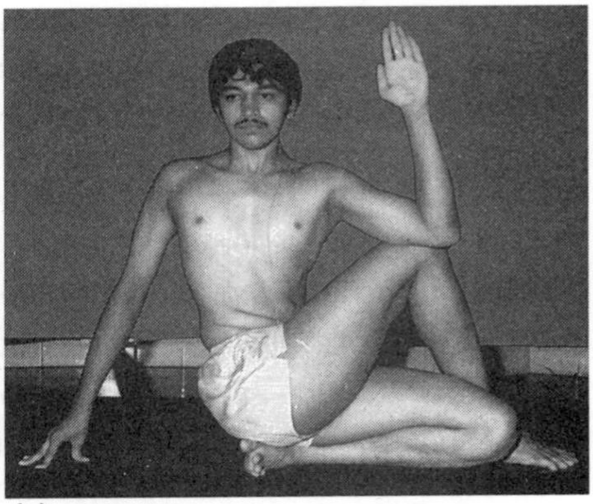
(b)

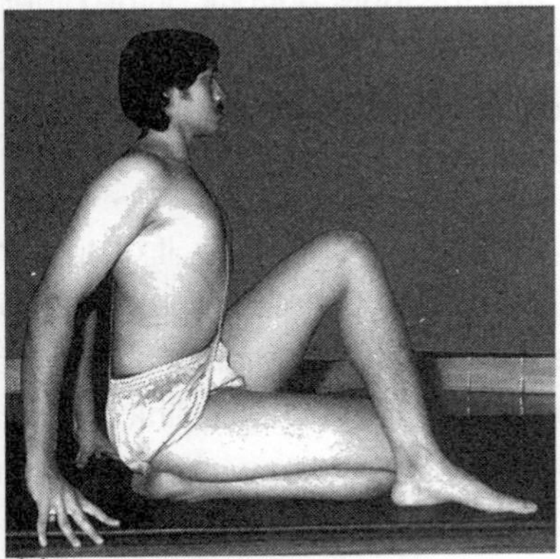
(c)

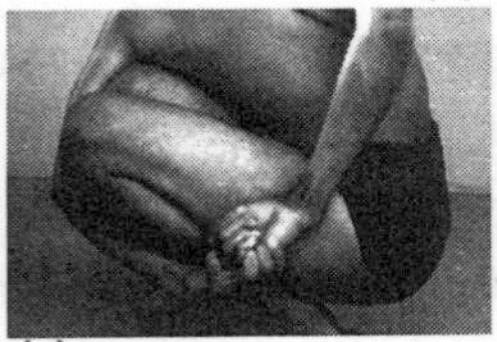
(e)

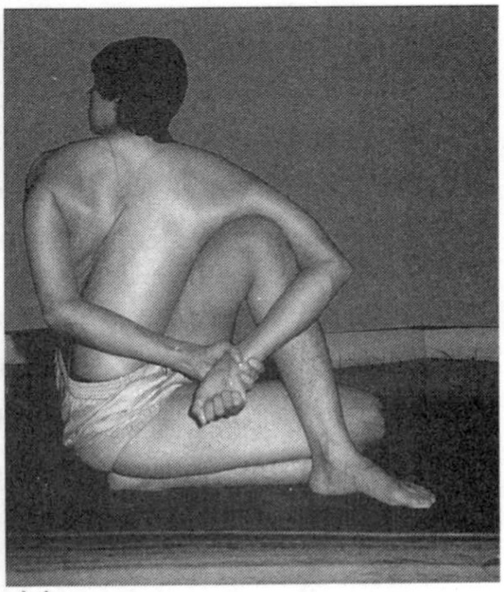
(d)

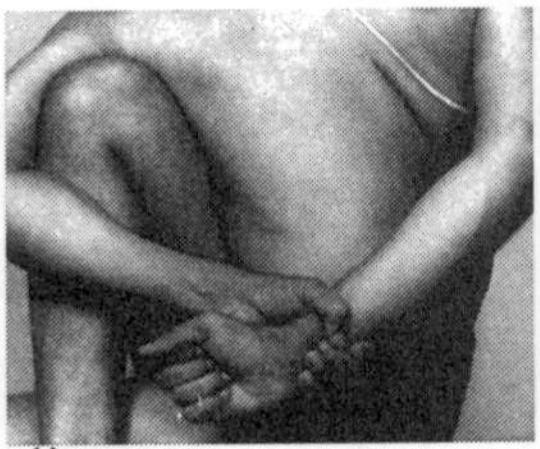
(f)

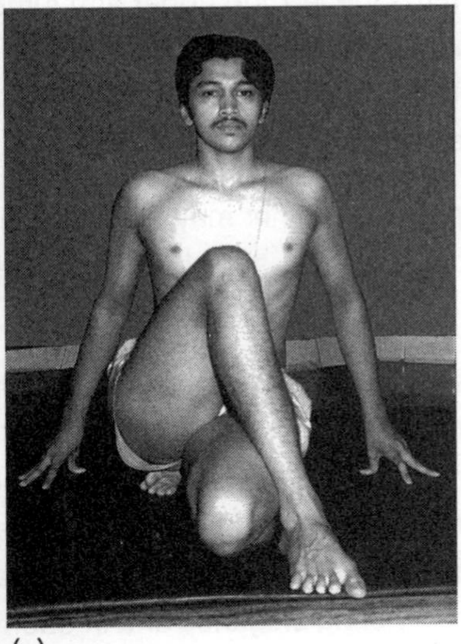
(g)

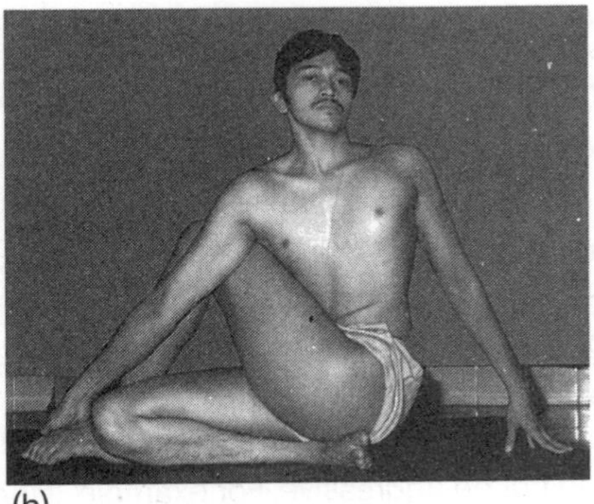
(h)

Plate n. 13 – *Ardha Matsyendrāsana* series

Similarly rest the ligaments of the knee to run parallel between the thigh and the calf muscles and cartilages resting in these positions. Normally they tilt on the leg on which one sits(g). These things have to be observed, noticed and rectified by the teachers of the advanced level.

The clue to this alignment is to lift the buttocks from the foot upwards, and then sit on the middle of the foot by placing the outer buttock on the heel and the inner buttock of the other on the mounds of the sole so that you are sitting on the median line of the foot. Do not lose the base when you take the arm to entwine behind the back or hold the left foot with the straight arm (h). Though it takes time for adjustment do not forget the base points.

This way learn to observe further when you take the hand over the leg. If disturbance takes place by readjustment, re-do so that the inner and outer knee ligaments are kept apart. Measure what space do the inner ligaments have with the outer ones, and maintain that space while doing this *āsana*. Now, carefully turn the head, without losing that balance, link the hands without disturbing the buttock on the foot or the big toe mound. Catch if there was any shift in the big toe mound and learn to readjust.

Observe how the forearm is turning. As it turns towards the leg, the upper arm turns in the opposite direction. Observe and feel the line of the forearm and the upper arm and touch the same area of the whole arm to follow without distracting the direction of the arms. This inter-connection and direction is the key towards obtaining alignment.

In the same way, one side of the spine may go up and the other may not. In the final *āsana* both sides of the spine should be parallel to each other as if the spinal column were in *Tāḍāsana* as far as possible.

Now watch and study the position of the pelvis. When one places one leg over the other, the pelvic girdle position changes for the *āsana*. Maintain its parallel position to the ground as you turn the upper arm in line to the lower arm. Commonly one side lifts up and the other side sinks and goes down. After entwining the arms, re-adjust the pelvis by creating room between the muscle and the bone as well as the skin. Adjust all the aspects of the geometry of the *āsana* within the body's anatomical and vital organic frame so that they bring elegance and freedom in the organs while in the *āsana*.

Do not be aggressive. For example, if the foundation has to become stronger and firmer in *Ardha Matsyendrāsana*, sit on the foot, measure the medial buttock bone so as to rest it on the middle of the arch. Do not move one way or the other. Keep the buttock bones in their position. Notice how the ligaments of the knee adjust. Then many other things find their right place.

When you go to the final pose, do not narrow the outer ligament of the knee. Question why the outer ligament narrows when the inner does not. With entwined arms, notice why the palm which grips (gripper) is dynamic and the other which is open (gripped) remains passive. Work out how to make the other respond to dynamism and positivity. While curling the knuckles on both hands, equal pressure has to be used. Measure and maintain the length of both the upper arms whether bent or straight. Similarly, measure one elbow with the other. Study the chest and spine when they go up as well as when they go down. This is learning, or call it re-learning through un-learning the wrong.

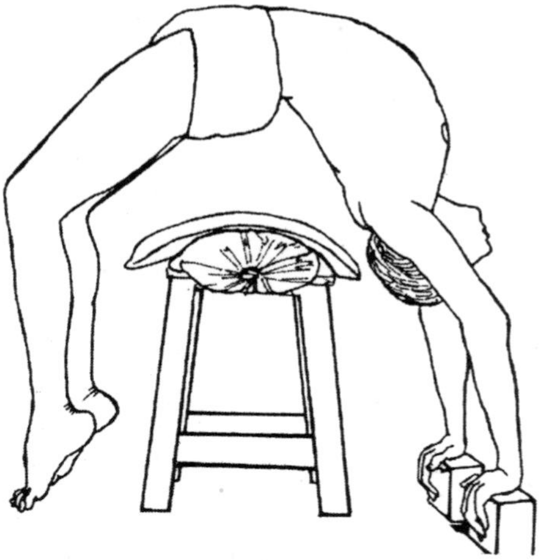

Plate n. 14 – *Ūrdhva Dhanurāsana* from a stool

ŪRDHVA DHANURĀSANA

Now I will explain this gradation in teaching in another *āsana, Ūrdhva Dhanurāsana.* First it is taught from support, lying on a stool, then by going up from the floor. When this comes, the teacher begins to teach back-bends from *Tāḍāsana.* Regarding dropping back from standing position, one has to find which part of the leg loses its grip and collapses. It may be that one calf muscle bends and collapses while curving backwards in the *āsana.* The muscle of the back leg should be in constant contact with the mind. If the contact is lost one loses control and bangs one's head or falls on the floor.

In order to stop the fall one has to co-ordinate the thigh muscles to the calves and calves to the thighs. Without the feel of the thigh one cannot control the calf, and without the calf one cannot control the thigh. This is the co-ordinated interaction which you have to use in all *āsana.*

One should see whether the calf muscles bend more or the thigh muscles bend more. If the thigh muscles are bent more they become shorter. When they shorten, the calf muscles bend too and cave in causing one to lose balance. To get that power into the calf muscle one has to watch from inside and ask, "Did I contract my thigh muscle? When I bend the knees, do I maintain the length of the thigh muscles? Do I maintain the steadiness in my knees?". All these points need to be studied.

The hamstring muscles in particular play a major role in this *āsana*. So if one pays attention directly to them, the calf muscles automatically develop resisting power. Confidence is built up in the legs and one learns to take the arms or the head back, further increasing the power and strength in the legs. Through this stage by stage curvature, the changes take place in the centre of gravity. Without changing the centre of gravity in the legs, one has to drop the arms to the floor. It is this sort of study that the senior students should be learning while practising.

GRADATION IN TEACHING

One should have a measured view of the length and width of the muscles and observe the reactions that come while doing various *āsana;* then the teacher has to bring his intelligence to co-ordinate the muscles to act and react. Then one can say that one is learning while practising.

You need to hold all the points in your mind (memory). The mind has to interact quickly at every other area and therefore reach every nook and corner of the body. When all these are well established, the teaching becomes easy. You can impart the knowledge to others.

Each day pay total attention to linking the missing points in two or three *āsana* and do the rest to keep in touch. Next day you can take another two *āsana* and work on them. In this way you study the changes that come in the cognisable and perceivable parts of the body in those *āsana*. Use this type of interchange in actions and reactions to proceed further. By this way one not only learns to make progress but also learns to mould the mind and ego.

Then go further and increase the sensitivity of intelligence to tap the subtle aspects of each *āsana*. This way you develop sensitivity and awareness. The foundation becomes stronger and stronger. In the beginning, the new students as well as the introductory teachers go aggressively. If the senior students still go on aggressively, it means that nothing has been learnt by them.

The balance and co-ordination in every movement and action in every *āsana* helps the *prāṇic* current to flow evenly. Unless one correctly adjusts the position of the *āsana*, *prāṇic* energy does not flow. It is a question of studying a few *āsana* which you think you can do well, of re-studying after adjustment, and comparing the understanding from the early practice to this new approach. Then work out and learn how to bring that feeling in other *āsana*. This is the way one has to progress, both in practice and teaching.

Senior teachers while teaching should show their up-coming students how to observe the parts that collapse. Make them observe by showing where things go wrong, or where the source of action loses its power. The teachers have to keep on asking and guiding, so the students become much more aware. This brings the growth of intellect in the students. First guide them from soma to psyche and then from psyche to soma. This is what Patañjali's friendliness is. Friendliness of the body with mind and mind with body as well as the interaction and co-ordination of one muscle with the other muscle.

Repeatedly practise with colleagues. Ask each other what the mistakes are. It is through this discussion and correction that one gets rich and right techniques. Without attempting on oneself, advising others about techniques has no meaning.

Hence, the senior teachers need to learn to observe and guide the juniors for their improvement.

Instead of seeing the mistakes and correcting then and there, better go home and work on those faults four or five times and then guide the students as to how these mistakes occur and later add one more point to learn. Do not worry about losing the students as psychologically you gain confidence and knowledge. Teach them by bringing their awareness on the visual mistakes that they can see. Ask them to first correct what they see on their own. If they are quick in correcting, then tell them how to correct what they cannot see. If the teachers progress, the students do too.

Teachers therefore need to practise in order to bring progress in themselves. Their *sādhanā* has to uplift them and enhance the expanse of awareness and consciousness gradually so that they proceed from *mṛdu* state to *ātma prasādanaṁ*. May you all cultivate this quality of seeing and feeling in order to become better teachers.

Teachers have to know the level or the standard of their students. Similarly while training teachers, the teacher-trainers have to be specific and limit the instructions according to the standard. There has to be a significant difference between each level of the teachers, such as levels I and II of Introductory and junior and senior of Intermediate and Avanced courses.

I have given the examples of *Taḍāsana, Sālamba Śīrṣāsana, Ardha Matsyendrāsana* and *Ūrdhva Dhanurāsana.* As a teacher, you need to work with each *āsana* in this manner. As a *mṛdu* teacher for the Introductory level, you need to give the understanding of the musculo-skeletal body and its movements, so a beginner begins to move at least the arms and legs. This is *ārambha-avasthā.*

Then you may further give progressive instructions so that the students begin to recognise and understand their own body movements and adjustments. The connative actions may be cognised by them so they begin to give some shape to their body. This is called *ghaṭa-avasthā.* The students at this stage are mediocre. They are *madhyama* students according to Patañjali.

Then the teachers have to teach the students of average to *adhimātra* level, in which they begin to connect their body with mind and energy. The depth of penetration increases. They are introduced to their intelligence through their bodies. Now they know where they lack or break their communication with the inner body and try to reach those areas so that they do not slip away from awareness. This is called *paricaya-avasthā.*

Then the teachers have to lead their students through further stages to the advanced level. The students have to be intensely intent or *tīvra saṁvegin.* The whole *āsana* has to be taught in such a way that it comes totally into the sphere of awareness. This is known as *niṣpatti-avasthā.*

Finally the teacher-trainers as well as the teacher-trainees have to proceed further on their own, since it is with their own efforts that they achieve the result which I named earlier as the fifth category, where the consciousness spreads all over. This is called *citta-prasādanam* or *ātma-prasādanam.* The spread of the body, the spread of the consciousness and the all-pervasive self remain parallel to each other, since there are no holes and no fissures. The subject is holy, the approach holistic, so that aspirants may come to experience the Self.

SECTION II

YOGA, HEALTH AND THERAPEUTICS

YOGA FOR OVERALL HEALTH*

Dhanyānāṁ uttamaṁ dākṣyam
dhanānāṁ uttamaṁśṛtam
lābhānām śreyamārogyam
sukhānāṁ tuṣṭiruttama.[1]

Talent is the best of blessings,
Wisdom is the rarest of treasures,
Health is the best of acquisitions,
Delight is the finest of joys.

Dharmārtha kāma mokṣāṇām ārogyam mūlamuttamam, says *āyurveda.*[2]

Whether one wants to follow the science of duty (*dharma* or religiousness) or to earn a livelihood *(artha)* or to enjoy life *(kāma)* or seek liberation *(mokṣa),* health is a must, as health is the wealth of everyone.

Upaniṣads proclaim that a weakling cannot enjoy the pleasures of the world nor become a master of the Self, *Nāyamātmā balahīnenalabhyaḥ.*

Thus, the importance of health has been stressed from time immemorial by the ancient seers and the sacred scriptures.

As healthy plants and trees alone yield fragrant flowers and tasteful fruits, similarly smiles and happiness blossom out like flowers and fruits from a healthy man.

Man is a triune of body, mind and soul. The body is the outer cover of the inner man. This body is called the *kṣetra* or the field, and the inner man, the soul – the dweller of the body – the *kṣetrajña.* The body and the soul are woven together through the thread of intelligence *(buddhi)* and the needle of consciousness.

* Courtesy All India Radio, Pune.
1 *Mahabharata* III.314.76.
2 *Caraka Samhitā.* See also *Aṣṭadaḷa Yogamālā,* vol. 1, p. 196.

Śarīramādyam khalu dharma sādhanam, says Kalidasa. The body is a very important and essential vehicle of man to carry out his duty and to follow a religious life. To unite the mind with the soul is the universal religion of mankind.

In order to unite the mind with the soul, the body, which is the foundation, has to be kept healthy.

The sages of lore divided this body, for the sake of convenience, into three tiers with five sheaths to convey the depth of the abode of man. Out of the three tiers, the first is known as the core of the body or the Self *(kāraṇa śarīra),* the second as the mental body *(sūkṣma śarīra)* and the last, the gross body or the physical body *(sthūla śarīra* or *kārya śarīra).*

These three bodies are interwoven from the skin to the self and from the self to the skin through the thread of intelligence so that they can interpenetrate as one single unit through the needle of consciousness or *citta.*

By nature, the body is inert, dull and sluggish; the mind, vibrant, active and dynamic, and self, luminous and illuminative. Practice of yoga destroys the sluggishness of the body and builds it up to become equal to that of the active and sensitive mind. Then both the body and the mind are made to transcend to the level of the illuminative self with perfect health in body, stability in mind and clarity in intelligence. The hands signifying *kārya śarīra* for *karma,* head signifying *sūkṣma śarīra* for *jñāna* and heart signifying *kāraṇa śarīra* for *bhakti,* are made to unite man into a holistic way of life.

If the mirror is clean, objects are clearly reflected. Similarly, practice of yoga removes the impurities of the body and causes the mind to reflect like the mirror, lighting the flame of wisdom which shines in the body, mind and self, so that they move and work in unison.

The body is one of the finest precise instruments on earth. It has about three hundred and odd joints, seven hundred and odd muscles. We do not know how many minor muscles and link muscles are in this machine. If the nervous system were stretched as a single thread, it would reach from Mumbai to London. If arteries, veins and capillaries are connected together, they run to one hundred thousand kilometres. The lungs are as broad as a tennis court supplying about two hundred and fifty millilitres of oxygen to the blood. The heart rhythmically beats about seventy times per minute pumping about five litres of blood per minute. This is enough to know how much one has to be vigilant to shape the body in order to possess good health.

Nature fortunately provides this precise instrument – the body – with means to adjust its rhythm to the turmoils of day-to-day pressures and environmental stress. It is also astonishing that in spite of imbalances created by the possessors of the body, it maintains its balance in spite of human overindulgence in satisfying their greedy wants. When the limits are overstepped, physical, physiological and psychological diseases set in. Prejudice, doubt and fear occupy the seat of the mind creating emotional disorders as psychosomatic diseases.

Health is generally understood as freedom from illness, but it is more than freedom from illness. Health is a perfect state of equilibrium and concord in the functions of joints, tissues, muscles, cells, nerves, glands, respiration, circulation, digestion, assimilation and elimination, and also a perfectly balanced disposition of mind.

Life is a combination of conscience, consciousness, intelligence, mind, senses of perception and organs of action. Health involves a tremendous communication with each and every part of man so that each cell communes with the other. This cannot be purchased in a market place. Health has to be earned with inspiration, sweat, and toil. Yoga does that.

Yoga has eight aspects known as *yama, niyama, āsana, prāṇāyāma, pratyāhāra, dhāraṇā, dhyāna* and *samādhi,* forming ethical, physical, mental, intellectual and spiritual disciplines. The first two aspects of yoga are from time immemorial, known as do's and don'ts or *rīti* and *nīti.* The next three are for progressive evolution of the practitioner and the last three are the wealth of yoga which comes by following the first five principles.

Yoga not only works and triggers the whole body but also develops and illumines the intelligence for the sight of the Self. It connects the anatomical and physiological bodies, as well as the mind and the soul of man. It deals with the structure of the body and proper functioning of the muscles with perfect flow of blood current in the blood vessels. It provides even distribution of bio-energy or life force, the very *prāṇa śakti,* and channels the mind to a state of calmness to face life without becoming a victim of circumstance and environment but as a master of them. Yoga starts from the health of the body and makes one climb the Everest of spiritual contentment, poise and peace.

Even if we compare yoga with other forms of exercises, it has its unique place. Yoga is a *sarvāṅga-sādhanā.* It unites the body, mind and soul of the *sādhaka* so that he experiences a complete and holistic state of being. It brings a proper synthesis of body-mind instrument. The other games or gym-exercises work only on certain parts of the body and hence they become *aṅgabhāga-sādhanā.* In this type of *sādhanā* certain parts are worked out and other parts are neglected and therefore it may cause *aṅgabhanga* – split or division affecting the body.

We have been bestowed by the Creator with one and only capital – the body – for a worthy and useful life. This body is the temple or the kingdom of man. As it is the essential duty of the dweller of the house to keep the house clean and surroundings tidy in order to live in peace, I think that it is the duty of a man or a woman to keep his or her temple – the body – healthy and clean. This is ethics, and ethics begins from here.

The first three aspects of yoga – *yama, niyama* and *āsana* – bring moral and ethical discipline into the organs of action, senses of perception and to the body and mind as a whole. Patañjali of course wants first that all beings acquire *śauca* and *santoṣa*. In modern terms, *śauca* means physical health and *santoṣa* means contentment. This is only the beginning of the yoga *sādhanā*, but this factor of yoga is essential if we are to reach the higher aspects of it, namely *tapas, svādhyāya* and *Īśvara praṇidhāna*. *Tapas* is the burning desire to practise with dedication, *svādhyāya* is paying attention to the whole of man, self-study from body to the self, and *Īśvara praṇidhāna* is surrender of oneself to God.

Āsana are innumerable in number. They cater to the needs of each individual according to constitution and condition. They have vertical, horizontal and circumferential movements which feed back through concentrated blood and energy supply to those areas of the body in need. *Āsana* such as *Śīrṣāsana, Dwi Pāda Viparīta Daṇḍāsana, Sarvāṅgāsana*[1] with their various cycles irrigate the braincells with a fresh supply of blood, refresh man and increase his power of concentration with the least strain. *Uttānāsana, Adho Mukha Śvānāsana, Padmāsana, Paśchimottānāsana* and *Halāsana* quieten the movement of the head and the heart creating poise within. *Jaṭhara Parivartanāsana, Pāśāsana, Ardha* and *Paripūrṇa Matsyendrāsana, Kapotāsana, Vṛśchikāsana, Upaviṣṭha Koṇāsana* and *Baddha Koṇāsana*[2] work on liver, kidneys, spleen, pancreas, intestines, urinary organs and the excretory system. In yoga each cell is observed, attended to and provided with the supply of pure blood and energy, so that the cells do their job profoundly before they die.

Prāṇāyāma, the science of respiration, has three functions, namely, inhalation, retention and exhalation. Inhalation is the intake of energy, retention is the distribution of energy and exhalation is the output of energy.

Prāṇāyāma too have varieties as *āsana*, such as *Ujjāyī, Viloma, Anuloma, Pratiloma, Bhrāmarī, Bhastrikā, Kapāla-bhāti, Sūrya Bhedana, Chandra Bhedana, Nāḍī Śodhana*,[3] etc. There are digital and non-digital *prāṇāyāma*. Non-digital *prāṇāyāma*, in which fingers do not control the flow of breath, have varieties which can be done in sitting as well as supine positions of the body.

---

[1] See *Light on Yoga*, Harper Collins, London.
[2] See *Light on Yoga*, Harper Collins, London.
[3] See *Light on Prāṇāyāma*, Harper Collins, London.

Again, *prāṇāyāma* in sitting positions can be done with *bandha* such as *Jālandhara, Uḍḍīyāna* and *Mūla,* and *mudrā* such as *Mahāmudrā, Ṣanmukhī mudrā* and *Aśvini mudrā.* The various *prāṇāyāma* energise different areas of the body. The depth, breadth and expanse of the breath touch new levels in different *prāṇāyāma.* The inhalation, exhalation and retention can be prolonged and qualitatively improved by practising various *prāṇāyāma.* The digital *prāṇāyāma,* in which the fingers are kept on the nose in order to control and channel the flow of breath, brings resonance and delicacy in the *nāḍī* of the body leading towards proper energy balance.[1]

Our life span is measured by the number of breaths occurring at about fifteen a minute. A proper rhythmic pattern of slow deep breathing soothes the nerves and checks emotional excitements. *Prāṇāyāma* helps the two tributaries – energy and consciousness – to flow into the river of tranquillity, so that one is able to withstand the present day trend towards stress, strain and speed. Thus, *āsana* and *prāṇāyāma* as fountains of health give a firm foundation for health. They also help in avoiding the hidden latent diseases which may surface later in life. Hence not only do they work as a therapeutic science but also as a preventive art.

The beauty of yoga is that it can be practised irrespective of whether one is young or old, male or female, healthy or unhealthy, poor or rich, undernourished or overnourished; but with one condition, that it has to be done half an hour before or four hours after food.

Know that an aggressor annexes a nation when it is weak and a thief burgles when the owner is careless. So also if one is careless the body becomes a breeding ground for diseases. Like the farmer who ploughs the uncultivated fallow land, removes the weeds, provides water and manure, sows the best of seeds, tends the crops and enjoys the best of harvest, *yama* and *niyama* plough the body, *āsana* removes toxins and symptoms of diseases, *prāṇāyāma* irrigates the body with energy and *pratyāhāra* tends the mind like a crop to enjoy the harvest of health, happiness and unalloyed peace in meditation. Then for the body and its dweller – the *kśetra* and the *kśetrajña* –, it becomes a heaven on earth.

[1] See *Light on Prāṇāyāma,* Harper Collins, London.

DIVINE HEALTH THROUGH YOGA

The prime concern of each and ever one is health – the health of the body and of the mind.

WHAT IS HEALTH?

Health is a state of distress-free, stress-free and unalloyed bliss in body, mind and soul.

Health does not mean just existence or freedom from disease. It is like a live wire, ever sensitive, ever vibrant and alert. It is like the running water of a river which is always fresh.

Good health is dependent upon one's heredity, body structure, broad understanding, family relationships and spiritual outlook.

WHY HEALTH?

Śarīramādyam khalu dharma sādhanam.

Body is the first and foremost instrument to perform *dharma* or duty of man as a human being.

Caraka, in the treatise on *āyurveda* declares, *dharmārtha kāma mokṣāṇām ārogyam mūlamuttamam.*

Health is the key to performing duty, earning wealth, or using life for enjoyment or for emancipation.

Upaniṣads proclaim, *nāyamātmā balahīnenalabhyaḥ.*

Self-realisation cannot be obtained by those who are weak.

The body, the embodiment and abode of the soul, is meant not for enjoyment but for emancipation. This nearest and dearest instrument of ours has to be used with discrimination to carry on the religious and virtuous duty that has been entrusted to us as responsible human beings – the evolved species on this earth. The health of the body and mind of human beings is important and without that one cannot carry on any duty or fulfil life's aims or ambitions. Even the realisation of the soul is impossible if one is weak in body. Whether to carry out *dharma* – duty, *karma* – action, or to have *darśana* – Self-realisation, health is the foundation. Therefore, in order to fulfil worldly or spiritual desires, the lower or higher aspects of life, basically one requires health.

HEALTH IS TO BE EARNED

Health or unhealth is in one's own hands. One needs the discrimination to choose.

Health is not a commodity to be bought and sold, but it has to be earned by inspiration and perspiration.

As a goldsmith heats gold to refine it, we have to bake our body, mind and intelligence through yoga to achieve health in body, mind and soul.

As a clean mirror reflects objects clearly, practice of yoga reflects health in oneself.

DISEASES

Diseases are classified as *ādhyātmika, ādhibhautika*, and *ādhidaivika roga* or *tāpa*.[1]

Ādhyātmika roga is self-induced. *Ādhibhautika* is from habits, wherein one imbalances the body mechanism and disturbs the ratio of the five elements of earth, water, fire, air and ether.

If the earth element is disturbed, it leads to constipation; water element, to frequent passing of urine and dropsy; fire element to ulcers, bleeding and burning sensation; air element to asthma, cough and bronchitis; while ether element towards rheumatism, atrophy and arthritis.

Ādhidaivika roga may be genetic or allergic. We call it, *prārabdha karma*.[2]

Patañjali says that sorrow, despair, tremor of the body, laboured breathing, overtake man's good health in the form of physical ailments; carelessness, idleness, indecision and sense gratification as mental ailments; living in the world of delusion as an intellectual ailment, and lack of perseverance and inability to maintain what has been obtained as spiritual diseases (*Y.S.,* I.30).

---

1 See this volume,The article "Is Yoga a Nature Cure?"

2 Merit or demerit from previous life to experience in the present life.

YOGA OFFERS A REMEDY

Practice of yoga destroys the impurities of body and mind, and radiates maturity in intelligence and wisdom from the core of the being, to function in unison with its vehicles; the body, the senses, the mind, the intelligence and the consciousness. (*Y.S.*, II.28).

Sufferings may be physical, emotional, intellectual or instinctive. Yoga is in a way, a remedial science also.

Yoga is a physico-physiological, physio-psychological and psycho-spiritual science and art, as it distinguishes diseases of body, mind and self, and shows remedies.

Body

Having spoken about health and disease, let us learn about our possession – the body.

The body is one of the finest instruments and the most complex apparatus. Even if it breaks down, it tries to repair the damage on its own. Practice of yoga accelerates the repairing process and helps to regain good health.

Know that our body has hundreds of joints, with hundreds and hundreds of muscles and hundreds of trillions of cells pieced together to form an organic system with the heart as the hub of the circulatory system. This is an extremely sturdy muscle operating continuously as an automatic pump, pumping blood at the rate of five ounces per beat covering sixty thousand miles of blood vessels. The body is such an instrument that it maintains and adjusts the frequency of the beats as occasion demands.

The metabolism is the major function of the body on which the health of the body depends totally. The various organs of the body such as liver, heart, spleen, kidney, function with co-ordination and co-operation. They are interdependent and, as a result, assist and support each other when the occasion arises. The source of this vitalism is the soul.

The most important organ, the brain, is made up of 10 billion cells needing 25% of the total oxygen supplied by the blood. I think that this is enough to prove the value of *Sālamba Śīrṣāsana* and *Sālamba Sarvāṅgāsana*.[1]

The bio-energy runs in the nerves which extend six thousand miles. Hence, the body is nothing but a network of nerve cells and fibre with energy travelling at the rate of two hundred miles an hour.

---

[1] See *Aṣṭadaḷa Yogamālā* vol 2, plate n. 5.

The nervous system has three layers – the peripheral, the autonomous and the central systems. The peripheral or the motor and sensory nerves get impulses from the organs of actions and the senses of perception. Skin transmits sensory impulses and the spindles of the muscles transmit the motor impulses. The autonomous nerves are influenced by mind, and the central nerves react through the discriminative intelligence. If the bones and marrow are towers of strength, muscles have the power to pull, and nerves the power to endure.

Let us see how yoga helps this God-designed body, through movements and postures to generate health in the musculo-skeletal, cardio-pulmonary, respiratory, circulatory, glandular, digestive, uro-genital and excretory systems.

YOGA

The word yoga has come from the verb *yujir* which means to unite, to join, to associate, to discipline, to attend to and to yoke the body and mind to the soul.

Saṁyoga yoga ityukto jīvatma paramātmanaḥ.[1]
Yoga means union of the individual soul with God.

Lord Krishna says, *yogaḥ karmasu kauśalaṁ* (*B.G.,* II.50).
Skillfulness in action is yoga.

Patañjali says, *yogaḥ citta vṛtti nirodhaḥ* (*Y.S.,* I.2).
Restraint of movements in consciousness is yoga.[2]

Yoga is like a ladder with eight stages; a chain with eight links. These are *yama, niyama, āsana, prāṇāyāma, pratyāhāra, dhāraṇā, dhyāna* and *samādhi.*

Yama* and *niyama

Yama and *niyama* are meant to cultivate good character. *Yama* guides us to discard violence, lying, stealing, lust and greed, whereas *niyama* teaches the ways of cleanliness, contentment, burning desire to develop purity and makes one study scriptures dealing with higher aspects of life and the art of surrender to God.

Āsana

Poise in body and peace in mind is the aim of us all. *Āsana* helps to reach this aim.

---

1 *Ahirbuḍha Samhitā.*
2 See the author's *Light on Aṣṭāṅga Yoga,* YOG, Mumbai, 1999.

Āsana means a posture, the positioning of the body in various forms with the total involvement of mind and self in order to keep the physical, physiological, psychological, intellectual and spiritual sheaths of man at the optimum level of health, equilibrium, harmony and balance.

Each *āsana* helps to create and generate energy. When one stays in the *āsana*, the energy is organised and distributed, and when one comes out of it with rhythm and grace, the generated and distributed energy does not dissipate. In this way, monitoring and managing the energy is *svāsthya* or good health according to *āyurveda*.

The body is like a railway track and train. If the bones represent the rails, joints act as fish-plates, making the muscles like the wheels of the train move in line with the bones for smooth movements. The train derails if the fish-plates are loose. Similarly, when the cartilages in our joints lose power, muscles move in different directions and cause ailments. Our spinal vertebrae are like the bogies of a train. As bogies are connected with vacuum pipes, our spinal vertebrae are created in such a way that they absorb jerks without colliding with each other. The driver of the train is the brain and the guard is the tail-bone. The guard cautions the driver, as circumstances demand, with green or red flags. When the running train derails, the bogies get mutilated due to the strong impact. Today the stress, strain and speed of modern living mutilate the cells, spinal disks, muscles and organs, introducing diseases such as ulcer, cancer, cardiac diseases, arthritis, anxiety, worry, distress, dissatisfaction and so forth. Therefore, while practising *āsana*, the attention is constantly drawn towards both brain and brawn in order to avoid such problems or accidents. The driver, the brain, has to remain alert, watchful and wakeful. The guard, the tail-bone, along with the sacrum, has to caution and control every movement of the body. Negligence on the part of either can damage.

Judicious practice of *āsana* lubricates the joints, creates mobility, increases the range of movement, brings strength, stamina, endurance and awareness in each and every muscle, joint and organ. It also rejuvenates the organs of the body, transmits energy, builds reflexes and resistant power preventing diseases and disturbances.

As one keeps one's house clean and tidy, we have to keep this body – the temple of the *ātman* – clean, tidy and fresh by bathing it in the pool of blood by an increasing or decreasing, rinsing or drying process through various *āsana* and at the same time, move *prāṇa* or bio-energy for distribution, recuperation and rejuvenation. Mastery of *āsana* brings perfect form in the body, grace, strength, compactness, hardness and a diamond-like brilliance in intelligence.

There are four stages in the practice of *āsana: āraṁbha-avasthā, ghaṭa-avasthā, paricaya-avasthā* and *niṣpatti-avasthā*. One begins with conative action, *(āraṁbha)*, cognises *(ghaṭa)*, then works with intelligence *(paricaya)* and after that becomes totally absorbed *(niṣpatti)*, losing the awareness of body, mind and intelligence, and lives with the core of the being. *Āsana* interpenetrates from the skin towards the self and outerpenetrates from the self towards the skin, touching the physical, mental, intellectual and spiritual bodies.

Āsana can be practised by all irrespective of race, creed, country, gender or age whether young or old, diseased or weak.

Āsana are called *sarvāṅga-sādhanā* or holistic *sādhanā* as they envelop man from the physical to the spiritual level, whereas the other types of *sādhanā* are *aṅgabhāga-sādhanā*, developing one part at the cost of the others.

Patients with serious problems are taken to the Intensive Care Unit. Similarly, the yogis gave us the use of props or supports to perform *āsana* if one is invalid. The method is called *yogakuruṇṭa*.

Prāṇāyāma

When the understanding, feeling and sensitivity of the action/interaction of the body, mind and breath comes to the *sādhaka* with the practice of *āsana*, the *prāṇāyāma-sādhanā* begins. *Prāṇāyāma* generates and distributes life energy to maintain youthfulness in the physiological body so that one grows old without the feeling of ageing.

As the physiological body is the bridge to cross over from the physical body towards the spiritual body, *prāṇāyāma* is the bridge to cross over from the physical and moral discipline towards mental and spiritual discipline.

Pratyāhāra, dhāraṇā, dhyāna* and *samādhi

By *pratyāhāra* - restraint of mind, intelligence is stabilised in order to move to *dhāraṇā*. Here oscillation and vacillation come to an end. Rays of attention radiate as *dhyāna*. Health shines without demarcation of body, mind and self. This is *samādhi* or *samādhāna sthithi* - an auspicious state of brilliance and divinity in health.

YOGA FOR STRESS-FREE LIFE

LIFE IN TURMOIL

We are living in the present rat race of life with an unnecessary creation of tension both within and around us. Because of this fast life, we are neglecting the body and the mind. The body and mind are beginning to pull each other in opposite directions, dissipating our energy. We do not know how to recharge our batteries of energy. We have become careless and callous.

Industrial development and urbanisation have no doubt triggered a fast life. Science and technology have given us the boons of physical comfort and leisure. But we do not allow our mind to pause and think. We throw ourselves mindlessly from one endeavour to another believing that speed and movement is all in life.

We seek entertainment and excitement on the T.V. screen and in the print media, but we forget the important criteria of how to use leisure time for our refinement and inner development and growth.

Movies bombard us with doses of violence. We read fiction, thrillers and murder mysteries day in and day out. However, reading the literature of high thinking and ideals has taken now a back seat in life.

Where is the time to think or ponder, to contemplate or introspect on the process of life? In the East we are a shade better. In the West there is the paradox of a communication upsurge going hand in hand with disastrous communication gaps. Husbands and wives have no time to talk to each other, parents have no time to communicate with their children.

The result is alienation from our near and dear ones and from the whole of society. This has built up violence in petty matters with all kinds of perversions and tensions bottling up which result in an escalating crime rate.

Here to our rescue comes the *sūtra* of *Pātañjala Yoga, yogaḥ citta vṛtti nirodhaḥ*[1] – The art of restraining the consciousness and of keeping in a state of restful motionlessness.

STRESS AND STRAIN

What is stress and strain? Stress is a forced extension, a force or a vacuum exerted on the body beyond endurance at a point of time. Strain is the overtaxing, injuring and exerting of mind or body or both. Tension may be physical, mental, intellectual or nervous. Strain and stress are often accompanied by muscular and intellectual tautness. Fatigue, both physical and mental, is another component. It can arise due to overacting or from a lack of it, or even due to boredom. Our educational system has proved to be a flop as more and more educated people, students, women, men comfortably placed in life complain, "We are bored stiff!". There is a wide spectrum of interests, games, music, arts, literature and natural beauty available, yet the main grievance is boredom. An individual who has cultivated himself would have a variety of interests to plunge into after work is over.

Fright and tension are not something new. It was there even in prehistoric time. Man was then and still is gripped by a "fight or flight" response. Our modern hectic life-styles have served to multiply them and invited them to mount up and pile upon us.

Life is not always a bed of roses. It contains pitfalls, pain and pleasure, happiness and unhappiness. Life has to be faced and what Patañjali describes as *kleṣa* – afflictions – have to be borne and have to be undergone with a patient and calm mind.

By burying our head in the sand like an ostrich, we cannot brush them aside or wish them away. It is our negative and escapist approach that puts the grindstone of anxiety and worry around our own neck. Patañjali expects yoga practitioners to prepare in advance for pains that might beset us.

Modern analytical therapists say that insecurity and anxiety is the fundamental cause of all neurosis. They strive to open up the unconscious to get to the cause. There are multiple causes that trigger tension, strain and stress. Anxiety may be due to insecurity or fear of the unknown and of what life will unfold before us.

Dread of the future, insecurity over whether the necessities and requirements of life will be met and fulfilled or not, and fear of losing what one has, worry mankind. These worries may build up around the house, food, the job, the circle of friends and relatives, the community, or the

[1] See the author's *Light on the Yoga Sūtras of Patañjali*, pp. 45-48.

fear of losing money, name and fame, as well as near and dear ones. Humans innately resist change for fear of insecurity. We tend to live in a familiar fixed standard and try to avoid accepting or even feeling what is beyond the known. The essence of life is relativity for a common man. Life inevitably oscillates, moves and changes between the known and the unknown. We are not ready to accept the flow of things or to study how to adapt and constructively build ourselves up. We are neither ready to face loneliness nor aloneness. We do not want either freedom or bondage. We do not allow life to "happen" and take shape.

Conflicts, opposition, clash of interests and ideas, collision of mutual ego, personal and collective, and limited understanding are all inevitable parts of life. They are like passing breezes, warm, hot, cold, soothing, unnerving, tolerable or intolerable. The individual takes them as a routine of life and conducts himself as well as his worldly affairs accordingly.

THE WAY OUT

Ancient sages, *ṛṣis* and seers, literature and scriptures set a great emphasis on what man does in this world in accordance with his past chain of *karma* and previous births. Their guidance is on how to construct ways and means for better living. For this they take us towards the yogic way of living. The approach of the western psychotherapeutics and that of the East with its "wisdom" is fundamentally different. Western techniques provide physical relaxation and superficial quietness.

This yogic approach is control of the movements of the mind. Mind is a great culprit. Self control will save many a situation, if the individual can retain his poise of mind, stay cool and be able to do the *sādhanā* without getting unduly perturbed or agitated. Having done what could be done, one is then prepared to await patiently the outcome or consequences of the action, whether they be a success, or partly success – partly failure, or bring suffering and want of comfort or pleasure.

Yoga believes in developing a strong fabric which will withstand the onslaughts of the fluctuations, the ups and downs, the pleasure and pain, or a mixed product of despair, hope, frustration, failure, triumph and so forth.

Yoga is a natural tranquilliser for the urges from within which we call "likes and dislikes". The discontent, frustration, disappointment, hopes, success, greed, ambition, sex and neediness in love veer round our expectations. All these situations are a part of normal daily life with its inevitable conflicts, oppositions, clash of interests and ideas, collision of mutual ego, limited or little understanding of the points of view of others. In the midst of hurry, and at times of stress or emergency, basic human values alter, latent impulses become more urgent. The conflict within the individual snowballs and gives rise to psychosomatic diseases.

YOGA COMES TO THE RESCUE

The first limb of yoga *(yama)* is a social virtue to observe in life while in contact with others. The second *(niyama)* is the individual discipline by which to improve oneself for the betterment of life. The third *(āsana)* is for maintenance of health and steadiness of mind. Health is a perfect balance of body, mind and soul, free from disease and at the same time protecting, sustaining and supporting the living cells to lead a positive, constructive and creative life. Life is a combination of consciousness, intelligence, mind, senses of perception and action. Mind is like a mirror receiving the aspirations of the self and acting through the senses for enjoyment and attainment. It has a dual role to play at both ends. It receives and acts for the impressions from the self to the senses, or from the senses to the self. If the mind acts without discriminative power, the body and the self become the abode of suffering. Hence, the practice of yoga purges the impurities of the body, bringing beauty, strength, firmness, calmness and clarity, revealing a happy disposition without creating any dualities between body, mind and self.

The fourth limb *(prāṇāyāma)* is the extension, expansion, prolongation, requisition, distribution of vital energy and consciousness to spread well in its field, the body and mind. It is said that where breath is, there the consciousness is. So correct *prāṇāyāmic* practices regulate man's habits, desires and actions, and act as a bridge in unifying the body, the mind and the self.

The fifth limb *(pratyāhāra)* brings the senses and mind under control and stops the dual functioning of the mind by diverting it from the enjoyment of pleasures towards the union of the Self. The last three limbs *(dhāraṇā, dhyāna* and *samādhi)*, are collectively termed as *saṁyama* meaning integration.

NEGATIVE LIFE

The supersonic speed in thinking and action drains the physical frame, tenses the nerves and taunts the intellect. If one cannot release these tensions and relax, one develops sleepless nights, which in turn affect the thinking faculty. Anxieties multiply, and doubts and incapacities set in. Attitudes of jealousy and malice develop. Then man becomes negative in his approach to life. He is evasive, reserved, indifferent, depressed, lazy, ill at ease and creates his own philosophy of illusion, seclusion and isolation. From these he switches to artificial ways of living. He gets addicted to tranquillisers, sleeping pills, alcohol and various other psychedelic drugs and an indiscriminate sexual life in order to find peace and happiness.

PRACTICAL AND POSITIVE REMEDY

In a person who sees life negatively, his eye-balls are unsteady or blink as if they have no contact within himself. The eyes work as the window of the brain and the ears for the mind. While practising yoga, he is made to contact his eyes with motion and action. He is also made to feel that his intelligence is in contact with the parts of the body through yogic practices. To focus his attention with his body, senses and mind, he is made to perform *āsana* like *Sālamba Śīrṣāsana*, *Adho Mukha Vṛkṣāsana*, *Viparīta Daṇḍāsana*, *Ūrdhva Dhanurāsana*, *Sālamba Sarvāṅgāsana*, *Halāsana*, *Setu Bandha Sarvāṅgāsana*.[1] For particulars regarding the *āsana*, see the author's *Light on Yoga*. to flush and irrigate the brain cells with oxygenated blood to invigourate him. As there is no one "wonder drug" for any one disease for all the time, so also the practices have to be varied and adapted to the states or conditions required of the day. The breathing techniques are taught only after mastering the above mentioned *āsana*, whereby the person is made to build up confidence in himself and hold the breath for short spells after inhalations, known as *Aṅtara Kumbhaka*. As he has no will power of his own, he has to be guided in such a way that he is made to develop will power without his awareness. By this type of training and observation, he is freed from states of depression and isolation to a life of joy and bliss. My teaching experience with such people has shown a definite and positive result. Like any other healing art or science, yoga too is a healing art and science.

The practitioners of yoga have learnt to listen to their bodies and discover their own biological nature and psychological needs. This is how yoga works. To start with it gradually induces one to look within oneself and from there to have a feeling of fearlessness to taste the superconscious or cosmic force.

---

1 See the author's *Light on Yoga*, Harper Collins, London.

YOGA DE-STRESSES THE STRESS

If stress creates distress, it is a symptom of suffering. If the type of distress is de-stressed, it is a means to health and happiness. Stress factors can either be acute in the form of loss of property or the death of a close one, unanticipated incidents that leave one helpless and hapless, or stress may be chronic due to financial worries, marital disharmony or dissatisfaction.

Both bring on physical, cellular and neuro-psychological fatigue syndrome, sweating, tremors, palpitation, bronchial asthma, peptic ulcer, psychological disturbances affecting the brain and mind with apprehensions, doubts, fears, biological imbalances, disharmony in the hypothalamus and autonomous nervous system as well as in glandular and immune systems.

The moment life begins to ebb, it is followed by stress. A positive stress is a life elixir. However the negative stress that arises from oppressive and destructive thoughts causes compulsive pressures, mental grumbling, lust, greed, strained physical efforts, occupational hazards, physical and mental agony, hyper or hypo tensions, sleeplessness, restlessness, anger, irritations, nervous breakdown, and ends up in strokes and cardiac problems. These factors indicate that one needs the necessary changes and adjustments in one's life style.

Over ambition to acquire position, fame or wealth by hook or crook, or hatred of fellow beings and colleagues or forcing beyond one's physical endurance, mental and intellectual capacities or hasty decisions, add further stress on one who is already under duress.

Modern life is also filled with tension on account of an unhealthy competitive mentality due to industrial development and fast life. No doubt science and technology has brought comforts, yet it is making one roam mindlessly from one thing to another without a pause or rest for the brain or mind. This hardens the cells of the brain and shakes the nerves. That makes one lose confidence in oneself and makes one live in a fear psychosis with flight or fight reaction.

If one makes up one's mind to come out of flight and fight, the only way left is to emerge from this situation and overcome the fear psychosis to gain back confidence. For this, yoga is the only way open to release the tension in the nervous system and lighten the tautness of the brain. Only if the cup or a vessel is empty, one can use it. Is this not so? When it is full, it cannot be used and remains as a worthless vessel. It is the same with our brain and mind.

Yoga is a holistic discipline wherein not only all the parts of the body are made to act skillfully and harmoniously but it also recreates attention and relaxation simultaneously in the brain and mind, and then helps in diffusing the intelligence from the head to the mind, organs of action, senses of perception and body to observe whether the bio- energy reached the cellular system for the cells to regenerate and produce fresh energy to coil into the nervous system.

The discipline of yoga not only acts as a shock absorber but also helps in rebuilding and reconstructing defensive energy to combat the destructive and the offensive energy that creates further strain and stress.

Actually, the western physio-therapeutics uses techniques to provide just muscular relaxation, while the yoga discipline works not only on muscular relaxation but also on the tendons, fibres, ligaments, cells, organic body, senses of perception, the nerves, the brain, the mind and the very consciousness so that they are made to remain passive and pensive. Yoga is much concerned with cellular quietness which lightens the brain to a bare minimum and makes it fit to bear stress and strain with comfort. As a result, the mind is quietened automatically.

Yoga gives clues on how stress is de-stressed. Patañjali speaks about stress in two *sūtra*. One is, *avidyā asmitā rāga dveṣa abhiniveśaḥ kleśāḥ* (*Y.S.*, II.3). The other is *vitarkā hiṁsādayaḥ kṛita kārita anumoditāḥ lobha krodha moha pūrvakaḥ mṛdu madhya adhimātraḥ duḥkha ajñāna anantaphalāḥ iti pratipakṣabhāvanam* (Y.S., II.34).

In the first of them, *avidyā* is defined as a perverted intelligence where the transient is considered as permanent, the impure as pure, pain as pleasure and sensual joy as spiritual bliss; *asmitā* is taking the instrument, the 'I' or the ego, as the core of the being, as true Self; *rāga* is desire that breeds attachment; *dveṣa* is the unfulfilment of desire igniting hatred and *abhiniveśa* is love of life and fear of death. All these are categorised as stress factors.

In the second *sūtra* it is said that perverse thoughts, emotions and actions result in endless ignorance and pain. They are caused on account of greed, anger and delusion with mild, medium or intensive degrees igniting one to act directly or through inducement or abettment.

Patañjali says that these perverted actions bring hoards of dis-eases, namely, *vyādhi, styāna, saṁśaya, pramāda, ālasya, avirati, bhrāntidarśana, alabdhabhūmikatva* and *anavisthitatva*.

It means that the nine impediments which obstruct a healthy life style are disease, sluggishness, doubt, carelessness, idleness, sense gratification, living in the world of delusion, not being able to hold on to what is undertaken and inability to maintain what one has achieved, distract the mind and the consciousness. Are they not the effects of wrong stress?

Again Patañjali speaks about the symptoms and classifies them as *duḥkha, daurmanasya, aṅgamejayatva* and *śvāsapraśvāsa*.

Besides the above nine diseases, symptoms like sorrow, despair, tremor of the body and laboured breathing further distract and add to psyco-somatic sufferings. All these are absolute stress symptoms.

See how beautifully Patañjali explains stress factors and their symptoms. Then he guides us on how to help ourselves to get rid of them through *yogasādhanā*.

Know that medicine works only on a short-term basis, while practice of yoga supports life in the long term, not only rejuvenating it but exhilarating it too.

The practice of certain groups of *āsana* and *prāṇāyāma* sequenced properly creates space inside the body and flushes out the impediments which block the blood from flowing in the blood vessels and clears the energy blocks in the nervous system, thus preparing man to bear the load with ease in the neuro- endocrine and immune system. Besides these, the eyes, the windows of the brain, and the ears, the windows of the mind, are made to relax during yogic practices which prepare us to develop calmness in the brain and mind, gradually releasing the practitioner from disturbance due to stress and strain for ever.

IS YOGA A NATURE CURE?*

Yoga is a holistic subject – oriental and very much original. It is a spiritual science having a healing touch. It is a *cikitsā śāstra* – the science of treatment – very close to nature cure. Nature cure is an objective way whereas yoga is a subjective process. In *prākṛtika cikitsā* – nature cure, the natural resources such as earth, water, fire, air and ether are utilised whereas in yogic *cikitsā* the very *prakṛti,* which is an embodiment of soul, is made use of. The treatment of yoga is not limited only to this visible body but also to the invisible body like the organs of action, senses of perception, mind, ego and intelligence.

The modern world traces the cause of diseases to stress, strain and speed as a mode of life and as such behavioural patterns have changed radically. Unhealthy competition, unfriendliness, envy and jealousy have become part of our nature. We say that we want to encourage youngsters to take to sports, but we are uprooting the very sporting nature and encourage them to develop "bad sportsmanship". Each one looks at the other with suspicion. No one trusts the other. One may speak sweetly, but the heart is full of arrogance and malice. We are polite on the outside but poisonous within. The love for work is lost. Unwillingness to work makes one feel that the work-load is very heavy. One gets exhausted easily because of the negative attitude. Selfish interest is the means and the end. Everyone wants to get rich, famous and successful quickly without any effort. "Work less and expect more!" has become the motto. No one has time to breathe, no one has time to relax. No one has the time to look back at past experiences, but everyone dreams of the fruits of the future. A man wants to grab the future. Everyone is in such a hurry that speed is God. And therefore stress and strain are inevitable. These three "S's" (speed, stress and strain) are destroying the mind of the human being.

Today, I am asked to speak on whether yoga can be a natural remedial treatment – *prākṛtika cikitsā* – for stress and strain. Do not expect a prescription of *āsana* and *prāṇāyāma* for stress and strain from me! We are supposed to find the root cause for stress and strain. The

---

* Speech given at a "Nature Cure and *Āyurveda*" conference, recently held by the *Karnataka Prakṛtika Parisad* in Bangalore.

disease has entered deep in and engulfed one and all. No more is it a symptomatic disease but it has become a chronic one. Just now, a few minutes back, someone said: "Do a few minutes of *Śavāsana*[1] and you will be free from stress and strain." How can *Śavāsana* be a treatment when the disease has penetrated deeply into the five sheaths of the body? *Śavāsana* could be a treatment merely for symptoms. How can the root cause be eradicated by doing *Śavāsana*? A person who is not pure in heart and mind, who not only cheats others but also himself and one who is avaricious and mints money by hoodwinking his fellow beings, can he do *Śavāsana*? One may relax the physical body but what about the mind and the intelligence? Can they be relaxed? Will the guilty conscience allow one to be peaceful? *Śavāsana* is easy to speak about but difficult to understand and harder to do. *Śavāsana* is to simulate the actual experience of death, i.e., complete stillness and silence. One has to live consciously like a dead body.[2] The *rajas* of the mind and the *tamas* of the body have to be conquered in order to remain in a *sāttvic* state. That is why *Śavāsana* comes at the end of practice. Have we sanctified and purified our body and mind to do *Śavāsana*? Have we sterilised, filtered and sanitised every cell of our body? Try to understand the cause of an unhealthy state! *Śavāsana* may give you relief from stress, strain and fatigue for a while, but can it be a permanent cure when stress and strain have gone deep into our system? Worry and anxiety lead one to heart-trouble and diabetes. How did the stress reach the core of our being, the heart and the liver? Why did these organs get affected?

It is time to look at the situation as a whole. Even Arjuna was not free from this so-called modern disease. Right on the battlefield, he developed tremors in his body. He felt as if the *Gāṇḍīva* (his bow) was slipping from his hand. He felt a burning sensation on the skin. He became unsteady physically as well as mentally and was in a confused state.[3] Are these not the symptoms of stress and strain? Lord Krishna could have asked him easily to do *Śavāsana,* but he did not do so. On the contrary, he changed Arjuna's mental attitude by making him understand the path of yoga by blending *karma, jñāna* and *bhakti* in it. Krishna did not medicate nor prescribe meditation. He made Arjuna face the situation boldly with clarity of intelligence and purity of conscience.

We too are supposed to learn the art of living. Our life is invaded by the three "S's": speed, stress and strain. Patañjali introduces three "W's": work, word and wisdom. Purity in work, clarity in word and sanctity in wisdom.

---

1 See *Aṣṭadaḷa Yogamālā* vol 2, plate n. 3.

2 See the author's *Light on Yoga, Light on Prāṇāyāma,* Harper Collins, London and specially *Aṣṭadala Yogamāla,* vol. 2, pp. 288-300.

3 *Bhagavad Gītā,* I.29-31.

We are all disturbed, perturbed and confused because of our own behaviour, our actions and our way of thinking. It seems that the words *sadācāra* (good and auspicious deeds and actions) and *sadvicāra* (good and auspicious thoughts) have become words to be found only in the dictionary.

From time immemorial, diseases have been traced to the three *tāpa* – distresses:

1 *Ādhyātmika* - Of body and mind
2 *Ādhibhautika* - Of the environment (allergy, virus, disease caused by insect bite, bacterial infection, water and air pollution).
3 *Ādhidaivika* - Genetic or hereditary diseases, accidents.

When the body is diseased, it is perceivable; when the mind is afflicted, it is felt. The diseases of the mind and body which come under the category of *ādhyātmika roga* are recognisable. But diseases which are *ādhibhautika* and *ādhidaivika* are caused by unknown factors which happen suddenly and we get caught in them. The causes of those are within us. We are responsible for all the three types of suffering on account of our own "doings".

Action is a reaction of thinking. No action is done without a thought. Unfortunately, these thoughts are very often improper and as a result, the action goes wrong. Perverse thoughts lead to perverse action. Lack of clarity in the way of thinking brings prejudices and biased attitudes. Polluted and morbid thoughts spoil the action. The action is then done with wrong intentions or induced or sanctioned by us with greed, malice, delusion and infatuation. These not only are painful to ourselves but also to others.

This causes life with endless sorrows and sufferings. Therefore, purity in action *(karmaśuddhi)* is very important. One needs to change the very mental attitude and develop mental equipoise. Yoga is the only remedy and solution.

Patañjali categorises the psychology behind action in three ways, namely *kṛta, kārita* and *anumodita*. *Kṛta* means done directly, *kārita* induced and *anumodita* is permitted to do. One either does or induces or gives permission for others to do. But we have all these three things within all of us. We are the enemies of ourselves. That is why Lord Krishna says in *Bhagavad Gītā*:

Uddharedātmanā'tmānaṁ nā'tmānamavasādayet |
ātmai'va hyātmano bandhur atmai'va ripurātmanaḥ || (*B.G.*, VI.5)

It means, we have to uplift ourselves with our own efforts by uplifting and purifying our mind. The pure and clean mind alone will uplift us and the impure and unclean mind will cause us to regress. We can be either friends to ourselves or enemies to ourselves. It depends on what we do.

We are the doers. Inner self-indulgence induces us to act and we ourselves sanction and justify our own acts. The organs of action are the doers. The senses of perception induce us to act and the mind gives its consent. The enemy is within us and not outside.

The organs of action are the most innocent. They never act on their own accord. The earth element is predominant in them. Their actions come under *kṛta*.

The organs of action are provoked *(kārita)* by the water element i.e., the senses of perception. The senses get allured easily and tempt the organs of action to act.

The mind, being the element of fire, gives consent, sanctions *(anumodita)* and permits itself to get tempted. The psychological forces and mental preparations behind these acts of *kṛta, kārita* and *anumodita* are within us. Yoga helps to control the organs of action, senses of perception and mind. Apparently the practitioner of yoga controls the three elements, earth, water and fire, and brings a change within.

Five elements exist in us in proportion in order to maintain a balance of sound health. Any imbalance in them causes diseases. The elemental body is criticised, ridiculed and undervalued by philosophers and spiritual people as an unfit instrument which is to be discarded. On the other hand the same elemental body is abused by commoners. Yogis are not supposed to either criticise or abuse the body but are supposed to realise what a great role it plays in mental and spiritual health.

Health depends upon the balance of these elements. Our behavioural pattern and mental attitude depend upon the elements. For instance if constipation, laziness, dullness and heaviness are connected mostly with the element of earth, dropsy, fear, frequency in urination, swelling, and obesity are connected with water element. Burning sensation, blisters, depression, sorrow, acidity, and anger are connected with the element of fire. Rheumatism, hysteria and shakiness are connected with the element of air, arthritis are connected with the element of ether. The *tridoṣa* – *vāta, pitta* and *śleṣma* – which are primarily elemental, cause such changes and disturbances.

The practice of *āsana* and *prāṇāyāma* controls these elements not for remedial purposes but in order to earn permanent health. In *āsana*, the body is placed in various positions. The act of positioning the body is done by *pṛthvi tattva* (earth element). After positioning, we reflect on what we have done. This act of reflection is an interaction of *āp tattva* (water element). As a reaction, we readjust and repose. This is *teja tattva* (fire element). Then we check whether our consciousness and intelligence are touching everywhere evenly and whether we are aware of each part. This act of reasoning comes from *vāyu tattva* (air element). Extension, expansion or contraction caused by diffusion of intelligence are movements within the body and they belong to *ākāśa tattva* (ether element).

As the doctor sterilises the needle before injecting to avoid infection, *āsana* too sterilises each cell. Various *āsana* are done to enable blood supply in abundance at one area by curtailing it at another. Allowing the blood to flush means to bring wetness, and curtailment of blood supply means bringing dryness. For instance in *Padmāsana*,[1] circulation is minimised in the lower limbs because of the peculiar positioning of the cross legs and maximised in the lower region of the spine. While doing *Sālamba Śīrṣāsana*,[2] venous blood is brought back to the heart and dryness to the legs whereas in *Tāḍāsana*[3] the blood supply increases in the legs. This process is a kind of sterilisation as one channels the circulation of blood.

In *āsana*, when one uses the power or weight on certain parts, it is done by the earth element. This element works on stability and firmness. The element of water is purification of blood current through sterilisation. The element of fire reacts and shapes each part of the body in that particular *āsana*. The element of air mobilises and brings movement as per requirement. The element of ether creates space for expansion or contraction according to the movement.

The inner energy is *prāṇa* and the consciousness is *prajñā*. *Prāṇa* and *prajñā* are twins. Energy and awareness go together. Wherever energy moves, awareness flows; and wherever awareness reaches, the energy moves. While performing an *āsana*, *prāṇa* and *prajñā* – the main instruments – are used to adjust the five elements. For instance, when one suffers from acidity, one may do *Paśchimottānāsana*[4] and other forward extensions to overcome the burning and vomiting sensation; but at the same time, one has to exhale in such a way that the energy is moved in the abdominal region and the abdomen is pacified consciously so that fire and air in that region are pacified.

One should know while doing the *āsana* where the power should be, where one should harden and where one should let loose, where one should have stability and where mobility. One should watch what sort of vibration is felt within the body. Why is there sensitivity at one place and insensitivity at another? One has to see whether the extension is away from the body or towards the body. With proper understanding, the elements are adjusted to remain in a balanced state.

The elasticity of the body is often considered the criterion for performing *āsana*. The parameter of elasticity does not provide the right way of judgement. Rather, it should be an adjustment of the elements.

---

1 See *Light on Yoga*, Harper Collins, London.
2 See plate n. 28.
3 See plate n. 27.
4 See *Aṣṭadaḷa Yogamālā* vol 2, plate n. 5.

The *Śiva Samhitā* (III.29) explains four stages of *prāṇāyāma*, namely: *āraṁbha-avasthā* (commencement), *ghaṭa-avasthā* (intent endeavour), *paricaya-avasthā* (intimate knowledge) and *niṣpatti-avasthā* (consummation) These stages exist not only in *prāṇāyāma* but also in other aspects of yoga, namely *yama, niyama, āsana, pratyāhāra, dhāraṇā, dhyāna* and *samādhi*.

When one begins to do *āsana*, first of all the attention is drawn towards their structure so that the required anatomical adjustments and movements are done. This is a conative action mainly done by muscles, bones and ligaments. This is *āraṁbha-avasthā*. Then the organs of perception and mind are involved to see how the *āsana* has been done. This is cognitive action. Though the mind can cognise, it cannot correct. One often understands that something is going wrong, but one is not sure what is going wrong and how and where to correct. The body performs without having clarity. This is *ghaṭa-avasthā*.

Then the body and the mind present the conative and cognitive observations to the intelligence to decide which is correct and which is incorrect. This introduction is *paricaya-avasthā*.

The intelligence has to touch all the parts of the body like the president of an international club. When all parts of the body work in unison, only then is there holistic health. This is called *niṣpatti-avasthā*.

There are varieties of *prāṇāyāma*. Just one type of *prāṇāyāma* is not at all sufficient to bring control over *prāṇa*. A labourer working in the factory will not gain strength unless he does *Ujjāyī prāṇāyāma*. At the same time, a labourer working near a furnace has to cool down his body and his system. He needs exhalation – *Bāhya Viloma* (exhalation with pauses), and *Śitāli prāṇāyāma*. Those who work in the field and take in a lot of dust need *Bhastrikā* and *Kapālabhāti*. Those who do a lot of brain work need digital *prāṇāyāma*. Those who are weak, aged, and have serious health problems need *Ujjāyī* and *Viloma* in *Śavāsana*. Those who feel low and depressed need *Abhyantara Viloma* (inhalation with pauses). How can we say that stress is the same for everyone? It depends upon the field they are working in. Obviously, therefore, *prāṇāyāma* has to be taught accordingly.

Yoga gives holistic health in this sense. Unless one is healthy in body, healthy in mind, healthy in intelligence and healthy in the very "I", one cannot enter the gates of the *antaryāmin* (the Lord within).

Āyurveda explains good health as *svāsthya.*[1] Yoga says, *svarupa-avasthā* (the seer dwelling in his true state) and when it comes to *āsana* it is said, *sthiratā* and *sukhatā* (firmness of body and steadiness of intelligence).

The meaning of health has to be understood in this broad sense. There should be *svāsthya, sthiratā, sukhatā* and *svarupatā.*

Health is life's alchemy. It is a very sensitive state of body and mind, like live wire. It is never static, but flows like the water of the river, ever fresh at every second. The health experienced and enjoyed in the past is not going to be of use in the present. Health has a forward flow and not a backward flow. Health is positive. One can always be healthier than one is. Maintaining health is a difficult and long process. However it does not take long to damage it. The nature of the body is to progress towards deterioration. Health has to oppose this deterioration. Therefore, the flow of health has to be straightened against the current of deterioration.

Stress and strain are not modern concepts of sickness. Patañjali had thought about them long ago. He speaks of *citta prasādanam: maitri karuṇā mudita upekṣānaṁ sukha duḥkha puṇya apuṇya viṣayaṇām bhāvanātaḥ cittaprasādanam.* (*Y.S.,* I.33), meaning, through cultivation of friendliness, compassion, joy and indifference towards pleasure and pain, virtue and vice, the consciousness becomes favourably disposed, serene and benevolent.

How can a man suffer from stress and strain if he has friendliness, compassion, joyous feelings and indifference to bad and evil? We have to know how to deal with ourselves when the external world disturbs us. How can a man suffer from stress and strain if he is friendly with those who are better off than him, compassionate towards those who are down-hearted, joyful towards those who are shining because of their own virtuous achievements and indifferent to those who are degraded and full of vices?

A man suffers from a heart-attack not only because of heavy workload but also because of emotional disturbances. How can there be health if the heart is full of jealousy, sorrow, passion, hatred and anxiety? How can there be health if a man cannot tolerate someone's progress, success and achievements? If there is no mental health, can there be physical health? If one channels the emotional and mental energy, where is there room for stress and strain?

Prakṛti is capable of giving enjoyment and emancipation. If one chooses to have enjoyment, then conflict is already created between *prakṛti* and *puruṣa*; but if one chooses have emancipation, then *prakṛti* becomes a servant of *puruṣa.*

---

1 *Sva* stands for oneself. *Stha* stands for stability. *Svāsthya* means to be stable within oneself – dwelling within oneself.

Under stress and strain one becomes a slave of *prakṛti.* That is how *prakṛti* exploits us by exploiting itself. But when *prakṛti* becomes a slave of *puruṣa,* the exploitation stops and a foundation is laid for emancipation.

Stress management is not today's discovery. It was thought of already in the Vedic period. The original definition of yoga is: *Saṁyoga yoga ityukto jīvātma paramātmanaḥ*[1] meaning, yoga is the union of the individual soul with the Universal Consciousness.

When one realises that one is part of the Universal Consciousness, this reduces the stress by half; but we do not want to accept this truth – the *jīvātma-paramātmaikyatā* (unity of individual soul and Universal Soul). The ego within us does not allow us to accept this universal truth. Since we cannot surrender to the universal truth, life becomes stressful. The next option if not *jīvātma-paramātmaikyatā,* it is *citta vṛtti nirodha.* Restraint of the movements of consciousness becomes important as movements and fluctuations cause stress on body, mind and intelligence.

Further there is prevention: *Heyam duḥkham anāgatam.* (*Y.S.,* II.16). According to Patañjali, the pains which are yet to come can be and are to be avoided. Prevention is inviting attention in order to increase defensive power.

The *Bhagavad Gītā* tells us how to reduce our stress and strain: *Samatvam yoga uchyate* and *Yogaḥ karmasu kauśalam,* i.e., have a state of mental equilibrium and perform a skilful act without anticipating the fruit.

Patañjali explains the ideology of skilful action using a different terminology. He asks us to avoid the *kṛta* (directly done), *kārita* (provoked) and *anumodita* (by consent) actions which ooze out like pus from the abscess of the mind. Avarice, anger and infatuation are the pus of the abscess of mind. When the pus is removed from the abscess, then it is important to allow the part to heal and dry. Similarly, in order to remove the absesses of the mind one has to avoid *kṛṣṇa karma* – evil acts – and *śukla kṛṣṇa karma* – the mixed acts –, and do *śukla karma* – good acts – to heal oneself. If one wants to remove even the last trace of the abscess, then the *karma* should be *aśukla akṛṣṇa* – the acts above good and evil, neither good nor evil. Lord Krishna calls them *niṣkāma karma* – the acts done without anticipating the fruit.

Some diseases are deep-rooted since the defect is in the genes. They cannot be vanquished easily. For instance, chronic asthma cannot be cured but its intensity can be reduced. Yogic science too recognises such diseases. The defect caused by the five afflictions cannot be conquered easily. First the defects caused by the five afflictions need to be reduced and attenuated.

---

1 *Ahirbuḍhna Samhitā.*

Avidyā and *asmitā* (want of knowledge and ego) are intellectual diseases. *Rāga* and *dveṣa* (attachment and aversion) are emotional. *Abhiniveśa* (clinging on to and the urge to live) is instinctive. If these diseases are not attended to and attenuated, then they entangle one in the web of sorrow and nothing else. Patañjali explains them as *pariṇāma duḥkha.* The afflictions are burnt out when there is a complete *karmaśuddhi* (purification of *karma*). *Karmaśuddhi* cccurs only by *cittaśuddhi* (purification of consciousness) and *cittaśuddhi* is only possible by *anuśāsanam,* i.e. discipline.

So, friends, *āyurveda* and *prākṛtika cikitsā* – nature cure – are objective treatments but *yoga cikitsā* is a subjective treatment. The principle of treatment is applicable to one and all whether it is in the *āyurvedic* or naturopathic way. But in the case of yoga the diseased has to do a lot of self-study. The patient has to search for the root cause of the disease which is hidden not only in the body but also in the mind, the ego and the intelligence. In the yogic way of treatment, the natural sources hidden within us alone are used and not the outside ones. It is in this sense a *prākṛtika cikitsā,* but the *prakṛti* which has engulfed the self is used as a means.

You all know about Bhīśmācārya. When he was totally injured in *Kurukṣetra,* he kept himself alive with sheer will power. He lay on a bed of arrows, known as *śarapañjara.* According to mythology, he was blessed by *icchā mṛtyu* (to die of his own will). But was it not a strain for him to lie on a bed of arrows? He preferred to lie in the same position. Why? Because he was supported by the arrows at the cardiac nerve. The ventricle of the heart was supported and that brought him a restful state though it was painful. I call it *Śarapañjarāsana.* In the Institute, those who suffer from cardiac problems are asked to do this *āsana* and they find great relief.

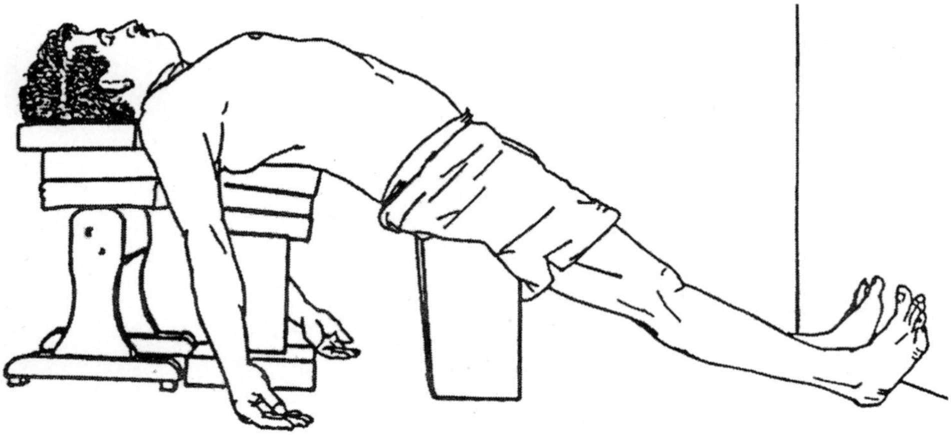

Plate n. 15 – *Śarapañjarāsana*

There are quite a few *āsana* and *prāṇāyāma* which can remove stress and strain and increase the capacity to bear stress as well as remove the state of distress. But what we basically require is dynamic, divine health. By practising *āsana* we realise how to balance the elemental body. By the practice of *prāṇāyāma* we understand how to balance the *prāṇaśakti.* The practice of *dhāraṇā* and *dhyāna* gives us *cittaśakti.* In *samādhi,* the rivers of *prāṇaśakti* and *cittaśakti* meet the sea of *ātmaśakti.* When one increases the *ātmabala* (power of the Self), then the question of stress and strain does not arise. Yoga gives *ātmabala.* From this power all one's actions are free from afflictions and fluctuations. This truly is health from all directions, in all dimensions, with complete perspective and depth.

CAN YOGA BE A THERAPY?

Therapy is a healing art used not only to combat disease but also to rehabilitate those who are afflicted with physical, organic, mental and social problems.

Can yoga help therapeutically to relieve and cure their sufferings so that they live with a healthy body and a happy disposition of mind?

The ancient healing art of yoga has stood and will stand as an unrivalled therapy for centuries. Basically yoga is not a therapy though healing is its sideline; it is mainly a spiritual healing science and art of uniting body, mind and soul as a single entity to merge finally in the Universal Soul.

According to *haṭha yoga*, diseases are man-made, man-invited as well as environmental and affected by natural imbalances. According to *Sāṁkhya, āyurveda* and yoga, imbalances take place and diseases set in when the soul conjuncts with nature. These imbalances are in the form of disease, weakness, sloth, indecision, carelessness, idleness, incontinence, illusion, disappointments, instability, distress, despair, body-infirmity and laboured breathing. Due to present day stress, strain and speed, these obstacles get aggravated in one's physico-mental health. Hence, Patañjali puts forward *aṣṭāṅga yoga* in order to live in the joy of health and tranquillity.

As science has advanced, and is still advancing, diseases multiply too. As modern comforts have facilitated life, the result has been that our body has become lazy; joints and muscles have lost movement, power and growth; and various systems like the respiratory, circulatory, digestive, glandular, urinary and eliminatory systems are rendered inefficient, these being but the vehicles of health of mind and harmony of the self.

Āsana plough the inner body and stimulate necessary supply of bio-energy and blood to irrigate each area of the body for efficient functioning. They also stimulate the diseased and affected parts by making each cell fulfil its function before it dies. *Prāṇāyāma* helps to store much vital energy as a reserve force to act when necessary. *Dhāraṇā* and *dhyāna* keep the mind calm and serene.

Thus, yoga not only acts as curative therapy but also as a preventive art in keeping the body healthy and firm, mind clear and clean with emotional stability so that the *sādhaka* is healthy both inside and outside. Patañjali has not forgotten social health too. He says that friendliness, compassion, delight, indifference towards happiness and sorrow, virtue and vice are the ingredients of social health.

Hence, yoga covers the inner field as well as the outer for a better, healthy, happy long life though its aim is freedom and beatitude *(mokṣa).*

YOGA – A METHODICAL SUBJECTIVE TREATMENT

Yoga has become a household word for its remedial utility as a curative and preventive science. The yogic method of treatment, however, cannot be put as a theory like other medicinal sciences. Though it is possible to describe in detail the *āsana* or *prāṇāyāma* for various ailments, it is not possible to prescribe precisely the set of *āsana* or *prāṇāyāma*. But, at the beginning of treatment, it is possible to give important basic *āsana* or *prāṇāyāma* with which to start.

Life being a forward movement, the quality of depth has to be changed as the patient progresses.

Often, the patients ask for the advice or opinion from yoga teachers as one does in the medical profession. Medical science is a recognised, conventional method of treatment. It has proved its results. A doctor, a medical practitioner, needs not suffer himself like the patient or take medicines to know their effects, because the science of medicine has proved them earlier by experiment. Even then, there are many problems, many diseases which have not yet been proved as curable and new experiments are carried out.

On the other hand, yogic science of treatment has now been undergoing tests and has proved to be of value. It has been recognised recently as an alternative method of healing science. In fact, it is a healing art having a science behind it, except that its laboratory is one's own body and the experiment is one's own practice.

I am often asked to give advice or the list of *āsana* if somebody is suffering from any particular disease. I may recommend the *āsana* in general terms. My guidance would be a tentative programme but not a definitive one. However, the teachers need to know the *āsana* thoroughly in order to know their applications, since they are face to face with the patients. Therefore, the teacher has to practise genuinely. In this sense it is a subjective science to have a subjective knowledge and subjective experience. One's own practice and the interpenetration in one's practice develop sensitivity in the practitioner. This subjective experience guides and leads one to deal with the treatment.

One may read books on medical science and medicine. One may know the effects of the medicines. One may buy the medicines from the medical shop and take them. But this does not make one either a doctor or a healer. Self-treatment may prove fatal. Similarly, one cannot acquire the knowledge of the treatment through yogic method by reading books on yoga or stealing someone's method of treatment without practising oneself and experiencing it.

While practising the *āsana*, the teachers have to develop prudence in order to have sensitivity and feeling. Teachers should be able to watch every change or transformation occuring within. While teaching or treating the patient, this prudence is of great help.

Therefore one has to observe oneself while practising as well as others who are practising. One should see how their body posture is in various *āsana*, how they work on themselves, how is their approach to the *āsana* when they perform. The teachers have to learn under the guidance of able teachers and then work at their own individual discretion.

Teachers need to develop a tremendous insight into their own practice. The majority of teachers practise with the brain – the intellect. Intellectual deliberation does not help in a practical, experiential subject. Yoga is an experiencing subject. As a teacher, when you practise your brain acts faster than the body. Therefore when you do *āsana*, certain actions, certain adjustments that have to be done are taken for granted as though you have already done them. For instance, you know the simple action that your legs need to be straight in a standing *āsana*. You may attempt this action of stretching the legs and they may remain fairly straight. But you do not reach the depth of it to find out where the source of action is or if the legs need to be straightened more, or which way the bottom of the feet, toes, heels, ankles, shins, knees, groins and spine contribute to that action. You tense your brain to stretch the legs. The more you tense, the more you think you have done your best. The body on the other hand is cunning. It says, "I have done it, I have stretched the legs", though this has not been done. The brain – the seat of the intelligence – acts strongly but the body does not react to the volition of the brain. And there, as a student, you miss the bus. The body does not do but the brain puts a tick mark to indicate that it has been done. Therefore you as a teacher need to make sure that your body puts the tick mark. The assurance has to come from your legs that they are definitely straight.

In order to understand this or to feel this, you have to learn to keep the brain in a non-tensed state. When the brain is in a non-tensed state, the imprints are received in a better way. You have to learn to see the body by the body. This is the first lesson in yoga. When that is learned, the effect of yoga is understood better.

This kind of insight and observation helps the teachers while treating patients. You as a teacher can see the patient, and whether it is the brain or the body which is acting. You have to tell the patient to keep the brain as an object and the body as a subject.

Perhaps it is more difficult for so-called intelligent people to treat the body as a subject, because they live in their heads. Often, it is a diseased brain rather than a diseased body. The yogi knows that his brain is from the bottom of his feet to the top of his head. An intellectual person thinks that he is only in his head and nowhere else. His intelligence cannot spread beyond the brain to inhabit the rest of his body. But the yogi says, "Diffuse that energy from the brain to the other parts of the body, so that the body and the brain may work in concord and the energy may be evenly balanced between the two." Here begins the healing process since the release of tension in the brain brings relaxation to the nerves.

If you as a patient have a stomach problem, you cannot dictate to it from the brain. The brain has to be tamed to become friendly and compassionate to the stomach. You need to tell the brain, "Oh! You, brain, relax". It is a kind of autosuggestion which takes away the tension of the brain. By lessening the brain tension, the stomach can endure the pain with ease. Thus, we have to learn to relax the brain and physiologically work on the abdominal organs. Then the brain too accepts the pain with tolerance. The energy used by the brain in the form of tension is transformed into healing energy to work on the stomach. Then the injury of the stomach starts healing.

Nevertheless, a stomach problem is a practical problem which has to be dealt practically. You need to see why there is pain: what happens when you are doing the various movements in various *āsana*, what mistakes you are making in your practice, how you are breathing when you are in that *āsana*, where the stress is while working, whether it is necessary to emphasise that part or whether it should be shifted elsewhere in order to nullify the strain. All of these things have to be seen in your practice, which helps you while treating others. You as a teacher need to watch your own practice and apply your experience in the form of technique on the patient.

Again, while treating the patient, you should know how to approach the afflicted part. Suppose you have a boil, does the doctor immediately pinch the head of your abscess to bring out the pus, or does he first clean the surrounding parts of the body? Again, if there is an internal cause creating the boil, is there any point just knocking the head off the boil? All you are going to do is get another one since the root of the boil is hidden. Similarly in yoga you cannot just knock on the point at which the ailment manifests itself. If you have a pain in your stomach, you should know the indirect parts connected with that ailment. You have to look at how the whole body is behaving. This requires common sense. You have to tone the other parts of the body before you directly touch the injured or affected area.

However, if the disease is fresh one can work from the spot directly. If it is a long standing problem, the teacher has to work from the other areas. The teacher has to tone the other healthy parts first, then attend to the affected part to make that healthy. That is how *āsana* has to be taught to the patients so that it serves a remedial purpose.

Never touch or stretch the injured or afflicted area directly. You need to know how to approach the affected area and work with it. First, train, tone and strengthen the surrounding areas before you work on the affected area. If you touch the affected area directly, the problem may get aggravated. Do not attribute this to the fault of yoga. The cause of pain should be known and the *āsana* are to be introduced judiciously to get rid of the pain. Deal with the muscles which are accessory to that painful area.

You, as a patient, need to have communication with the teacher. Tell your teacher if you feel uncomfortable in the afflicted area. Then nothing goes amiss. The teacher and the patient have to co-ordinate and co-operate.

As I said earlier that you have to watch the brain, as a teacher, you should observe the eyes of the patients also. If the patient clenches the eyes, know that something is going wrong in your adjustments. If you see a relaxed face, soft in the temples, know that the adjustments you made are in the right direction.

Observation and insight are the key points for the teachers while undertaking the responsibility of teaching *āsana* as a treatment. They should know which *āsana* are to be taught and how to help the patient in that *āsana* in order to bring proper effect. One has to practise, experiment with oneself, develop sensitivity, experience oneself before treating others. There needs to be a total involvement of the teacher.

YOGIC THERAPY

Yoga is a spiritual science which has beer gi:ted to us by our ancient *ṛṣis* for the final emancipation. But these days the science of yoga has become a popular subject as a preventive and a curative measure for human suffering. The doubt arises in the common man's mind, as to whether yoga really cures the diseases. This doubt is due to the fact that we have narrowed the meaning of the word "cure". To cure means to free, to liberate from bondage. A disease is that which puts the body and mind in bondage creating uneasiness. When one does not feel "at ease" one is said to be diseased and this is the bondage.

Life is full of pleasure, pain, tension, stress and strain. Man is affected by inner and outer environments, social structures, competition and never ending struggles. He is afflicted within himself by anxieties, worries, desires, lust, anger, greed, aversion, hatred, temptations and so on. Modern living has changed simple life into a complexity and affected the consciousness, whereby it has lost its simplicity and originality. This is how life gets too complicated, mixed, fabricated, soiled and scattered.

Yogic methods gives the maximum and the minutest techniques for the cure of a soiled body and mind. In this sense, yoga is therapy. Therapy is treatment. The treatment for a disorderly mental and physical condition or disease by remedial techniques is called therapy.

Diseases are categorised mainly in three types, *ādhyātmika*, *ādhibhautika* and *ādhidaivika*. *Ādhyātma* means the one which covers the Self. The body and mind cover the Self. The diseases of these coverings – the body and the mind – are called *ādhyātmika* diseases. *Ādhibhautika* disease is that which is caused by the matter of living beings, derived and produced from five elements, namely earth, water, fire, air and ether. Therefore, the diseases caused by flood and draught (water), fire *(agni)* or food poisoning come under this category. *Ādhidaivika* disease is one which is caused by the super-natural and divine bodies, the movements of planets and so on.

Lord Krishna in the *Bhagavad Gītā* gives five causes for the accomplishment of any action:

Adhiṣṭhānam tathā kartā kāraṇam ca pṛthagvidhaṁ
vividhāśca pṛthakceṣṭā daivam chaivātra pañchamaṁ (XVIII.14).

The body *(adhiṣṭhāna),* the doer *(kartā),* the five organs of perception as well as the intelligence, ego and mind, and the five organs of action are the causes or factors (*kāraṇa*). But above all there is *daivam* or destiny, which is nothing but the effect of previous *karma*.

Patañjali helps us with yogic method to eradicate this root cause of diseases by bringing cleanliness in the body *(śarīraśuddhi),* cleanlines in the mind *(manaḥśuddhi),* purity in action *(karmaśuddhi),* purity in the consciousness *(cittaśuddhi)* and, as a result of these, there is *ātmaśuddhi* or purification of the Self.

Patañjali says that yoga is a science of preventing suffering. *Heyam duḥkham anāgatam* (*Y.S.,* II.16), meaning, the pain which is yet to come can be avoided through *aṣṭāṅga yoga* on a preventive level as well as on a curative level.

The body is the outer sheath of the self. This body is unable to bear the slightest of pains but hankers for repeated pleasures. The mind as an inner sheath of the body gets easily enamoured and becomes negative if it cannot indulge in pleasure. The *āsana-prāṇāyāma* therapy is effective on the body-mind apparatus. Yoga, like *āyurveda*, accepts two ways of treatment, called *śodhanavidhi* – the method of purification, and *śamanavidhi* – the method of pacification. Though *āsana-prāṇāyāma* therapy falls mainly under the method of pacification, yet it plays both roles.

The organic body machine functions on the biochemicals which exist in the humours *(doṣa),* constituents or ingredients *(dhātu)* and excretions *(mala).* The five elements constitute the chemical universe outside as well as a mini-universe in the body. The *āsana-prāṇāyāma* are not to be prescribed as medicine but performed by the body through description. Here, the description means a complete or thorough technique of *āsana* and *prāṇāyāma.* In order to generate the products of five elements towards health, one needs to perform them very correctly with precise actions and adjustments. As the consciousness gets involved in practice, change in the biochemical substance of the body takes place through proper blood circulation and metabolism. That is how *aṣṭāṅga yoga* works as a natural medicine. Through *prāṇāyāma*, the *prāṇa* within the body is vitalised for dynamic psychological growth.

In medicine the drugs act on the body and the body reacts to the drugs, and the disease is eradicated. The drug is a chemical substance which reacts on the bio-chemistry of the body. Similarly, the *āsana-prāṇāyāma* reacts on the organic body in a like manner to those therapies with elements like calcium, zinc, vitamins, enzymes, etc., in which the body chemicals are vitalised.

While performing *āsana-prāṇāyāma,* the application of intelligence in utilisation of the "body-mind substance" brings the effeotive change. The *āsana-prāṇāyāma* is performed by a living person who animates the chemistry of the body by infusing bio-energy into it. The body does not borrow the substance but brings the required effect by producing physio-chemical substances and bio-chemical changes in the organs, hormones, blood contents and so on.

A common man understands *āsana* as a posture in which the *sādhaka* stays comfortably with cessation of all *vṛtti* and stays with mental poise.

Sthira sukham āsanam (*Y.S.,* II.46).

What is perfection in *āsana?*

1. Firmness in the body
2. Steadiness in the intelligence,
3. Benevolence in the consciousness
4. Ceasing of the efforts,
5. Body and mind totally merging or assuming the infinite form of the Seer.
6. Finally, the ending of dualities and differentiation in the levels of body and mind processes.

Until these are experienced, the efforts have to be continued. The ideal state in *āsana,* mentioned above by Patañjali, is found when the *sādhaka* is at a point of perfection where the questions of disease, unhealth, pain and problems do not arise. From this angle one can use this art and science as a therapy.

Therefore, the *sādhaka* has to do the *sādhanā* as *tapas* to reach the above mentioned perfection. The method of doing *āsana* involves action which ultimately leads towards passivity. *Āsana* consists of the actions or movements such as rubbing, squeezing, freezing, pacifying, activating, stimulating, supporting, soothing, penetrating, narrowing, spreading, fixing, warming and cooling. The *āsana-prāṇāyāma* is sensitively grafted on the body. The movements consist of contortion, contraction, expansion, extension, circumduction and abduction. Again, there are vertical, horizontal, circular, spiral and circumferential movements. The practice of various *āsana* penetrates the physiological body depthwise, widthwise and lengthwise. The penetration of *āsana* must reach from the outer body towards the inner body from all directions; and at the same time, the body, along with mind and breath, holds the *āsana* in a required and effective way. Each *āsana* with six aspects, namely, quality, potentiality, intensity, effectuality, substantiality and "relishability", works on the body in specific capacities. The grouping of *āsana* is done on this basis alone. Therefore, one cannot expect quick relief by yogic treatment, since the body and mind have to undergo the change as an effect of *āsana-prāṇāyāma* mechanism.

The *āsana-prāṇāyāma* therapy is administered according to the root cause of diagnosed disease though the visible and peripheral symptoms are not neglected, since these symptoms need an immediate pacification. The order and sequence of *āsana-prāṇāyāma* on every disease is charted on the basis of anatomical structures, physiological functioning, intensity, purifying and pacifying capacity, the stage of disease, the age and the basic constitution as well as the combination of diseases and disorders of the patient.

While doing *āsana*, one has to undergo the three stages in performance, namely

1) Beginning of the *āsana* to reach the *āsana (ārambha),*
2) Remaining in the *āsana (sthiti),*
3) Concluding the *āsana* to regain normal position of the body *(visarjana).*

All these three stages have therapeutic value and psychological effect.

Besides these three stages and breathing techniques, the utilisation and involvement of a particular part of the body varies. In the same *āsana* the activation of certain parts and relaxation of certain parts differ according to the disease. Each stage of *āsana* and *prāṇāyāma,* whether intermediate or final, can yield something as a therapy. Each action and movement by the body, as well as the stability and establishment of the body are significant and important. The vital breath is circulated and perambulated through the system by a proper mechanism of inhalation, exhalation and retention.

The *āsana* is performed in different ways to bring the expected and required effect. One has to know where the impetus should be and where the gravitational centre must be. One must know where, when and how the energy should be diffused, infused and instilled.

Āsana work to hyperactivate the slothful parts of physiology which establishes the balance in the inner body tension, and they also work to hypoactivate some parts of physiology towards the same end. A hypoactive physiological part amounts to hypertension in some other parts of the body. *Āsana* brings this inner balance so that no part is tensed. Various *āsana* are meant to serve a variety of psycho-physiological and neuro-physiological needs. They work as desired on the corresponding glands and organs by particular breathing patterns. In fact it is the bio-energy through the breathing mechanism that animates and operates the whole human mechanism playing a vital role in maintaining the body in various postures.

While doing *prāṇāyāmic* inhalation and exhalation, the first part of breath, the middle breath, the end breath, the holding of breath, the length of breath and its velocity, and the required volume of the breath are taken into account. With *prāṇāyāma*, the cells of the body are planted and cultured in the right way. *Prāṇāyāma* energises the body and the mind to flow with the breath for proper distribution and utilisation. The varieties of *prāṇāyāma* serve the body, mind, intelligence and *citta* in spiritual pursuit bringing the required changes at physical, biological, physiological, psychological, moral and spiritual levels.

This is how the *āsana-prāṇāyāma* method works as a preventive and curative measure. By the practice of *āsana* and *prāṇāyāma*, the body and mind are cleansed and purified and one thinks of *omkāra-japa* for the *citta* to become devotional. This cleanliness, purity and devotion sanctifies the body, mind and *citta* to reach the state of *samādhi*.

Therefore, while using the word "therapy", I do not make the meaning narrow or parochial. On the contrary I take it comprehensively, extensively and expansively so that the aim of *cittaśuddhi* is attained.

The *vṛtti-sārupyam* of *dṛṣṭā* (Seer) itself is the state of "disease"; whereas the *svarūpa-avasthā*[1] of *drṣṭā* is a state of "at-ease". In this state the bondages are broken. The Seer is freed from the bindings of *prakṛti*. Hence, yoga therapy is not merely a therapy of diseases of the body and mind but is a therapy of *citta* or consciousness.

Yoga is the oldest, the greatest, the finest and the ultimate therapy in this sense.

---

1 *Sva* means one's own, *rūpa* means form, *avasthā* means state. When the Seer remains in his own true form and pure state, it is called *svarūpa-avasthā*.

THE MEETING POINT OF ANCIENT WISDOM AND MODERN SCIENCE*

This is my first visit to Berlin. Some of you have taken to the practice of yoga recently and I am sure you must have a little background of what yoga is. I will say what little I know about this subject, as you would like to ask me questions after my introduction.

Yoga is undoubtedly a spiritual subject, with the aim of making the conciousness come into contact with the seer, who is within us; health is just a by-product of this process. When we take to the practices of yoga, health automatically follows. Yoga is not a medicine to gulp or swallow, it is a way to maintain a healthy long life. It is a preventive art which frees one from future ailments that may arise, and it is a science as it acts as a curative system on an unhealthy person in order to make him healthy.

It is a preventive subject, wherein the entire human system, namely, the circulatory, the digestive, the urinary, the excretory, the nervous and the glandular systems are all kept in a healthy state for their perfect functioning. This is the meaning of real health. In this state, the practitioner forgets his body and pays attention more towards the growth of the mind and intelligence. Also it covers the physical, physiological, physio-psychological, psycho-intellectual and spiritual subjects.

Ill health, according to the yogic texts, appears as pain, unhappiness, ficklemindedness, trembling or shaking in the body, heavy or laboured breathing, which act as symptoms of various ailments and eat away one's energy physically and mentally as well as spiritually.

According to our science of health, these manifestations are intimately linked to physical, physiological, mental and spiritual diseases. All ailments, obstacles and impediments for health come under the three categories known as *ādhyātmika, ādhibhautika* and *ādhidaivika* afflictions *(tāpa),* and have to be combatted through penance *(tapas).*

---

* Press conference in Berlin, October 1996, organised by the Medical Chamber of Berlin, by Dr. Ellis Huber (President of the Medical Chamber of Berlin) with Hermann Traitteur (Medical practitioner and board member of the B.K.S. Iyengar Yoga Association of Germany).

Ādhyātmika tāpa comes due to self-abuse or self-amuse by which lots of diseases are invited such as AIDS, HIV, etc. Instances of self-abuse may cause diseases to incubate early or after months or years, or even after generations, and the *ādhyātmika tāpa* becomes *ādhidaivika tāpa*. Genetic and hereditary problems also come under these categories.

The *ādhibhautika* diseases are due to the imbalance of the five elements, namely earth, water, fire, air and ether, and their atomic structures, namely smell or odour, taste, form, touch and sound. As we are made up of these five elements, we have to balance these inner five elements with the cosmic elements. Yoga teaches us how to balance these five elements of the body with the five elements of the universe. If there is an imbalance between the elements in our system and of the outer atmospheric elements, disturbing changes takes place in the persons. Then the defensive strength which has not been built up in our system allows diseases to appear. These we call environmental or pollution-caused diseases.

The third one is *ādhidaivika*. We, the yoga practitioners, believe in *karma* (actions). Each action has a reaction, and this reaction is the product, the fruit or the effect of that action in the form of health or disease, joy or sorrow, pain or pleasure, or evil or good.

Today modern scientists test the genes. This third type of disease, known as *ādhidaivika*, has an unknown origin. The genetic problems or allergies with no cause or reason come under this category. The yogis call it *pariṇāma duḥkha*. These diseases are the consequences of the various actions of past lives.

With these three types of diseases as a basis, the yogis found ways and means to build up a science to fight the diseases that already exist in the body and to protect from those which are waiting to appear at a later date.

From soma to psyche, it is a psychosomatic science. You can change the soma or body through the mind or the mind through body. Using the body for transforming the mind or vice versa, the mind and body come closer to each other and understand each other. This understanding between body and mind is the sign of good health.

The various *āsana* filter our blood, improve its biochemistry, generate tremendous bio-energy and keep one healthy. Health is a very difficult word to describe. Health is not like still water. As electricity is generated when the water is flowing with force, similarly health is a dynamic force. Therefore, the word health can be used as a sign but it cannot be described in specific terms. It is like an electric current. Today to say exactly what health is, we can take the example of a river. If a person is taking a dip in a river, the water is fresh and whenever he ducks in, he dips into new water. Similarly health flows dynamically, electrically, moment to moment, changing the entire system existing in the human body. In this sense, there is no regression in health. It cannot regress, but only progress.

It is said in yogic science that the senses of perception are controlled by the mind, and mind is controlled by the nerves. So the master for the entire human system for good health and happiness is the nervous system. The science which studies the nervous system and the mind is known as neuropsychology or psychoneurology. Neuro may disturb the psyche, psyche may disturb the neuro.

The peripheral, autonomous and central nervous systems are also described in the yogic science as *piṅgalā, iḍā* and *suṣumṇā*. *Piṅgalā* stands for the functions like the peripheral nerves. *Iḍā* is the autonomous nervous system and it is semi-controllable. *Suṣumna* is the central nervous system. Peripheral nerves work on the organs and senses, the autonomous nervous system works on the mind and the central nervous system on the discriminatory power of the intelligence. The Eastern scientists knew not only the solar-plexus *(sūrya nāḍī),* but also the lunar-plexus *(candra nāḍī).* One heats the body and the other cools it. Today the hypothalamus is considered to regulate body temperature.

The yogis discovered years ago that the solar plexus *(sūrya cakra)* is in the navel area and the lunar plexus *(candra cakra)* is at the back of the brain, and they also knew very well that the network of *sūrya nāḍī* and *candra nāḍī* are spread throughout the body. Now modern science explains how sympathetic and parasympathetic nervous systems too are spread throughout the body. *Sūrya nāḍī* corresponds to the sympathetic nervous system and *candra nāḍī* corresponds to the parasympathetic nervous system. The techniques of *prāṇāyāma* were developed on these concepts. Still water cannot be used to generate energy, but flowing water can. The yogis found out various postures to circulate the entire blood supply, to filter it in each and every *āsana*, and in the breathing process they channelled and restrained the inbreath and the outbreath to produce and generate bio-energy in the system through *prāṇāyāma.* That is why the technique of *prāṇāyāma* came in order to improve the health of the body, as energy alone is what maintains good health. Thus, the techniques of *āsana* and *prāṇāyāma* came to enhance biochemistry and bioenergy so that man lives in unison with the body, mind and self. That is the entire gamut of yogic science and philosophy.

As a therapy, yoga is a healing art and a healing science. It is not a medicine, hence it cannot be bracketed with alternative medicine. It is a self-energising, self-monitoring and self-generating process, which has to be understood and followed individually.

Yogic practices fight diseases from our defensive energy, which we build up through *sādhanā* and the methodology of treating the various ailments. All diseases may be dormant in the beginning, then they may be attenuated, then sometimes active, sometimes passive, and later fully active. When we treat the patients, we explain the way of living moods and behaviour that has to be followed as far as possible and then use various methodologies in yogic postures to bring relief in them. If the disease is very active, we work from the peripheral body, if it is passive and active, we go deep inside the physiological body, when it is attenuated we go towards the mind and when it is dormant, we go to the very source. So *āsana* and *prāṇāyāma* work from the source to the periphery and from the periphery to the source, according to the growth of disease.

I have worked with various diseases, from acidity to cardiac ailments. Even people who have gone bypass surgery, open heart surgery, have recovered and expressed their gratitude to yoga.

I am glad now that at least the German scientists have come forward to do some research work. Yoga is a subjectively experienced health science. Medicine is an objective science, and this is the time where the subjective science and the objective science or the subjective and experienced observance and the objective referential knowledge can come close together. If these two are brought together, future generations will experience the best health.

We are dependent upon subjective observation, without survey records, but building up health in harmony. Medical science cannot convert objective into subjective science and as yogis we are not able to convert the subjective into an objective science. This is the first time I think that we are meeting and I hope this acts as a ground to bring the objective knowledge of medicine to the subjective experience of yoga, so that perfect health is gained by the combination of these two sciences.

Medical science is doing a good job on how to make unhealthy people healthy, but not one scientist has come forward to show how a healthy man might not become unhealthy at all. I think yoga is the only subject which makes man healthy throughout his life. It is the yogic science which speaks of preventive ways. Since one does not know what type of diseases are in store, one has to develop defensive strengths for the future, so that offensive diseases may not enter into one's system. *Heyaṁ duḥkham anāgatam* (*Y.S.,* II.16). Patañjali says that one will not know at what time the pains and sorrows come. He wants us to prepare from now on so that they are kept aside.

Scientists have to give their thoughts on research work in the field of yoga on various ailments and how the healing process takes place through yoga, and yogis too should get the feel of modern science to use in yogic methods. Medical science however is still not coming forward. If they do it, I am sure that in the 21st century there will be tremendous peace in each and every individual. If one individual is content because of the health and peace due to the practice of yoga, others are also tempted. People want contentment, health and peace. Contentment is like a river which makes the surrounding areas wet and green. Similarly, the river of contentment flows from one person to another, causing more and more people to have health and peace through yoga practice. The message is passed on automatically as the river flows naturally to reach its goal, the sea.

There is no fight for peace, but there is a fight for the eradication of disease.

Today one takes pills to sleep and pills to wake up. Yoga says nothing of that sort. It says to face the stress and strain of disease with the right action, right study and right discretion. With right understanding, the illness factors will never touch the person who regularly practises *āsana* and *prāṇāyāma,* which cleanse the nerves and store energy.

The currents flow naturally and hence there will be no disease. Yogic science makes the energy flow in the right channels. Imagine how much effort has to be put to filter the 10,000 kilometres of the nervous system in the body.

I was invited as a chief guest to speak and teach at the first conference on alternative medicine and yoga which was held in Moscow, in 1989. I think that was the starting point. Now other conferences take place on this subject and I hope that concrete steps will emerge soon.

Today I am very happy that we as yoga teachers and you as body-scientists co-operate with each other to study and survey the effect of yoga on blood pressure, hypertension, hypotension, glandular disturbances, hormonal disfunctioning, and so forth.

If yoga and medicine work together on the patients, the acceleration of recovery will be faster and hence, both can go hand in hand. If both yoga and medicine are administered and monitored, the patient may be able to shed the side effects of medicines and may come out with new energy and new life.

If we work together, suffering can be minimised to a very great extent. That is my feeling. If yoga and medicine go together, confidence sets in and man can experience unalloyed health and bliss.

SECTION III

ĀYURVEDA

PARALLELISM BETWEEN YOGA AND *ĀYURVEDA**

Yoga has become a popular subject these days as a preventive and curative measure, but doubt arises in a common man's mind as to whether yoga really cures diseases. In many cases, yes, but I say with emphasis that there is no doubt regarding the fact that yoga changes the life of a human being and thus brings health. Here, I am trying to interpret the *Yoga Sūtra* of Patañjali in the style of *āyurvedic* treatment.

Though there are two opinions regarding Patañjali and Caraka, whether they are one and the same person or different, I see a great similarity in them. Patañjali is not less than any physician and surgeon. The only difference is that Patañjali treats the consciousness *(citta)* and Caraka treats the body. According to Patañjali, the consciousness, the mind, is the ground which needs the treatment. According to *āyurveda*, the body in which the soul dwells (living body) needs the treatment.

Patañjali gives the maximum and the minutest techniques for the cure of a soiled consciousness, and Caraka, similarly, provides various methods of treatment for the soiled body.

Disease is that state when one does not feel "at ease". The art of leading a life "at ease" is health.

Normally, we find life full of pressure, pain, tension, stress and strain. Man is affected by environment, social structures, life-taking competitions and never-ending struggles. He is afflicted (polluted) within himself by anxieties, worries, desires, lust, anger, greed, aversion, hatred, temptations and so on. Modern living has changed simple life into complexity and affected consciousness, and therefore it has lost its simplicity and originality. It is getting too complicated, mixed, fabricated, soiled and scattered.

Let us see how Patañjali deals with the problems and gives the solution, and where he comes near to *āyurvedic* science of treatment. The embodied or empirical soul called *jīvātman*

---

* From *Iyengar, His Life and Work*, Timeless Book, USA, 1987, pp. 139-158.

has dressed and ornamented itself with intelligence, ego, mind, five senses of perception, five organs of action, five gross elements and five subtle elements. According to both yoga and *āyurveda,* the empirical soul has decorated itself with sixteen qualities, namely:

1. happiness *(sukha),*
2. unhappiness *(duḥkha),*
3. desire *(icchā),*
4. aversion *(dveṣa),*
5. cheerful efforts to secure the objective *(pratyaya),*
6. vital energy which keeps the body alive *(prāṇa),*
7. vital energy which keeps the body-machine intact *(apāna),*
8. blinking of eyes – opening *(umeṣa),*
9. blinking of eyes – closing *(nimeṣa),*
10. intelligence having the power of discriminative discernment *(buddhi),*
11. will power, the determination to carry on the work *(manōsaṁkalpa),*
12. power of reason *(vicāraṇā),*
13. memory *(smṛti),*
14. power of intelligence to know the objective world *(vijñānam),*
15. apprehension of clear and clean knowledge of the knowable *(adhyavasāya),*
16. the achievement of ends: experience and emancipation *(viṣayopalabdhi).*

The *jīvātmā,* however, identifies itself with its dress, decoration and ornaments and gets lost, and this is its disease. Patañjali brings back the empirical soul to the trans-empirical state.

The diseased self identifies itself with the seen. The disease is *vṛtti* (mental modifications) and *kleśa* (afflictions). The five mental modifications are real perception, false perception, fanciful or imaginary knowledge, sleep and memory; and the five afflictions are lack of spiritual wisdom, egoism, attachment towards pleasure, aversion to pain and clinging to life.

The afflictions are causes for the modifications to become diseased.

The five modifications and afflictions are basically nurtured by the three qualities of primordial matter: illumination, activity and inertia, which are known as *sattva, rajas* and *tamas.* These three qualities in different proportions activate the consciousness to undergo the modifications and afflictions. Similarly, *āyurveda* holds the *tridoṣa* or three humours of the body: *vāta, pitta* and *kapha,* responsible for causing disease. Almost all diseases are considered *tridoṣika.*

Let me put this *tridoṣa* concept in short.[1] The three humours of the body support the structure of the body and maintain its metabolism. The *vāta* represents nerve force and comprehends all the phenomena that come under the central, sympathetic, parasympathetic and peripheral nervous systems. It is a dynamic, vital and inherent force that exists in the cells. It is an energy force that circulates the blood and lymph and stimulates the nerves. The *pitta* maintains metabolism in the system and generates body heat (thermogenesis). It is the base for all chemical activities. It is the sustaining fire for metabolic activities. The *kapha* regulates heat and preserves body fluids, lubricates the joints, builds tissues, produces energy and brings firmness of limbs.

Derangement in the function of the three humours gives rise to disease. The *tridoṣa* in their pathogenic state vitiate seven constituents: chyle, blood, flesh, bone, bone-marrow and semen. These constituents go into an inbalanced state causing disease.

When the humours are in a balanced state forming a proper constitutional structure, it is called a state of *dhātu sāmyatā* (balanced constituents), and it is a healthy state of body. Similarly, according to yoga, when the three constituents of nature are in an acquiescent and balanced state, it is called *sāmya-avasthā,* which is an expected goal. At this stage, the Self abides in its own nature (*Yoga Sūtra,* I.3).

Since disease is due to a disturbance in the humours, it could be either mono-*doṣika,* bi-*doṣika* or tri-*doṣika.* In fact, if one gets disturbed, the other two are affected. Since the vitiation is in different proportions, almost all the diseases are categorised into five types:

1. *vātaja,*
2. *pittaja,*
3. *kaphaja,*
4. *vāta-pittaja, pitta-kaphaja, kapha-vātaja,*
5. *sannipātaja* or *tridoṣaja.*

Hence, the diseases, modifications and afflictions are mainly of five types.

According to yoga, the seat of *sattvaguṇa* is from head to heart, that of *rajōguṇa* from heart to navel, and that of *tamōguṇa* from navel to feet. According to *āyurveda* the location of *kapha* is from head to heart, that of *pitta,* from heart to navel and that of *vāta,* from navel to feet.

---

[1] See also the author's *Aṣṭadaḷa Yogamālā,* vol. 2, p. 315.

Yoga is eight-limbed and so is called *aṣṭāṅga yoga*, and *āyurveda* also has eight branches and is called *aṣṭāṅga āyurveda*. The eight limbs of yoga are:

1. self-restraints *(yama)*,
2. fixed practices *(niyama)*,
3. postures *(āsana)*,
4. regulation of energy through breath control *(prāṇāyāma)*,
5. quietening the senses *(pratyāhāra)*,
6. attention *(dhāraṇa)*,
7. meditation *(dhyāna)*,
8. absorption *(samādhi)*.

The branches of *āyurveda* are:

1. surgery *(śalya)*,
2. diseases of eyes, ears, nose and throat *(śālakya)*,
3. the body treatment through medicine *(kāya-cikitsā)*,
4. treatment of mental diseases *(bhūta-vidyā)*,
5. midwifery and diseases of children *(kaumāra bhṛtya)*,
6. toxicology *(agada tantra)*,
7. science of prolongation of life *(rasāyana)*,
8. means of securing vigour *(vājīkaraṇa tantra)*.

Now let us see the method of treatment according to both sciences.

Patañjali advises two remedial methods for restraining mental modifications and burning the afflictions. They are practice *(abhyāsa)* and detachment *(vairāgya)*. *Abhyāsa* is the practice of the eight aspects or petals of yoga, and *vairāgya* is reducing oneself to a state of desirelessness. *Abhyāsa* is an evolutionary method and *vairāgya* an involutionary method.

In *āyurveda* there are two remedial methods: *śodhana*, the cleansing or purifying method, and *śamana*, the pacifying method. *Śodhana* is a drastic method where *śamana* is a mild method. *Abhyāsa* is also a mild treatment which can be lenient and soft while treating the patient. That is why *aṣṭāṅga yoga* is applicable to all. Neither *śamana* medicine nor *aṣṭāṅga yoga* harm or show any adverse effects.

Śodhana treatment brings drastic change but at the same time is harmful as it can uproot the humours if used wrongly and frequently. If it is not utilised at all, then it also causes problems in the body; so Caraka explains that it should be used very carefully. Patañjali also warns against using *vairāgya* as a remedial measure, as a sudden drastic change may uproot the *sādhaka*. First, he wants *abhyāsa* to be done positively and renunciation to be introduced accordingly with proper measures. Therefore, the doses of five types of *vairāgya* are introduced slowly in five stages so they work on the body and mind very delicately but definitely. They are:

1. *yatamāna* – disengaging the senses from action,
2. *vyatireka* – keeping away from desire,
3. *ekendriya* – stilling the mind,
4. *vaśīkāra* – mastery of desire,
5. *paravairāgya* – supreme detachment.

Disengaging the senses from enjoyment and controlling them with continuous effort is *yatamāna*. Then thoughtfully controlling the desires which cause obstruction in the path of Self-realisation is called *vyatireka*. Though the five organs of action and five organs of perception are entirely withdrawn from the external world, feeble desires remain in causal form in the eleventh sense – the mind. To withdraw the mind from all the desires is *ekendriya*. To remain completely detached from worldly and heavenly desires is *vaśīkāra*. *Paravairāgya* is the highest form of renunciation in which nothing is desired except the soul. Like *vairāgya*, the *śodhana vidhi* or purifying method is also applied in five stages:

1. *vamana* – emission,
2. *virecana* – purgation,
3. *basti* – enemata,
4. *śirovirecana* – enema to head,
5. *raktamokṣaṇa* – blood letting.

According to my understanding, the *abhyāsa* and *vairāgya* are curative measures similar to the *śamana vidhi* and *śodhana vidhi* of *āyurveda*.

Modern days are days of pills, tablets and capsules. Multi-vitamin pills are claimed to be equal to nourishing food by the medical world.

Naturally the mind of an average man is also trained to question in a similar manner. The question may be, "Mr. Iyengar, is there any pill or capsule which we can take to reach emancipation?" I say, "Yes", emphatically, "take four capsules every day, namely faith *(śraddhā)*, vigour *(vīrya)*, memory *(smṛti)* and complete absorption in the practice of yoga with full attention *(samādhi prajñā)*, without missing a day and you will be a liberated soul" (*Y.S.*, I.20).

This *sūtra* has a therapeutic value.

Now some may ask whether these capsules should be taken along with water or milk. In *āyurveda* there is *anupāna*. *Anupāna* is that which is taken along with the main medicine to bring proper and immediate effect. It is also meant for lessening the side effects of vital drugs which could be dangerous and harmful.

Patañjali calls the *anupāna*, "profound meditation on God or *Īśvara praṇidhāna*" (*Y.S.*, I.23).

There is a story in the *Bhāgavatam*. The Queen Satyabhama[1] asks Lord Krishna why he considers the *gopi*[2] his best *bhakta* – devotees. Lord Krishna says that he will reply later. One day, Lord Krishna complains of acute and severe chest pain. The doctors attend to him but they give the opinion that it is incurable as their medicine fails to give any relief. Then Krishna himself, being the Almighty, says that the medicine given by the doctors is absolutely a right treatment but somehow the *anupāna* is not correct. Naturally, the Queen asks him what they should give as *anupāna:* milk, juice or *tulasi* water. He says that the dust of the feet is the best *anupāna* for the disease. Naturally, all the queens are taken aback and Nārada gets puzzled knowing very well that nobody will give the dust of their feet to the Lord of the Universe. Krishna sends Nārada to Gokul, and the *gopi* come running to enquire about the well-being of Krishna. Nārada says that Krishna has an acute chest pain and needs the dust of the feet as *anupāna*. The *gopi*, best among all the *bhakta*, immediately give the dust of their feet and tell Nārada to take it as early as possible so that their Lord will soon be relieved from the pains.

After taking the *anupāna*, Krishna feels hale and hearty and tells the queens that this is the love of *the bhaktan* who do not mind giving anything to the Lord. So this *Īśvara praṇidhāna* is the best *anupāna* to be taken with the above-mentioned capsules.

However, the consciousness cannot get rid of modifications and afflictions so easily as it is a chronic disease of the patient. Chronic disease makes the patient weak; he loses his power to resist to a considerable extent and becomes vulnerable. Each disease tends to be accompanied by other diseases which come as side-effects or after-effects.

Similarly, the afflictions and modifications are accompanied by *citta vikṣepa* (impediments): diseases *(vyādhi)*, sluggishness *(styāna)*, doubt *(saṁśaya)*, carelessness *(pramāda)*, idleness *(ālasya)*, sense-gratification *(avirati)*, living in the world of illusion *(bhrāntidarśana)*, inability to hold on to what is undertaken *(alabdhabhūmikatva)*, inability to maintain progress *(anavasthitatva)*, sorrows *(duḥkha)*, despair *(daurmanasya)*, tremor of the body *(aṅgamejayatva)*, heavy breathing *(śvāsapraśvāsa)*. These obstacles and distractions harm the *citta*.

---

1 One of the eight wives of Lord Krishna.
2 Herdswomen

Does Patañjali give any preventive measures? Yes. The preventive measure is *ekatatvābhyāsa*, the single-minded effort to continue with yogic practices.

In *āyurveda*, there are certain medicines which are meant for external application. These are known as *bahir-parimārjana*. They are applied in the form of *snehana* (oleation), *svedana* (sudation or steam treatment), *pradeha* (application of ointment), *pariśeka* (poultice or affusion) and *mardana* (massage). These are the external means to affect the inner body.

Patañjali gives an equal treatment with *citta prasādanam* to bring the internal change in *citta*. Many times we have to change our behaviour and approach towards the external world for our own good. These treatments cultivate the mind to tread on the yogic path smoothly. They are as follows:

1. *maitrī* – cultivation of friendliness towards those who are happy,
2. *karuṇā* – cultivation of compassion towards those who are in sorrow,
3. *muditā* – cultivation of joy towards those who are virtuous,
4. *upekṣā* – cultivation of indifference or neutrality towards those who are full of vices.

If this is an external means, then Patañjali gives the internal means or *antaḥ-parimārjana*. According to *āyurveda*, medicine taken orally or internally for cure or relief from diseases is called *antaḥ-parimārjana*. *Parimārjana* is cleaning, cleansing or washing. In *āyurveda* the treatment is to wash and clean the *doṣa*, and in yoga to wash and clean the *triguṇa* out of which the *citta* is made. The internal means are as follows:

1. Bringing calmness and quietness with the retention of breath after exhalation.
2. Total involvement with application, dedication and devotion in an interesting object, tasting the essence of calmness and steadiness emanating therefrom.
3. Contemplating on a sorrowless luminous effulgent light.
4. Contemplating on men of illumination who are free from desires and attachments.
5. Studying, recollecting and contemplating during the wakeful state, the experiences of dream-filled and dreamless sleepy states.
6. Contemplating on a thing which is conducive and pleasing to steadiness of mind. (*Y.S.*, I.34-39).

These are the various methods of concentration and contemplation utilised and applied to bring calmness, quietness, steadiness and serenity of the mind.

At this stage, the aspirant of yoga is considered to be at the stage of well-being because the mental modifications have been made feeble, attenuated in order to undergo *samāpatti*. The consciousness becomes highly sensitive, choiceless, pure and stainless. It becomes crystal clear. Such a crystal-like consciousness enables revelation of the knower, knowable and the instrument of knowing by holding them as a substrate. This is called *samāpatti* or consumation.

In *āyurveda*, *svāsthya* means to be healthy physically, psychologically and spiritually. *Āyurveda* helps to bring health of the body so that the patient develops his own talents to progress as far as mental and spiritual aspects are concerned. For this purpose, *āyurveda* gives the treatment called *rasāyana* or *ojaskar* treatment. *Rasāyana* means the treatment which controls the ageing process, increases vitality, prevents diseases, brings health and yields long life. It is like a tonic. *Ojas* adds vitality and increases resistance power to combat diseases. These treatments are meant to bring *svāsthya* or equilibrium in man so that he leads the worldly as well as spiritual life in a disciplined way.

Yoga brings the consciousness to a state of *tatstha* (becoming stable) and *tadañjanatā*[1] (taking or acquiring the shape of seen or known). These are the states in which the consciousness totally remains in the object presented to it and appears completely in the shape of the object. These objects could be either subtle elements or gross elements (objects of the world) or the organs of perception or even the self. At this stage consciousness needs some tonic. Patañjali introduces these tonics *(rasāyana)* for the steadiness, silence, placidity and clarity in intelligence *(samāpatti)* in the form of *savitarkā*, *nirvitarkā*, *savicārā*, *nirvicārā* – deliberative contemplation, super-deliberative contemplation, reflective contemplation and super-reflective contemplation.

Āyurveda is not interested merely in treating the person to get rid of disease, but further it wants to establish health in the body; so rehabilitation and rejuvenation also are part of the treatment to bring a full stop to further treatment.

In yoga, Patañjali feeds a proper diet to consciousness with *sabīja samādhi* (seeded *samādhi*). When *citta* develops the spiritual light of intelligence filled with unalloyed wisdom, glowing with truth and reality, then the question of rehabilitation or rejuvenation arises, which Patañjali answers with the state of *nirbīja samādhi* (seedless *samādhi*).

Citta expresses itself in five planes according to the proportions in which the *triguṇa* exist. These planes are:

1. *mūḍha* – forgetful mind,
2. *kṣipta* – wandering mind,
3. *vikṣipta* – alternate states of steadiness and distraction of the mind,

---

1 *Kṣīṇavṛtteḥ abhijātasya iva maṇeḥ grahītṛ grahaṇa grāhyeṣu tatstha tadañjanatā samāpattiḥ* (*Y.S.*, I.41). The yogi realises that the knower, the instrument of knowing and the known are one, himself, the seer. Like a pure transparent jewel, he reflects an unsullied purity.

4. *ekāgra* – one-pointedness of the mind,
5. *niruddha* – restrained mind.

The above mentioned treatment in *Samādhi Pāda* is for the patients who fall into the category of *ekāgra* and *niruddha*. Patañjali gives treatment to those who belong to the first three categories.

In *āyurveda* the patient is examined to assess the *bala* (strength and vitality) and *doṣa* (morbidity of three humours) to give required treatment. The constitution of the patient is measured by assessing the *bala* and *doṣa*, and accordingly the patient is classified into three divisions: *pravara* (high), *madhya* (medium) and *avara* (low). This also decides the intensity or mildness of the ailment.

Has Patañjali not done it?

Patañjali portrays distinctly different levels of aspirants as feeble, average and keen, besides the supremely enthusiastic. Here Patañjali asks the aspirant to weigh himself up and assess his constitution and strength. If *āyurveda* pathologically finds out the morbidity of *tridoṣa*, yoga finds out the morbidity of *triguṇa*. Yoga gives five capsules (*śraddhā*, etc.) and asks the aspirant to find out whether he can digest them, as they work with those for whom there is less morbidity and more purity in the *triguṇa*.

If *triguṇa* are very much in a morbid state, the capsules have to be changed, and they are, *tapaḥ svādhyāya Īśvara praṇidhānāni kriyā yogaḥ* (*Y.S.*, II.1).

This capsule is called *kriyā yoga* which is three-layered or thrice-coated by *tapas* (self-discipline or a burning desire with devotion to reach perfection), *svādhyāya* (self-study or study of oneself from the body to the Self) and *Īśvara praṇidhāna* (total surrender of oneself to God). The *triguṇa* reach the morbid state because the web of afflictions covers them. Afflictions are mainly five in number: lack of spiritual wisdom – *avidyā*, egoism – *asmitā*, attachment towards pleasure – *rāga*, aversion to pain – *dveṣa* – and clinging to life – *abhiniveśa*.

All these change the very simple and pure nature of original mind and make it complicated. As the diseases weaken the strength of man by increasing the morbidity of *tridoṣa*, so also afflictions weaken the strength of consciousness by increasing the morbidity of *triguṇa*. In *āyurveda*, the *vāta* is considered to be the strongest prime *doṣa* on which depends the health of a person. The *vāta* creates disease in a state of agitation and aggravation, and restores health too, when it is in a balanced state. In yoga, it is the *sattvaguṇa*. When *sattva* becomes weak, it is dominated by other *guṇa* and man is caught in afflictions, but when *sattva* is strengthened or when it becomes predominant, man is free from afflictions.

How are the afflictions to be eradicated? *Pratiprasava* and *dhyāna* are the two methods. *Pratiprasava* (involution) is counter-activation and *dhyāna* is meditation. The subtle afflictions are destroyed at the time of final deliverance with counter-activation, and the mental modifications are annihilated and silenced by involution of the senses throug meditation. The counter-activation – *pratiprasava* –is *śodhana-vidhi* (purifying method) and meditation – *dhyāna* – is *śamana-vidhi* (pacifying method).

In *āyurveda*, the diseases are categorised in four parts: adventitious – *āgantuka*, physical – *śārīrika*, mental – *mānasika* – and natural – *svābhāvika*.

The adventitious are those caused from external factors such as bites, injuries, accidents and so on, while the physical and mental diseases are commonly known to all. The *svābhāvika* are natural diseases which cover birth (the very birth itself and the constitutional weakness by birth), old age, death, natural hunger, thirst and sleep.

Here the view is very clear. Patañjali calls *pañca vṛtti* (five modifications) and *pañca kleśa* (five afflictions) natural diseases since the conjunction between the seer and the seen exist from time immemorial.

Now general treatment given for these is as follows:

1. adventitious is treated surgically,
2. physical is treated medically,
3. mental is treated psychologically,
4. natural is treated spiritually.

In yogic treatment, the same method is followed.

The afflictions are the root cause of *karma*. The afflictions have to be eradicated only by *karmaśuddhi* (purification of action). The consciousness gets affected by afflictions, and the pure consciousness becomes the fabricated consciousness. This is adventitious disease which needs surgical operation. Operation is a drastic treatment; Patañjali's operation is *pratiprasava* (counter-activation or involution). The *vṛtti* are natural diseases which need a treatment such as meditation.

Avidyā, or lack of spiritual wisdom, is the root cause of afflictions. *Avidyā* is the product of predominant *tamōguṇa*. It has to be treated. To uncover the *sattvaguṇa*, which is covered by *tamōguṇa*, the *sattvaguṇa* itself has to be operated on. This operation is called *vivekakhyāti*. The instrument used to perform this operation is the *aṣṭāṅga yoga* (eight-petalled yoga).

Patañjali is a perfect pathologist. He does not give superficial treatments; he first takes pathological tests to find out the root cause of the disease. Thus, he declares that it is the pleasant and unpleasant experiences of the mundane or celestial world which are ultimately painful, causing sorrow, as sorrow is the cause of disease. The painful experience is due to the contradictory functions of the *triguṇa*, and that is the cause of disease. Therefore, the pains have to be avoided, and Patañjali takes responsibility for curing disease by applying the yogic method.

For therapeutics, four factors are necessary: the physician, the medicament, the attendant and the patient. Patañjali fulfils these requirements. In the yogic path, Patañjali himself is the physician, the science of yoga is the medicament, the teacher teaching yoga is the attendant and the student is the patient.

The physician is expected to be excellent in medical knowledge, having practical experience, dexterity and purity. He should know all the drugs, their suitability, their multiple forms and potency. So also while treating the patient, it is necessary on the part of a *guru* (attendant) to have the knowledge of *āsana* and *prāṇāyāma*, the performance, the multi-effects and multi-forms in order to apply them as medicine.

Patañjali vividly and clearly knew the conjunction between the seer and seen as the cause of disease. This union has to be avoided. Therefore, Patañjali dissects the human being in order to get a clear picture of *dṛśya* and *dṛṣṭrā* (*Y.S.*, II.18 & 19). He makes the seer *(dṛṣṭrā)* aware of the truth that the seen *(dṛśya)* exists for the sake of the seer to lead him to abide in his pure state of existence.

He declares that *aṣṭāṅga yoga* is the only cure of this disease. It includes all those curative measures used in *āyurveda*. It is meant for cleansing *śarīra* and *citta* so that one attains the state of *aśuddhikṣaya* (cleansing-purification) and *jñānadīpti* (adding *ojas* to *jñāna*).

The kindled consciousness *(jñānadīpti)* and the discriminative discernment *(vivekakhyāti)* are the state of health of *citta* – consciousness.

In *aṣṭāṅga yoga*, the *yama-niyama* are moral principles. When one does not follow these moral-health principles, disease sets in. It is called *vitarka-bādhana*. *Vitarka* is not *viśeṣa tarka*, as it is in *Samādhi Pāda*, but *viparīta tarka*.[1] It is the way of thinking in a topsy-turvy manner. For

---

[1] Those who do not know *Sanskrit* may get puzzled with the word *vitarka*, which is refered in *sūtra* I.17. It is the first step of *samprajñāta samādhi*. It is also referred in *sūtra* II.33-34 for the dubious thinking which is of questionable value. Therefore the *sūtra* says, *vitarkā hiṁsādayaḥ*. *Vitarka* has two meanings. The prefix *vi* stands for *viśeṣa* and *viparīta*, whereas *tarka* means to think, to ponder, to reason, to speculate. When the thinking, reasoning or deliberation is done specially for *samādhi* in order to come to accurate conclusion, it is *viśeṣa tarka*. When the

cont over . .

instance, the *sādhaka* knows that he is supposed to follow the principles of *yama* led by Patañjali. But because of perverse thinking, his thoughts remain based on violence, untruth, stealing, non-celibacy and covetousness. The deliberation on thoughts proceeds on these opposite ways of thinking. This kind of perverted or contrary thinking is an obstruction to the human mental faculty. This does not lead towards constructive thoughts, but destructive or controversial thoughts in a wrong way. *Bādhana* is to get possessed by such thoughts. The *vitarka-bādhana* is a kind of infectious disease of *citta* which does not allow it to keep its moral health. The cure for this disease is *pratipakṣa bhāvanam*. This is *śamana vidhi;* a process of counteracting *vitarka*, or improper thoughts, with *tarka*, or proper thoughts. The proper thoughts eradicate improper thoughts and naturally the *citta* regains its moral state.

Āsana is a cure for physical, mental and spiritual disease. By conquering the *āsana,* one can effortlessly tread on the path of yoga, as one's body and mind totally merge or assume the infinite form of the seer. The *āsana* put an end to the dualities and differentiations between the trio – body, mind and self.

Prāṇāyāma removes the veil covering the light of knowledge and increases the *bala* or strength of the *citta;* for it to become competent to tread on this path.

Pratyāhāra is the conquest of senses of perception. This is the health of the senses. The disease of perceptual organs is to go after objects and indulge in them. The indulgence causes indigestion. The medicine for indigestion is *laṅghana* (lightening) or *karṣana* (attenuating). Fasting comes under *laṅghana*. The organs of perception have to go on a fast. *Laṅghana* has both varieties of treatment, the *śodhana* (purificatory) and *śamana* (pacificatory).

In *pratyāhāra*, the organs of perception are withdrawn. The objects are vomitted *(emesis)* through the organs. The enema is given so even in the form of memory the residue does not remain. But such a drastic change may show adverse effect. So the treatment of pacification is given along with the practice of *āsana* and *prāṇāyāma*. The organs of perception learn to remain on a strict diet through the practice of *āsana* and *prāṇāyāma,* and finally they do a complete fast.

Dhāraṇā, dhyāna and *samādhi* are like *rasāyana*. *Rasāyana* in *āyurveda* means treatment to arrest the ageing process, prevent disease, increase vitality and bring longevity along with health. Are these three limbs extending their helping hand? *Dhāraṇā* is focussing the attention.

---

cont . . .

thinking, reasoning or speculation is done deliberately in an opposite way, or contrary to the rules, it is called *viparīta tarka*. This way of deliberation is based on wrong principles. This is definitely due to the unethical or impaired mental faculty where the person thinks in an immoral, unethical or illogical way. Patañjali points out perverted thinking as *vitarka*, which are opposite to the principles of *yama* and *niyama*.

Dhāraṇā makes *citta* potent, like *rasāyana. Dhyāna* is a continuous flow of attention which increases the vitality of *citta. Samādhi* is a state in which the consciousness *(citta)* merges in the object of meditation, i.e. the Seer. This is a state of total consummation of *citta.* The seen in its pure state remains parallel to the seer. This results in abiding in his own state.

Medicine is meant to bring physical and mental health. The *rasāyana* is given when the patient is free from disease. *Rasāyana* is not a medicine but a tonic. It is a treatment given to a healthy man to remain healthy. The last three limbs of yoga, called *trayi*, are the *rasāyana* for those who have gained health by practising the first five limbs *(pūrvasādhanā).*

In *āyurveda*, before starting the treatment of the five-fold elimination therapies *(śodhana vidhi),* the patient is prepared for elimination. This pre-preparation is called *pūrva karma.* This *pūrva karma* includes *snehana* (oleation) and *svedana* (fomentation and sudation). *Snehana* is oiling the body using ghee, oil, etc. This is given as an oral treatment, as an oil-enema or as a skin massage, and it arrests the agitating *vāta. Svedana* is a treatment in which the patient is made to perspire or sweat.

The *pūrvāṅgas* of *aṣṭāṅga yoga*, namely, *yama, niyama, āsana, prāṇāyāma* and *pratyāhāra* are the *pūrva karma.* By these the body and consciousness are prepared to become a fit instrument undergoing changes known as restraining modification, trance modification and one-pointed modification *(nirodha, samādhi* and *ekāgratā).* The practice of the last three limbs is to bring a total transformation by eliminating the dual state in body, mind and self. That is why these limbs are called *rasāyana* – tonics to the consciousness.

Finally, the consciousness (seen) reaches the healthy state of exaltation and becomes as pure as the seer. Both being pure, remain aloof and unmingled and in the indivisible state of existence.

DIFFERENCE IN TREATMENT OF YOGA AND *ĀYURVEDA**

The mystic, the esoteric and spiritual aspects of the age old wisdom of our sages and *ṛṣis* are in our *vedic* texts and scriptures. Neither were therapy and healing neglected by these wise men, since health was a primary requirement. Yoga is currently in the forefront of the therapeutic revolution, healing and curing, and then restoring full health in order to preserve it throughout the span of life. Fortunately now the hidden treasury is slowly being unlocked.

We have in addition the frame of *āsana* and *prāṇāyāma* as well as the discipline of *yama* and *niyama* to serve in quest of physical well-being, mental peace and poise so that we may explore the spiritual consciousness. The strands of yoga and of the structure of consciousness have been superbly codified in Patañjali's aphorisms *(Yoga Sūtra).*

If I am expansive in praise of the wide and varied application of yoga practices in medico-therapeutics, it should not be misconstrued as the assertions of the ego. I have been involved in yoga for long years, and have been able to penetrate deep into this "therapeutic yoga" by my experimentation, experience and the insight I acquired through them. I am neither a medical man nor an *āyurvedic* physician. I am an ardent yoga *sādhaka*. I have written on *āsana*, *prāṇāyāma*, yoga *sūtra* and yoga related subjects, and its philosophy.

I have successfully treated persons suffering from hypertension, blood-pressure, insomnia, cardiac troubles, diabetes, arthritis, rheumatism, spondylitis, ruptured spine, persons experiencing excruciating pains when mentally depressed. Men of medicine who had thrown their hands up in despair, sufferers who had confined themselves to bed came to me for solace. In response I studied yoga for remedial measures. In my yoga therapeutic class, you have seen how we work, though there are cries of agony at that moment. Then you have also seen how they move freely without trauma and are happy whereas the specialists had pronounced, "No hope for improvement". We have to innovate props for the modification in *āsana* to get the right results.

---

* Lecture given at the Ramāmaṇi Iyengar Memorial Yoga Institute, 1997.

A person who had developed an almost freakish stoop had drugged himself with pain killers. Ankylosing spondylitis (bamboo spine) is said to be a genetic affliction and regarded as incurable. At one stage the person could not even lie down on his back, rocking like a see-saw. After one year of painful yogic practices, his solid mass became mobile, the suffering and pain became less. His whole family is now doing yoga and one of his sons has become a reputed yoga teacher.

Yoga and *āyurveda* are two streams that intermingle in our ancient literature. They are naturopathic treatments but with action. The exterior and the interior manifestations tend to interact, react, fuse and work as opposite forces integrating and disintegrating the cells to keep life process progressing or regressing. There is a striking similarity in yoga and *āyurveda* in the diagnosis of health and disease at all levels. Both have a philosophy for life-giving and sustaining processes.

The doctrine of yoga was established in harmony with natural law. The three principal qualities or the *guṇa,* namely *tamas, rajas* and *sattva,* recognised by the science of yoga, run parallel to the three humours or *tridoṣa,* namely *vāta, pitta* and *śleṣma,* recognised by the science of *āyurveda.*

Yoga goes to the core and treats *citta* while *āyurveda* treats the body. If yoga seeks to purify the soiled consciousness, *āyurveda* prescribes methods and modes for treating the soiled body. *Śauca* and the elimination of *mala* (body toxins) as well as modulations of the psyche in quest of deeper insight form today's psychosomatic science.

Both yoga and *āyurveda* have adopted *Sāṁkhya* cosmogony. The cosmos consists of two primary entities, *puruṣa* – the life principle, and *prakṛti* – nature. The third entity yoga adds to *Sāṁkhya* philosophy, is the cosmic or universal soul, the *Īśvara.*

Tridoṣa, the three factors of *āyurveda,* have no adequate English equivalents; therefore they are loosely translated as wind *(vāta),* bile *(pitta)* and phlegm *(kapha* or *śleṣma).* Wind, bile and phlegm are the air, fire and water, having approximate connotation with anabolic, metabolic and catabolic principles.

Yoga moves around the main pivots of body, mind and soul and the three tendencies of *tāmasic, rājasic* and *sāttvic guṇa.* The aim of yoga is to return the *triguṇa* to equilibrium and that of the *āyurveda,* to restore the *tridoṣa* to balance. The *triguṇa* concept is pivotal to yoga as the *tridoṣa* concept is pivotal to *āyurveda.*

Disease is that state when one does not feel "at ease", and the art of leading a life "at ease" is health.

Āyurveda defines a healthy person as one who has healthy digestion, whose bodily humours are in a state of equilibrium and in whom the vital fluids course in their normal state and quantity, accompanied by normal processes of secretion, organic function and intellect. To sum up, it is the balance of *tamas, rajas* and *sattva* of yoga and *vāta, pitta* and *kapha* of *āyurveda* which lead to health and well being.

The criteria and concepts of disease or ill health cover a vast expanse according to yoga as well as *āyurveda*. The causes for diseases could be *āgantuka* (extraneous), *śāririka* (bodily), *mānasika* (mental) and *svābhāvika* (natural) or deranged humours and vitiated modulations *(vṛtti)* of mind. The causes could be emotional such as anger, grief, fear, joy, envy, jealousy, malice and pride. All these emotional inbalances impinge on each other causing a lot of confusion, and therefore, the body, mind and intelligence seem to be in a mess.

Then how does the sphere of treatment of yoga and *āyurveda* differ?

According to yoga, disease has to be eradicated by removing the causes of sorrow and through the control of consciousness so that consciousness identifies with the Seer *(svarūpa-avasthā)*.

The accent in yoga is on arresting the mental modifications *(vṛtti nirodha)*, whereas the accent in Āyurveda is to arrest disease *(roga nirodha)*. The focus of yoga is on the use of the body, mind and intelligence (the very substratum itself). While the focus of *āyurveda* is on the use of *dravya* (substratum of properties).

The *triguṇa* and *tridoṣa* are pervasive and there is no situation where one or the other is absent. There is not one single living being that can be found to be *monoguṇic* or *monodoṣic*. Likewise there is no such thing as perfect balance in the *guṇa* or *doṣa*. The whole of humanity is under the influence of the *triguṇa* or *tridoṣa*.

Only in a state of beatitude does a yogi bring equilibrium in the *guṇa* and *doṣa (sāmya-avasthā)*.

Yoga and *āyurveda* are identically and potently holistic in their application and approach. Every individual is an autonomous entity in the complex of his body, mind and soul. Health is perpetually in a state of flux. Both health and disease are dynamic.

Man being a *cikitsā puruṣa,* yoga and *āyurveda* are *cikitsā śāstra* (therapeutic sciences). Yoga treats *citta* (intelligence, ego and mind) and *āyurveda* treats the body and the phase of mind which is in contact with the body. Both lay emphasis on a code of conduct and personal hygiene. If *āyurveda* calls it *sadvṛtti,* yoga calls it *yama* and *niyama.*

Each *āsana* and *prāṇāyāma* have a therapeutic value. They are administered according to the root cause of the diagnosed disease. The sequence of *āsana* and *prāṇāyāma* on every disease is charted on the basis of anatomical structure, physiological functioning, progressive intensity, purifying and pacifying capacity, the stage of the disease and the capacity and mentality of the patients as well as their age. Both enhance immunity and resistance to disease. Lord Krishna, in the *Bhagavad Gītā,* says that the average person has very little control over his physical, mental and emotional health.

The spine being the central column for the nervous system, the weight of the body has to be harmoniously distributed along the thirty-three articulations of the vertebral column. It has seven cervical, twelve thoracic, five lumbar, five sacral and four coccygeal vertebrae, giving room for countless movements of the body.

The vertebral column forms space and one creates space in the vertebral column. The rib cage with the floating ribs help lateral movements of the spine and make to breath deeper and longer.

Hence, I would like to stress once again that the application of yoga therapeutics is of vital concern to our country, fitting within our economic constraints.

The West has taken the lead in applying yoga in arthritis, rheumatism, cardiac complaints, arteriosclerosis, high blood pressure and so on.

With the help of modern medical science one can work with tests of how yoga and *āyurveda* help in the eradication of ill-health and building up of dynamic health.

YOGA AND *ĀYURVEDA*

Yoga begins from the mind and *āyurveda* from the body. They appear to differ at the starting point, though both have a spiritual base and have the same goal – the realisation of the Self. They are the gift and heritage coming from the wisdom of the ancient sages and *ṛṣis*. However, both *śāstra* primarily aim at gaining physical and mental health. There is a striking resemblance in the three-dimensional approach of *yoga śāstra* and *āyurveda śāstra*.

Yoga speaks of *triguṇa*, the qualities of nature –*sattva, rajas* and *tamas*, which interplay with *puruṣa* and *prakṛti*, while *āyurveda* speaks in terms of the *tridoṣa*, namely *vāta, pitta* and *kapha*, which interplay with body constitution and metabolism. When vitiated, they cause diseases of the body and mind.

A weakling cannot reach the soul or God. *Nāyamātmā balahīnenalabhyaḥ*, so says the *Mundakopaniṣad*. Therefore, one needs to strengthen the body, mind and self. Both yoga and *āyurveda* say that diseases are caused on account of the misidentification of *prakṛti* – nature or object – with *puruṣa* – the seer or subject. *Draṣṭdṛśayoḥ saṁyogoḥ heyahetuḥ* (*Y.S.*, II.17). The root cause of pain is the association of seer *(puruṣa)* with seen *(prakṛti)* and remedy lies in their dissociation.

Āyurveda however restricts itself to remedial measures against the diseases of the body, whereas yoga deals in depth since its duty is to find the root cause of all the diseases, problems and afflictions of body, mind, intelligence, ego and consciousness. Yoga thinks of the ultimate remedy which seems to be drastic and that is dissociation – in other words, emancipation.

Yoga demands more will power while the advantage in *āyurveda* is that you can take medicine to build up strength and then gain will power by turning towards yoga. Yoga demands individual efforts, therefore it is subjective. *Āyurveda* prescribes medicines which one can take effortlessly, therefore it is objective.

In *āyurveda* the seven *dhātu*, namely, chyle *(rasa)*, blood *(rakta)*, flesh *(māṁsa)*, fat *(meda)*, bones *(asthi)*, marrow *(majjā)*, and semen or ovum *(śukra* or *śoṇita)*, and three *doṣa*, namely, wind *(vāyu),* bile *(pitta),* phlegm *(śleṣma),* plus *mala* (toxins) play a role in both health or disease. Yoga too accepts the cause of disease as vitiation and disturbance in these ingredients and humours of the body, but looks beyond.

Fluctuations such as direct perception, misperception, misconception, sleep and memory, and afflictions like want of knowledge, pride, attachment, hatred and fear of death draw the mind and self towards desires. It seems as though the self is getting mixed up with the thoughts which come in the form of fluctuations and afflictions – *vṛtti sārūpyam itaratra.* This wrong identification of self with thoughts creates the imbalance in body, mind and consciousness. The self is caught in objects or things as desires.

Desires *(vāsanā)* get aggravated according to Patañjali, which he expresses in aphorism – *vitarkā hiṁsādayaḥ kṛta kāritā anumoditā lobha krodha moha pūrvakā mṛdu madhya adhimātrā duḥkha ajñāna ananta phalā iti pratispakṣa bhāvanam* (*Y.S.,* II.34). Greed, anger and delusion induce or abet and aggravate sufferings in mild, moderate or intense forms or may remain dormant, attenuated, fluctuating or active. Actions done directly, indirectly, or abated bring diseases and pains in the form of self afflicted, elemental disturbances as well as those which are genetic, allergic or due to destiny.

The ailments are lack of interest, doubt, carelessness, laziness, sensual gratification, mistaken notion, missing the point or inability to hold on to one type of *sādhanā,* and inability to maintain the achieved state. They are nine in number, affecting not only the nine gates[1] of man but the body and consciousness also. These pains bring physical, mental, intellectual and spiritual unhealthiness which is further aggravated by despair, weakness of the mind, tremor of the body and laboured breathing.

Yoga and *āyurveda* are both preventive and curative sciences. Both have two methods of treatment, to purify and to pacify *(śodhana* and *śamana).*

According to *āyurveda,* the gate of health in man is the digestive system, on which the health of other systems depends. According to yoga, the gates of health are the respiratory and circulatory systems. If these two systems are kept healthy and clean, the other systems,the digestive, nervous, glandular and excretory systems do their jobs without hindrances and pacify the subliminal impressions. Both *āyurveda* and yoga accept the theory of *karma* and the role that *karma* plays as the cause of disease. But *āyurveda* does not go in depth to cleanse the *karma* since it is not its subject matter. However, for yoga it is important to deal in depth with *karma* since yoga wants to eradicate disease from its very base.

---

[1] The nine gates known as *navadvāra* are the two nostrils, two ears, two eyes, mouth, generative and excretory organs (*Śvetāśvara Upaniṣad,* III.18). For more details, see *Aṣṭadaḷa Yogamālā,* vol. 1, p. 120.

Patañjali emphasises that our past *karma* play their role in forming and framing our life fabric and explains how to face them. Though the body seems to be the source and springboard for all actions, it is the afflicted *citta* that is the cause behind each action.

Thus Patañjali puts the theory of *karma* in three *sūtra*. *Kleṣamūlaḥ karmāśayo dṛṣṭādṛṣṭa janma vedanīyaḥ* (*Y.S.*, II.12), meaning, good and bad actions leave their impressions in the subconscious mind which afflict in the present life according to the degree of merits and demerits of actions. This may be categorised as *ādhidaivika tāpa*. *Satimule tadvipāko jātyāyurbhogāḥ* (*Y.S.*, II.13), meaning, the seed of the past lives actions sows itself in this life, defining birth, span of life, and what one has to undergo in the experiences of this life. This is the seed of *ādhibhautika tāpa*. And lastly, *te hlāda paritāpa phalāḥ puṇyāpuṇya hetutvāt* (*Y.S.*, II.14), meaning, class of birth, span of life and experiences whether pleasant or unpleasant or mixed are the fruits of our good and bad actions from our previous lives. This is *ādhāytmika tāpa*.

Through regular practice of yoga, it is possible to overcome the three *tāpa* as yoga develops discriminative power in the doer.[1] It strengthens the will power and intelligence to increase the potentiality of discriminative power so that, through this power, he frees himself from aims and goals, and lives a state of *tadā dṛṣṭuḥ svarūpe avasthānam*.[2]

1 *Kṛtārthaṁ prati naṣṭam api anaṣṭaṁ tadanya sādhāraṇatvāt*, the relationship with nature ceases for emancipated beings, its purpose having been fulfilled, but its processes continue to affect others. (*Y.S.*, II.22). *Sva svāmi śaktyoḥ svarūpopalabdhi hetuḥ saṁyogaḥ*, the conjunction of the seer with the seen is for the seer to discover his own true nature. (*Y.S.*, II.23).

2 *Y.S.*, I.3. Then, the seer dwells in his own true splendour.

YOGA: HEALTH AND BEYOND

Today we are living in a most health-conscious era. The world is overflowing with medical systems, therapies, treatments and medicines. Over the media, electronic and otherwise, across the laboratories, in the hospitals, medical schools, professional periodicals and popular platforms, there is a frantic search for health. This concern for health may appear laudable; but on deeper examination it appears to be more of an endeavour to combat disease than an authentic quest for dynamic health. The quest is more disease-oriented than dynamic health-oriented. Health is something that cannot be gathered from others or bought across counters. It has to be earned through one's own efforts and discipline.

Medical science has grown by leaps and bounds. New medicines and cures continue to flood the market. New surgical inventions have almost become a spare-part industry. Yet, the diseases and strains are growing rapidly, and in terms of mundane health and happiness, let alone spiritual fulfilment, we are not better off than our forefathers. If anything, we are much worse off. The crime rate is increasing, drug addiction is growing alarmingly, and morality in public life has come to mean 'not being found out'. The citadel of morality and the nursery of love, affection, sympathy, compassion, sacrifice, character and right values of life have become a nightmarishly insecure edifice.

The root cause of all this is the old fashioned term selfishness. The modern world is governed by consumerism – a mad rush for instant pleasure gratification. This is so in every field. The modern motto is: "Enjoy and pay later!" Children become addicted to sweets, drugs, crime and pornography even before they reach their teens. Fast food, against all medical wisdom, is spreading from country to country and continent to continent. The massive developments in science and technology have become subservient to the senses and not the intellect. Men have set themselves up as little tinpot gods, but in reality, man has become a consuming and devouring biped. The more developed the country, the higher the consumption. Ethics have no place in the quality of life; they are not a valued item in the list of goods and services.

In this world, where "things are falling apart", yoga dominates as one of the alternative therapies in combating diseases and the strains of modern life. Its cures continue to surprise us and its promises ever seem to grow. Among the educated and the discerning, yoga has become a household word. Much is expected from yoga, yoga teachers and yoga masters. Will yoga meet this challenge? Can yoga meet this challenge?

The opening of the floodgates of yoga has led to the entry of misguided enthusiasts, half-baked experts and downright charlatans. Various limbs and techniques of yoga have been wrenched away from their context and yoga has been tortured to yield instant results. Yoga threatens to become one more commodity in the consumer supermarket, one more drug, one more imaginary hope. Instead of uplifting man and mankind from the moral morass, it may become corrupted, lose its power, purity and dignity surviving only to cater fitfully to pleasurable satisfactions. If yoga is meant only to cure disease or for pleasurable gratification, then it loses its right to be called yoga. The tragedy is that there is little understanding of how yoga helps in building physical and mental health and as to what the final goal of this health is. The yogic process, the yogic path and the yogic destination cannot be separated. If the final vision is lost, the path and process become murky, leading nowhere. If we understand this, we will appreciate the contributions of yoga to permanent health, happiness and tranquillity.

Yoga means the union of the self with the Divine. When the modifications of the *citta* cease, the self surfaces in its real nature *(Y.S.,* I.2 and I.3).[1] Patañjali states that the practice of the eight aspects of yoga removes impurities and brings forth the light of discrimination (*Y.S.,* II.28).[2] These eight aspects can be divided into three types of *sādhanā: Yama, niyama, āsana, prāṇāyāma* and *pratyāhāra* as *bahiraṅga sādhanā; pratyāhāra, dhāraṇā* and *dhyāna* as *antarāṅga sādhanā* and *samādhi* as *antarātma sādhanā. Pratyāhāra* – withdrawal of the senses – is a twilight zone between *bahiraṅga* and *antarāṅga sādhanā.* The foundations of *yama* and *niyama* are best laid in the home through proper examples and impressions – *saṁskāra.* The last three subtle aspects of yoga, namely *dhāraṇā, dhyāna* and *samādhi* require a certain level of intellectual understanding, emotional stability and purity that qualifies and enables one to practise them. For the vast majority, yoga practice and teaching has to begin with *āsana* and *prāṇāyāma,* which act as character building during and after the practice. Health and ethics of the body are the precondition for mental, intellectual and spiritual health. When harmony and synthesis are developed together in body, mind and self, then, I say, that is real health.

---

1 *Yogaścittavṛtti nirodhaḥ,* yoga is the cessation of the modifications of consciousness. (*Y.S.,* I.2). *Tadā draṣṭuḥ svarūpe'vasthānam,* then the seer dwells in his own true splendour. (*Y.S.,* I.3). Refer to *Light on the Yoga Sūtras of Patañjali,* B.K.S. Iyengar, Harper Collins, London.

2 *Yogāṅgānuṣṭhānāt aśuddhikṣaye jñānadīptiḥ āvivekakhyāteḥ,* by dedicated practice of the various aspects of yoga impurities are destroyed: the crown of wisdom radiates in glory. (*Y.S.,* II.28).

Āyurveda, the ancient Indian medical system, is considered the fifth *veda* and is a sister discipline of yoga sharing the same cosmogony or metaphysical framework and, to some extent, similar objectives. It shares with yoga the concept of *puruṣa* and *mūlaprakṛti*. *Mahat* or cosmic intelligence leads to the evolution of *citta* (a combination of mind, intelligence and ego), *pañca mahābhūta* (five elements): *pṛthvi* (earth), *āp* (water), *tej* (fire), *vāyu* (air) and *ākāśa* (ether); *pañca tanmātra* (five infra-atomic structures): *gandha* (smell), *rasa* (taste), *rūpa* (form), *sparśa* (touch), *śabda* (sound); *pañca jñānendriya* (five senses of perception): ears, nose, tongue, eyes and skin, and *pañca karmendriya* (five organs of action): arms, legs, speech, genital and excretory organs.[1]

Āyurveda deals with *svāsthya* (health) which revolves around the concept of the *tri-doṣa* (three humours)[2], *tri-mala*[3] (three impurities), *sapta-dhātu*[4] (seven constituents) and finally *ojas* (vitality or essence). The *āyurvedic* concept of health is a dynamic equilibrium which depends on the life cycle (childhood to old age), yearly cycle (seasons) and daily cycle (day and night). Health is concerned with purification (removal of impurities), the equilibrium of the three *doṣa* (wind, heat and phlegm) and the seven *dhātu* (chyle, blood, flesh, fat, bones, marrow and semen) as well as excretion of three *mala* (faeces, urine, sweat). The mind plays a very important role in reaching the cause and cure of diseases which are brought on by *ādhidaivika* (supernatural) factors, *ādhibhautika* (caused by one's environment) factors and *ādhyatmic* (self-inflicted) factors. Apart from preventive measures, *āyurveda* has its own pharmacology and the *pañca karma* system. And yoga has its own.

The diagnosis of physical and mental diseases, their prevention and cure requires, apart from the objective knowledge of anatomy, physiology and psychology, also a humane touch and experiential knowledge of *āsana*, *prāṇāyāma* and *dhyāna*. In yoga we do not have to induct anything from outside. All material creation is a manifestation of the *pañca mahābhūta*. Therefore the human body, which is made up of the *mahābhūta*, is a miniuniverse. The use of the limbs in *āsana*, *prāṇāyāma* and *dhyāna* and the play of consciousness bring about the required cellular, chemical and organic changes through *pañca vāyu* as they interact with *pañca mahābhūta*. Our great ancient sages discovered these natural techniques of preventing and curing diseases to reaching emancipation and freedom. All kinds of diseases can be prevented, controlled and

---

1 See the author's *Light on the Yoga Sūtras of Patañjali*, table n. 15, Harper Collins, London).

2 The three *doṣa* are *vāta* (wind), *pitta* (heat) and *śleṣma* (phlegm). See in this volume, "Parallelism Between Yoga and *Āyurveda*", and vol. 2, p. 315.

3 The *mala* are *mūtra* (urine), *pūrisa* (faeces), and *sveda* (sweat).

4 The seven *dhātu* are: 1. *rasa* (chyle, including lymph); 2. *rakta* (blood and specially the haemoglobin function of it); 3. *māṁsa* (muscle tissue); 4. *meda* (fat or adipose tissue); 5. *asthi* (bone tissue); 6. *majjā* (marrow) and 7. *śukra* (semen – specially the sperm in male and ovum in female).

cured by yoga through strengthening the concerned organs, their functioning and interrelationships, provided the one affected and afflicted uses his will power and discretion and practises yoga sincerely and honestly.

The whole *aṣṭāṅga yoga* and each of its aspects is concerned with purification (*Y.S.,* II.28). In the *niyama, śuddhi* is specifically mentioned as *śauca* and *tapas,* in which the physical and moral impurities are removed (*Y.S.,* II.41 & 43). *Āsana* and *prāṇāyāma* help to balance the *tridoṣa* and restore the balance between the *saptadhātu. Dhyāna* teaches the mind, intelligence and consciousness to remain in a passive and pensive state.

The modus operandi of *pañca mahābhūta* in *āsana* and *prāṇāyāma* can only be briefly touched on here. When limbs are placed in an *āsana,* the *pṛthvi tattva* starts functioning. Some parts are heavily placed, e.g. the legs in standing poses, head in *Sālamba Śīrṣāsana,* or shoulders in *Sālamba Sarvāṅgāsana.*[1] The *āp* element controlled properly can increase or decrease the flow of blood and other fluids. *Tej,* the fire element, manifests in the form of the heat produced in the body. *Jaṭharāgni* – the digestive fire, which is weak in modern man, can be easily increased through *āsana* and *prāṇāyāma* leading to better appetite and digestion. The *vāyu,* which consists of five *prāṇa*[2] and five *upaprāṇa,*[3] can again be properly balanced. The *vāyu* element is also concerned with touch. The *karmendriya* and *jñānendriya* provide the feedback for correct positions, movements and experiences. The sensations through the skin, muscles and joints guide us in the performance of *āsana* and *prāṇāyāma.* The touch of *prāṇa* in the nostrils during *prāṇāyāma* introduces the sense of what meditation is. The *āsana* basically deals with the extension, contraction, expansion, flexion and rotation of the limbs, moulding the required space in the *āsana.* Yoga strengthens the subtlest element *ākāśa* and then takes us beyond. *Uthitta Trikoṇāsana*[4] is not just placing the limbs in a particular order, it is a search for the infinite in the finite.

Unlike *āyurveda,* yoga deals not just with predominantly surfacing or expressed diseases. According to yogic science, disease may be dormant, attenuated, alternating or fully developed (*Y.S.,* II.4).[5]

---

1 See *Light on Yoga,* Harper Collins, London.
2 *Prāṇa, apāna, vyāna, udāna* and *samāna.*
3 *Nāga, kūrma, kṛkara, devadatta* and *dhanaṁjaya.*
4 See plate n. 25.
5 *Avidyā kṣetram uttareṣāṁ prasupta tanu vicchinna udārāṇām,* lack of true knowledge is the source of all pains and sorrow whether dormant, attenuated, interrupted or fully active. (*Y.S.,* II.4). The *sūtra* numbers are as in *Light on the Yoga Sūtras of Patañjali,* Harper Collins, London.

As lack of knowledge is the breeding ground for afflictions, so also for the diseases. The afflictions could be in any of the four phases, namely dormant, attenuated, alternated or active state. Similarly, the diseases can be *prasupta*, hidden or dormant, waiting to surface in due course of time as cancer may be diagnosed at a later stage. The diseases could be in a mild or attenuated state, such as cancer detected at an early stage, which is curable to a great extent. The diseases could be alternating, one coming into the foreground while another goes into the background. For instance, the main disease could be arthritis but the patient suffers from malaria or diarrhoea which needs immediate attention. Or the disease may surface predominantly as cancer or AIDS.

Āsana constructs and destroys the cells balancing the metabolism. It balances the hormones by correcting the underfunctioning or overfunctioning of the glands. During *prāṇāyāma*, in the inhalation *(pūraka)*, the energy is drawn in for the construction of the cells, while with retention *(kumbhaka)*, the energy is distributed evenly throughout the body, and with exhalation *(rechaka)* the energy is made to reach those parts of the body by releasing tension in the physiological organs, nerves and mind. Inverted *āsana* not only help the venous blood flow towards the heart but activise the internal organs when they impede the flow of blood and energy so that the circulation of blood is nowhere hampered.

Huge stones obstruct the flow of water in a river, so that the water recedes and then flows on circumventing the obstruction. A similar action happens while doing *āsana* or *prāṇāyāma*, as the different areas or various organs are placed in such a way that they remain in a compact situation, which causes the energy to perambulate and circumnavigate each area, each cell and each organ. In each āsana actions like scraping, rubbing, rinsing, squeezing, massaging, spreading, activating, stimulating, pacifying, attenuating, solidifying, liquefying, supporting, fixing, warming and cooling take place. The *āsana* penetrates the depth, width and length of the physiological body. There are curative *āsana*, recuperative *āsana*, strenuous, irritating *āsana*, soothing *āsana*, pacifying *āsana* and so on. Of course, all these *āsana* are required as in medicine, that may be bitter, sweet or tasteless as required.

Yoga is an adjustive science. It does not mean it is a compromising science. It adjusts with the inner body and mind according to need and condition. Health is a moving, dynamic equilibrium requiring adjustments all along the journey of life, through the seasons and the days and the many unanticipated variations in weather, food and social life. Health is like a river, ever flowing, ever fresh, ever pure. Disease is but a form of stagnation. Health is like a live wire, charged with energy which can only be experienced and not seen.

Yoga is the basic health science in a profound and comprehensive sense. Naturopathy and *āyurvedic* treatments can be terminated after some time. But yoga can only end in yoga (union) or *kaivalya.* Yoga goes beyond the *doṣa* and *dhātu* of *āyurveda* and deals with the three *guṇa* – *sattva, rajas* and *tamas.* Yoga is a subjective science that touches the roots of existential human problems.[1] It deals with the *kleśa*[2] and *vṛtti*[3] that affect the body and the mind. Patañjali offers the symptoms[4] that accompany the nine *antaraya* (impediments) that disturb the *citta.*[5] Patañjali holds out the glorious promise that the sorrow yet to come[6] shall be removed.

Yoga is a precise science which deals with the physical, physiological, mental, intellectual and spiritual dimensions of man. According to *yoga śāstra,* man is made up of five *koṣa* (sheaths), namely *annamaya, prāṇamaya, manomaya, vijñānamaya* and *ānandamaya.* Beyond the *koṣa* is the eternal witness – *puruṣa.* The *āsana* and *prāṇāyāma* start with the grosser and move on to the subtler *koṣa.* As our practice continues with faith and vigour, depth and reverence, we penetrate the *koṣa* further and further in each *āsana* and in each *prāṇāyāma,* in each session and every time, finally purifying and transcending them. For the learned intellectuals, the discourses appeal to them. But for the majority of the people, they are of little use. The mind is ordinarily the prisoner of the senses and the intelligence is the prisoner of the mind. But before taming the mind and the intelligence, one has to tame the senses. For this yoga has to be done as a *vrata* (vow) or *tapas* (penance). The unabated *tamas* of the body and the *rajas* of the mind cannot allow the intelligence to become *sāttvic.* There cannot be *citta vṛtti nirodha* – cessation of the movements within consciousness – without *snāyu vṛtti nirodha* – cessation of the movements within the cells and nerves.

However, the foregoing should not be interpreted as an endorsement of the mind-body-self trichotomy. Certainly, mind and body vanish when the soul withdraws from them. In each and every *āsana* and *prāṇāyāma,* at each and every moment, mind, intelligence and consciousness

---

1 *Pariṇāma tāpa saṁskāra duḥkaiḥ guṇavṛtti virodhāt ca duḥkham eva sarvaṁ vivekinaḥ,* the wise man knows that owing to fluctuations, the qualities of nature and subliminal impressions, even pleasant experiences are tinged with sorrow, and he keeps aloof from them. (*Y.S.,* II.15).

2 *Avidyā asmitā rāga dveṣa abhiniveśaḥ kleśaḥ,* the five afflictons which disturb the equilibrium of consciousness are: ignorance or lack of wisdom, ego, pride of the ego or the sense of 'I', attachment to pleasure, aversion to pain, fear of death and clinging to life. (*Y.S.,* II.3).

3 *Vṛttayaḥ pañcatayyaḥ kliṣṭā akliṣṭāḥ,* the movements of consciousness are fivefold. They may be cognizable or non-cognizable, painful or non-painful. (*Y.S.,* I.5).

4 *Duḥkha daurmanasya aṅgamejayatva śvāsapraśvāsāḥ vikṣepa sahabhuvaḥ,* sorrow, despair, unsteadiness of the body and irregular breathing further distract the *citta.* (*Y.S.,* I.31).

5 *Vyādhi styāna saṁśaya pramāda ālasya avirati bhrāntidarśana alabdhabhūmikatva anavasthitatvāni cittavikṣepaḥ te antarāyāḥ,* these obstacles are disease, inertia, doubt, heedlessness, laziness, indiscipline of the senses, erroneous views, lack of perseverance and backsliding. (*Y.S.,* I.30).

6 *Heyaṁ duḥkham anāgatam,* the pains which are yet to come can be and are to be avoided. (*Y.S.,* III.16).

are, or should be, involved. In the present state of objective science, we know very little about the interface between body, mind and self. *Āsana* and *prāṇāyāma* bridge the gap between physiological and psychological bodies, and make the practitioner cross over towards the Self. Then the psychological and spiritual dimensions of *āsana* and *prāṇāyāma* will be justly appreciated. Till then, sadly, *āsana* and *prāṇāyāma* will be considered as physical practices by armchair-yogis shirking from *tapas*.

Āsana and *prāṇāyāma* are the form of *tapas* to reach the highest. Disjointed from *yama* and *niyama*, deflected from *samādhi* and *kaivalya*, offering instant benefits, they become yogic pills, which like other pills offer temporary relief and false hopes. The yogic path is arduous and the yogic journey is long.[1] Done with faith, zeal and discrimination,[2] both the journey and the destination will be richly rewarding. Let us not limit yoga to just one more therapy. It deals with *bhava roga* (existential disease), the conjunction between *jīva* and *ātma* or *prakṛti* and *puruṣa*.[3] Mundane physiological and mental cures are but the by-products of the *sādhanā*. Health is a form of *siddhi*.[4] When yoga is practised this way, then and then only, in this disease-ridden and chaotic world, can man have health, joy and serenity.

---

1 *Sa tu dīrghakāla nairantarya satkāra āsevitaḥ dṛḍhabhūmiḥ*, long, uninterrupted, alert practice is the firm foundation for restraining the fluctuations. (*Y.S.*, I.14).

2 *Śraddhā vīrya smṛti samādhiprajñā pūrvakaḥ itareṣām*, practice must be pursued with trust, confidence, vigour, keen memory and power of absorption to break this spiritual complacency. (*Y.S.*, I.20).

3 *Draṣṭṛdṛśyayoḥ saṁyogaḥ heyahetuḥ*, the cause of pain is the association or identification of the seer *(ātmā)* with the seen *(prakṛti)* and the remedy lies in their dissociation. (*Y.S.*, II.17).

4 *Rūpa lāvaṇya bala vajra saṁhananatvāni kāyasaṁpat*, perfection of the body consists of beauty of form, grace, strength, compactness, and the hardness and brilliance of a diamond. (*Y.S.*, III.47).

SECTION IV

YOGA AND DIFFERENT DIMENSIONS

YOGA AND OLD AGE*

Our philosophers have proclaimed, from time immemorial, that *prakṛti* (nature) is transient and changes from moment to moment whereas the *ātman* or the soul is eternal and unchangeable. The individual soul, which is a part of the Universal Soul, dwells within the body from birth to death. However, while the body undergoes constant change, the individual soul remains unaffected.

Our body is made up of the five elements of nature, namely, earth, water, fire, air and ether with their infra-atomic structural counterparts which are smell, taste, form, touch and sound. *Mahat*, cosmic intelligence, is the first principle of nature. It transforms into consciousness in each individual. Thus, as the body is made up of five elements of nature, it constantly transforms and is therefore transient.

Ageing is a natural phenomenon. It is growth from childhood to adolescence, to middle age and to old age. It is a change from one phase of life to another phase although the owner remains the same.

The fragrance of life in each of us begins to dry out as we age, similar to a sapling which grows into a healthy gigantic tree bearing tasty fruits each year and then withers away.

I am also ageing but my yogic practice, for hours together, is very regular like the rising and the setting of the sun. I began yoga when I was sixteen to free myself from my sickly existence. I gained good health after four years of regular practice and this encouraged me to share my knowledge of yoga with people who are suffering – as I did. I have relentlessly worked to make yoga attractive and appealing and have carried the message of "yoga for health in body and peace in mind" throughout the world and am glad that now yoga is considered as a form of alternative medicine.

---

* Talk given for Senior Citizens and published in *Yoga Rahasya*, vol. 3, no. 1.

I have gained sixty years of bonus life because of my regular practice, therefore I am not afraid of death. I am ready to embrace death with ease because through yoga I made life worthy for myself and for others. I still continue with my early practices so that I can have a natural, majestic and noble death. I have given my own example to encourage people of my age group to take to yoga.

I feel that old age is a blessing which brings with it a great deal of respect from youth, provided one pays attention to keep oneself healthy and is not dependent upon others like a parasite. At this age, one should reflect on one's thoughts and one's actions. One should guide one's family and friends so that they do not commit the same mistakes as oneself, which acted as a stumbling block in one's progress through life.

God has given us this body to evolve in the spiritual world and it is meant to serve one's self as well as one's surroundings.

The body ages but the soul does not. When one is aged the mind fuels a negative attitude towards life. By the power of will over mind, old age can be lived benevolently through yogic practices.

Yoga is an art, a science and has a philosophy too. It begins with the body, cultures the mind and leads the practitioner to experience the fragrance of the unbiased or unalloyed bliss within and without.

Yoga keeps the two main gates of health, the respiratory and the circulatory systems, fit and maintains health in each and every cell of the body.

Health is not a product that can be bought in a medical store. It has to be earned. Health is dynamic like live charcoal and its purifying force should constantly burn the toxins that are created in the body. This purifying force can be generated by will power, determination, attention, application and devotion in order to supply the much-needed energy to the trillions of cells which sustain health.

The physiological organs like the lungs, liver, spleen, pancreas, intestines, have to be exercised in a similar manner by flexion, extension and circumduction of the anatomical body. *Yogāsana* and *prāṇāyāma* work on both the physiological and anatomical bodies. They help one voluntarily to alter the blood supply to the organs. They keep the cells and the nerves of the body as well as the respiratory, circulatory, digestive, endocrine, reproductive and excretory systems in a healthy state and make them function in harmony.

When the body is healthy, the mind – which is otherwise preoccupied with the body – gets freed from the body. The mind can then move closer towards the soul in order to enable one to surrender oneself to God.

Old age is the right time to devote our thoughts to God. Yet because of ill-health, which generally accompanies old age, we the aged have to continue to work out for poise in body and peace in mind. Practice of yoga gives us these things and prepares us to surrender our breath force to God and to merge with the Universal Soul. It is the right of all in our old age to embrace God towards which end nature guides us. So, practise yoga, keep the body and mind free and ready for surrender to the Lord of Time in order to embrace the Timeless – that is the freedom which is termed as Death.

In old age the philosophy of the body is more important than the philosophy of the soul. Lust, greed, anger, are at a lower ebb. The philosophy of the soul is a must to all. But in order to be independent in life in old age, the philosophy of body is essential.

The capital we are born with, the human body, remains unutilised by most of us! Often, it is used for enjoyment and not emancipation. Yoga teaches us how to use it for the right purpose. In old age the mind may gravitate towards emancipation but the body does not allow. Body becomes an enemy. In order to make the body gravitate towards emancipation, one has to practise yoga.

YOGA AND I

Growing old is a natural phenomenon. For me old age has come gracefully and I enjoy this period which helps me to accept the inevitable and live with it in beauty and freedom.

I am still active, practising yoga daily with religiousness and determination and guiding those who come to me for physical health and strength, mental poise and spiritual serenity. Yoga is life and life is yoga for me.

While young, I was afflicted with tuberculosis and in those days there were no remedies. I was told by the medical profession that I might live to the age of sixteen or seventeen years.

Though I was not fit for yoga at that time, I thank yoga for it has embraced me. I practised reluctantly as my body was not pliable but stiff as a poker as my time then had for years been spent lying on a bed. Finally, like a leech sucking blood, I had to cling to yoga in order to taste the nectar of health. I cultivated yoga and yoga cultivated me.

At last the joy of activity set in me after four years of practice and I have been graced with a bonus life since 1938. Then I made up my mind to use this God-given bonus life to help my brothers and sisters of this world to live in good health through yoga. This is what I did, am doing and I like to do, as long as He keeps me on this planet, as a service to my Lord. I wish to leave this planet, when the call comes from Him, not only nobly but majestically.

It is He who gave me birth. It is He who led me on the yogic path. It is His will when He wants me to return to Him.

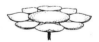

YOGA AND DANCE*

I am neither an artist nor simply a yogi, but a lover of art. I have loved to live in the art of yoga with constant practice for the past fifty years and would like to continue for years to come.

Sages of India discovered that man is made up of physical, mental and spiritual bodies. In order to develop and purify the three layers of body, mind and self systematically, rhythmically and uniformly and make life beautiful they introduced yoga in the form of the art of living – *jīvana-kalā*.

This art of living – *jīvana-kalā* – was brought under the umbrella of *dharma* – science of duty – in order to maintain religiousness and purity in the art of living and the life of human beings. Religion was meant to bring homogeneity and cohesion in man and his society.

Several arts in the name of religion were introduced as cultural, spiritual and sacred in order to lead us from evolution to liberation. They are meant to uplift and elevate man from lower tendencies to higher goals so that his life becomes useful, fruitful and complete. This is how the *jīvana-kalā* was meant to transform us towards *jīvana-muktan*.

The six principal arts recognised by sages are:

1) *yogikā* – yoga,
2) *māllikā* – wrestling, weight lifting, boxing, etc.
3) *dhānuṣya* – archery, military training,
4) *nāṭya* – dance, drama, acting,
5) *sāngitikā* – music (vocal, instrumental, orchestra), poetry,
6) *vyāvahārika* – social behavioural patterns, politics, economics and agriculture.

Each one reveals truth, perfection and beauty, and hence the gamut of art is termed as

---

* December 1982.

satyam-śivam-sundaram (truth, purity, beauty).

Art is not only nature's beauty but goes beyond nature. Its purpose is meant to be educative, aesthetic, moral, impressive, instructive, intellectual, protective, clear and divine in one who is involved in it, and through him in society. Art is an expression of harmony and beauty in one's way of living. It is a craft wrought between nature, people and environment. It is not a fantasy but it is a wonder of life. Art is a discovery of the relationship between life and its context. It is a path chosen by one according to one's choice – *svadharma* – and mental attitude – *manodharma* – as well as according to inclination – *ābhilāṣā* – and improvisation – *kalpanā*. It has to be striven for with a constant love of labour in order to refine one's own thoughts and actions and then to taste the fragrance and delicacy of presentation.

We have numerous arts such as basic, useful, creative, liberal, manual, healing, sculpture, painting, photography, architecture, music and dance.

No doubt art appears individualistic in application, taste, flavour and delicacy, yet in depth it is impersonal. It is unity in diversity. As truth, perfection and beauty are universal and vibrant, so is art. Each time it is practised and repeated, a new awareness sets in and a new field of discovery crops up.

Patañjali indicates the main key for learning art in one *sūtra* as *pratyakṣānumānāgamāḥ pramāṇāni,*[1] direct perception, cognition, inference, proposition, scriptural authority and power of understanding in the chosen art are the channels for art. Though the *sūtra* explains one of the five mental modifications – *pramāṇa,* the *pramāṇa* is meant to bring clarity in intelligence by acquiring knowledge. Art has to be learnt with this *pramāṇa vṛtti* so that this modification leads to mastery over the art. When an artist follows the chosen art single-mindedly, then he is trying to reach its zenith – which is the aim of all arts. Opening all the gates of finite art and touching the point beyond the finite is the end of art.

Without discipline one cannot develop art. This disciplined development leads one to freedom. According to Patañjali the disciplines of yoga are *yama, niyama, āsana, prāṇāyāma, pratyāhāra, dhāraṇā, dhyāna* and *samādhi*. They deal with the moral, physical, physiological, psychological, mental and spiritual disciplines. Actually the end of discipline is *samādhi* or freedom from the contact of pain at all levels. Without these disciplines, an artist may not grow in stature. He may get physically exhausted in the stress and strain of creativity inviting bodily diseases, lack of interest, indecision, illusion and lack of perseverance which retard his faculties to think

1 *Y.S.,* I.17.

and act clearly. Disciplined practice of yoga develops a sound body with a sound mind, so that the artist and the yogi can keep head and heart open without fanaticism in order to get the best from the art.

Art is of two types. One is *bhoga-kalā* and the other is *yoga-kalā*. *Bhoga-kalā* belongs to the senses. It is pleasure seeking and may end up in mere entertainment. *Yoga-kalā* demands intensity in *sādhanā* and its field is spirituality – *adhyātma*. A balanced blend of both is essential, otherwise one ends up with sensual satisfaction and the other with the isolation of himself.

Foundation in yoga and dance or in any art comes only by a long uninterrupted devoted practice. From this one may well understand how many years one can take to master an art.

From a cursory observation of yoga and dance, they appear as divergent arts. When they are studied carefully, one realises that they meet at several points as if they are akin to each other. Yoga is the sublimation of all emotions with a disciplined practice, whereas dance is the artful display of emotions.

Kalidasa says in his drama *Vikramorvśīyam* that dance, opera, ballet and drama are sources of entertainment for all men and women of diverse tastes at one and the same time. Sage Patañjali says that the art of yoga gives good shape of the body and brings beauty, valour and lustre. A careful study and keen insight of these two systems of art will not take long to draw inferences of similarity when they are performed and presented side by side. Differences are seen in dress, costumes and gesture, but the rest of the presentation and expression mostly remain the same.

Yoga being the root of all art,[1] it is complementary and supplementary to dance. Practice of yoga develops a keen mind, alert eye, proportionate division of limbs, good features and good voice. It brings agility, swiftness and elegance in movement, repose and reflection *(laya)*.

Often it is observed that the active life of a dancer remains short due to exhaustion and ageing. The practice of yoga will build up stamina with proper circulation and supply of nourishment through the blood stream and help dancers maintain their quality of presentation for many more years.

Is it a coincidence that the Lord of yoga is Lord Shiva – bestower of happiness – and the Lord of dance is the same Lord Shiva in the form of Naṭarāja – the king of dancers? Similarly, is it again a coincidence that Patañjali, the master of yoga, is also the master of dance[2] and is

---

[1] See the author's *The Art of Yoga,* Harper Collins, London, pp. 3-20.
[2] See *Aṣṭadaḷa Yogamālā,* vol. 1, pp. 200-201.

considered as *guru* for both arts? Hence, as students of yoga and dance, we pay homage to Lord Naṭarāja and Patañjali, as both of them gave these arts, yoga and dance, for cultural growth and at the same time to savour the nectar of spiritual life.

It can be easily noticed from the preceding points that yoga and dance sprang up from the loins of the common Deity with the sole object of making man and woman realise within themselves supreme peace and God realisation.

Both need *rūpa, lāvaṇya* and *bala* to climb to the ultimate in art.

Yoga is a subjective expression of an experienced feeling. Dance is expression through the artful display of the emotions, gestures and comportment of an experienced yogi.

Yoga is action. Outwardly it is static but dynamic within, whereas, dance is motion and dynamic throughout.

Yoga is beauty in action and dance is beauty in motion.

Yoga has three types of movements – *tīvra* (intense), *madhyama* (medium) and *mṛdu* (soft). So too in dance there are *tāṇḍava* (vigourous), *lāsya* (soft and slow) with *abhinaya,*[1] *bhāva*[2] and *rasa.*[3]

As yoga has innumerable *āsana*, so are there *karaṇa* in dance, which are nothing but yogic *āsana*.

Yoga looks to the formless devoid of attributes or qualities *(nirguṇabrahma)*. Dance looks at it with form and attributes *(saguṇabrahma)*.

Yoga is a path of involution and renunciation – *nivṛtti mārga*, whereas dance is the path of evolution and acceptance of all creation – *pravṛtti mārga*. However, the paths of *karma, bhakti* and *jñāna* are blended beautifully in both the arts.

For a yogi it is important to treat his body as the temple of the soul and each movement is the *mantra* or the *japa*. Each adjustment is the *artha* or the meaning of the movement and each experience is *bhāvanā* or feeling. So also in the dance which is known as *Bharatanāṭyam, bha* stands for *bhāva* or expression, or mood, *ra* stands for *rāga* or melody and *ta* for *tāla* or rhythm.

---

1 Gesture, action or emotional expression.

2 Disposition and feeling.

3 The feeling or sentiment prevailing in a taste or a character. Concerning the *navarasa*, see *Aṣṭadaḷa Yogamālā*, vol. 2, pp. 264-265.

The yogi comes himself to the altar, all alone, in body and mind, simple and innocent, delighting in purity and tranquillity of the soul. In dance, one has to depend upon outside help and with dexterous mind express purity and tranquillity.

A yogi uses both sides of the body evenly whereas dancers mostly use one side. So the charm, grace and versatility are missing on the other side. Yoga is a *sarvāṅga-sādhanā* and dance is a *aṅgabhāga-sādhanā*.

Yoga develops a fine body, brings a smiling face, a sweet voice, clear eyes, clean mind, firm legs and abounding health. Dancers need all these to uṣe the mouth for music, hands to convey meaning, eyes to express feelings and feet for firmness and rhythm. So yoga is a great help for dance.

Yoga is the merging of *prakṛti* with *puruṣa* and in dance it is the expression of *Nāyaka nāyaki*, i.e., merging *puruṣa* with *prakṛti*.

Yoga is a subjective presentation displaying position, gesture and expression in the *āsana, prāṇāyāma* and *dhyāna*. It is an internal experience and feeling of integrating the body, the senses, the mind and the intelligence with the self. Dance is an external expression of thoughts, passions and actions. The six characteristics of desire, anger, ambition, love, pride and jealousy are considered as the enemies for the growth of spiritual knowledge in yoga, and the yogi controls and sublimates them by friendliness *(maitri)*, compassion *(karuṇā)*, delight *(muditā)* and indifference *(upekṣā)*. The above mentioned six characteristics are considered in dance as companions for expressing the varied sentiments of man's feelings. These six basic emotions are converted as *navarasa* into erotic *(śringāra)*, comic *(hāsya)*, pathetic *(karuṇā)*, heroic *(vīra)*, furious *(raudra)*, fearful *(bhayānaka)*, marvellous *(adbhuta)*, revolting *(bibhatsa)* and peaceful or meditative *(śānta)*. Yoga is a dynamic internal experience of oneself and dance imitates the inner experience of the yogi externally for one to see.

Thus, both yoga and dance glow from the immortal forms of the soul expressing themselves through the mortal frame – the body –, the temple of the soul and the abode of God consciousness.

YOGA AND DIET*

It is said that, "As you sow, so shall you reap"; the yogis say, "As you eat, so you think". Hence diet and yoga should go hand in hand.

For any student of yoga or any other spiritual aspirant, it is common knowledge that pure diet is absolutely necessary for the development of the body and the mind and the enlightenment of the self. All results of actions are dependent on the causes themselves. If the cause is righteous, the result ensuing therefrom is bound to be righteous. Therefore, the character of a man is determined by the food he eats and the way he eats. Every morsel of food is for the service of the Divine; thus no impure element can ever be accepted in this holy sacrament. The importance of pure *sāttvic* food is emphasised in all yogic texts for the yoga practitioner. Neither the physical health of the body nor mental quietude can ever be achieved by exciting, harmful food or flesh. Yoga teaches that the primary principle is to take food not for the sake of the pleasure of the senses but for the nourishment of the soul within. The food must be natural to the constitution of man. Animal foods disturb the harmony of the total well-being of the individual. Any disturbance caused by wrong food reacts on the thinking power and thus creates confusion and delusion. This brings about restlessness of the body and mind which hinders spiritual progress.

Yoga aims at disciplining the body and mind. Health of the body and mind depends on the observance of the laws of right living. According to the creation of our teeth and intestines by nature, the human being is herbivorous and frugivorous. Thus, any other food is against the law of nature. Similarly, man being an intellectual creation, his system does not require flesh and meat. Physical health is dependent on the food we take. If we are not conscious and careful about the nourishment of the body, we impoverish the whole system.

The body is the temple of God in which the holiest of the Holy dwells. How can any impurity be admitted into this pure Temple? This body is the vehicle of the Divine to manifest himself in his true glory. If the blood stream is polluted by the blood of animals, no light can ever

---

* World Vegetarian Congress, 1957.

shine in the function of the intellectual heart and thus this Divine Temple is darkened. Even if due to ignorance the body is weakened and disturbed by wrong food, yoga points the way of establishing equilibrium and restoring normalcy. By the persistent practice of yoga the instincts are refined and gradually man moves towards higher knowledge. In his ignorance, if he considers animal food is essential for the strength of the body, he begins to realise through yogic practice that he was under a delusion and illusion and therefore now he cannot entertain the idea of consuming flesh or non-vegetarian food.

Yoga is a perfect practical science on its own. It is one of the basic philosophies of India which can rightly be termed as a real necessity in man's daily walk of life. Health is a universal science and therefore yoga is a universal culture. Through its practice man realises the importance of dietetics for the well-being and progress of each and every individual.

The ultimate aim of yoga is to achieve union with God – enjoying the unalloyed peace from within. To achieve this aim, several paths have been advocated. They are, namely, *rāja mārga, haṭha mārga, bhakti mārga, jñāna mārga, karma mārga* and so on. All these paths ultimately lead to the one goal – Self-realisation. Just as there are different paths to reach the peak of a mountain, one easy, the other tedious, one long and the other short, but all leading to the peak, so also in yoga these paths, though they seem to be different, lead to the same and only goal – Self-realisation. The seemingly different paths are just to suit one's mental tastes and environment. One of the basic principles for all these paths is that the vegetarian diet keeps the mind clean and pure.

Practice of yoga prevents our body from decay and cures many of our disabilities. It is also the best and unrivalled system for the prevention of diseases. Yoga is as old as civilisation and yet it fits well for our own modern times in helping to maintain and sustain sound health which is absolutely necessary for pleasure or for emancipation. It is now a proven fact that food plays a major part in the prevention of diseases and curing of ailments.

Nowadays some who are sincere in the practice of spiritual discipline or *ātmavidyā*, are unfortunately afraid to give a thought to the perfection of their own bodies, lest they should become body conscious. The body is the temple of the soul, an instrument to take us nearer to the goal of realisation. It seems a pity that such persons who are endeavouring to advance spiritually, fear that they may fall back in their advancement. Here, the fear itself is a hindrance and retards their aim in life. It is not that one who is in search of Truth has to neglect the body. So let me assure the sincere aspirants that body perfection through pure nourishment and the principles of "right living" is very essential. The *ṛṣis* and sages of the past explained more about *ātmavidyā* than about *śārīravidyā*. That does not mean that they neglected the body. They were training their students in *āsana* and *prāṇāyāma* and also in social virtues from their childhood so that they could enjoy sound health.

It is easy to forget the body when it is in perfect condition. When there is illness, pain or discomfort, it is then that we become body conscious and spiritual progress is hindered. All the yogic accessories point to the highest moral and spiritual purpose and goal. Though sage Patañjali nowhere explains directly about food, I feel that it is covered in his epitomes of *yama* and *niyama*. Non-violence, non-killing, non-stealing, truthfulness, continence and non-covetousness, cleanliness, prayers, contentment, persevering practice, kindness to all and complete surrender to the Will of God are the essence of the individual virtuous qualities. These build the moral character of the student of yoga which remains as proof from the dawn of civilisation that vegetarian diet is considered the best for human development.

Everyone wants peace. The body is like a nation. An aggressor takes advantage of a nation to annex it, seeing its weakness. In the same way, diseases attack our system and create unhappiness and misery in place of happiness, peace and love.

To climb the "Everest of bliss", yoga and vegetarianism go together like the two wings of a bird which flies higher and higher to prove its strength and bliss.

VIEWS ON DIET*

I have never written or spoken about diet for the practitioners of yoga although the whole world writes or states that a practitioner of yoga should live on nourishing food. It is easy to speak on food when everything is easily available. I came from a poor family and to get a square meal a day was itself a great luxury. I have lived on tap water in my early days. So, I know the value of food.

Today, God has given me plenty but I cannot abuse it. My diet depends upon my practice for the day. My food would have changed yesterday if my practice were to be severe today. For me, the practice is more important than the diet. The discipline of yoga disciplines my food habits. It is not the discipline of my food habits that disciplines my yogic practice. Many of you may have realised that you cannot perform the *āsana* as well as you intended to if you eat a little more of a particular type of food. So each time, one has to think and discriminate to determine 'what is good food'. There is no single theory about which food is good for the practice of yoga.

Food should be congenial to your practice and the brain. If you eat a lot of chillies then you may feel discomfort in your abdomen or a burning sensation in the chest that aggravates when you perform backbends such as *Ūrdhva Dhanurāsana, Kapotāsana, Vṛśchikāsana.*[1] You may even have to sacrifice your practice on that particular day. If you eat heavy and sweet food that takes time to digest, then you snore and sleep during your practice, and the practice may end with ignorance.

Instead of pondering over food, eat only when you are hungry. It is the mind which needs tasty food. The body is more honest than the mind. The body refuses food when it does not want it. That is why you vomit or get diarrhoea and expel unwanted and unassimilated food. Avoid that food which you know does not suit your body. Do not eat food that is unwanted and unpalatable. The mind likes to have tasty food. At least, the mind is honest at that time. The same mind prevents you from touching certain kinds of food that will not be congenial to the system.

---

* From *Yogatarañga*, Thane, February 1996.

[1] See *Light on Yoga*, Harper Collins, London.

For example, milk is considered to be very good for health. It gives you energy and *ojas* but the same milk is bad when you have phlegm or when you have diarrhoea. Moreover when you see somebody who is hungry and does not have anything to eat, then to drink that *sāttvic* milk is also non-*sāttvic*, since you are enjoying it when someone else is dying of hunger.

When you feel thirsty and ask for water, can this thirst for water be quenched by anything else? Even alcohol cannot quench thirst. Your friends may offer you orange juice but you would prefer only water. Water alone is the right food at that moment as it quenches thirst whereas orange juice kills your thirst and alcohol kills your hunger. Do not load yourself with food and disturb your digestion and metabolism and tire your body. You have overeaten if you are unable to digest your food within six hours.

The question that often arises is about vegetarianism and non-vegetarianism. The *Upaniṣads* state *annamayaṁhi saumyamanaḥ*. It means, the mind is formed by the food. The mind has the ability to think, and therefore you have to find out for yourself what is right food. Consume only that food which keeps your mind alert and awake to think rightfully and at the same time brings poise and peace within.

We need discipline and courage to tread the yogic path and therefore the food which we take should strengthen our mind towards our goal. Varying the food means varying the process of the mind. Different foods create different attitudes. Although no diet was recommended for physical health, the yogis say that the moment you go to the spiritual level then the dietary system follows – "as you eat so shall you reap". You have to be very careful that your thinking processes are not diverted due to various qualities of food. So the practitioners of yoga are advised that in order to avoid any deviation in one's thinking process one must not change food from day to day. One needs tremendous discipline and strength to follow one type of food for several days with no variety. The practitioners of yoga were not allowed to eat food for the sake of taste but for the sake of sustenance and for the practice of yoga. Rich food is not the key to health but the way the food is assimilated into the system is the golden key that unlocks the gates of health, of the body, of the intelligence and of the self.

I do not think that you can do yoga if you only eat rich nourishing food. A real practitioner of yoga needs very little food. For him, yoga itself is food. Yoga itself is nourishing. Yoga itself is life and energy.

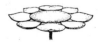

FOOD

Life and the movement of mind are dependent upon the food one consumes. As the food is, so is the mind.

Food is to be treated as medicine as well as the sustainer of the body and life. Food certainly is to be taken to act as a medicine so that it nourishes the vital organs of the body to function properly, healthily and harmoniously. Food should not be eaten to put undue stress on the vital organs. If we are fond of tasty food, we have to remember that we are inviting many diseases to rest in the abode of our bodies. Eating and drinking unethically without having control is not only an unhealthy diet but also an immoral way of consuming and it becomes nothing but poison to the body, mind and self. A clean body is an aid for a pure mind. So, right wholesome food should be chosen which gives all nutrient values to the system. This is clean food.

As it is not possible to express the feeling of experiences such as joy and sorrow, pleasure and pain, contentment and discontentment, fulfilment and non-fulfilment, similarly it is impossible to deal with food as each one's system has its own cycle of functioning in digestion and assimilation. Though general lines on what is wholesome could be given, yet each has to find out his diet according to his physical ability to digest and assimilate.

Food has various tastes. It may be sweet, sour, saline, bitter, pungent or astringent. Avoid the food which is sharp, sour, pungent, hot and oily. It has to be free from flesh. Eat that which is pleasing, nutritive, easily digestible and assimilated by the system. Do not overeat or eat fast. Be moderate. Moderation in food according to yoga texts is to fill half the stomach with solid food, one quarter with water and leave the next quarter empty for the digestive energy to move freely so that it mixes and blends well for digestion.

Normally food is of four types. It can be (a) masticated or chewed, (b) sucked, (c) licked and (d) drunk. These four types of food can be classified into three classes, namely, *sāttvic, rājasic* and *tāmasic* foods.

Sāttvic food is that which increases the span of life, brings purity and cheerfulness in thought, and is agreeable to the body, mind and soul. The food that is bitter, sour, saline, spicy, pungent, dry, burning hot, brings unpleasantness and grief. This is *rājasic* food while the one that is stale, tasteless, stinking or cooked several times is *tāmasic*.

Choose the food that supplies the needs of the body, namely, oxygen, hydrogen, nitrogen, carbon, chlorine, fluorine, phosphorus, iron, calcium, potassium, magnesium, sodium, manganese, sulphur and other trace elements.

Balanced food is that which contains building materials in the form of minerals, fuel and energy; i.e. protein, carbohydrates and fat. Natural food such as vegetables, fruits, pounded rice, wheat and water is the right diet.

Movement of body depends upon life force. Life force depends upon the intake of wholesome food. It is said in the *Upaniṣads* that mind is made up by solid food, vital energy by liquid food and the intelligence in speech by fat. This solid, liquid and fat food is divided into sixteen parts. Out of the sixteen parts, ten parts become the grossest, five parts the middling and one part the subtlest. Through solid food, the grossest becomes the faeces, the middling the flesh, and the subtlest the mind. Out of the liquid part, the grossest becomes urine, middling,the blood and the subtlest – the life force or energy. Out of fat, the grossest becomes the bone, the middling the marrow and the subtlest the speech.

Table 1.- Need of food for body, mind, *prāṇa* and *vāk*

Form of food	After digestion, division into sixteen parts		
	Grossest 10/16	Middling 5/16	Subtlest 1/16
Solid	Faeces	Flesh	Mind
Liquid	Urine	Blood	Life-force
Fat	Bone	Bone-marrow	Speech *(vāk)*

Thus, food becomes the Lord of speech, Lord of energy and cause for the tranquillity of the mind. So, it must be taken as an oblation to the various energies such as *prāṇa*, *apāna*, *vyāna*, *udāna* and *samāna* and lastly to Brahma – the highest cosmic energy.

The *Upaniṣads* further say that word is knowledge. Speech is the expression of knowledge. In order to express, mind is needed. So mind is greater than speech. Will is greater than mind. Greater than will is intelligence, greater than intelligence is contemplation. Greater than contemplation is understanding. Greater than understanding is strength and faith. In order to obtain strength and faith physically, morally, mentally, intellectually and spiritually, food is essential. Hence, food is Brahma. In order to realise the Self, food is the key for building up character and contentment. Hence, careful thought is essential in choosing food for the evolution of oneself.

SECTION V

ON TEACHING

ADDRESS TO THE CERTIFIED TEACHERS*

How should I address you? Fellow travellers, fellow sufferers? My children? Or would-be yoga teachers?

Yoga is a spiritual subject. You are all re-born through the practice of yoga, apart from your biological birth. As children belong to their parents biologically, you all belong to me spiritually as my children on the yogic path. Through my guidance in yoga, you are all my "spiritual children". You are all re-born with a new approach towards life emotionally, intellectually and spiritually. I consider you as spiritual children as I have imparted to you the yogic touch of spiritual well-being. I called you fellow travellers. I being a parent and you being children, we all have to enjoy or suffer together while travelling on this path.

Responsibility has to be taken by children to live in and bear with the surrounding situation and at the same time respect aged parents. Similarly, you as my spiritual children have to know your responsibilities, face all your shortcomings and respect the teachers who are senior to you.

All of you started yoga in 1968. At that time only eleven individuals came to me for undergoing training in yogic discipline. As a father with a small group then, I never dreamt that this subject would spread so fast and so many would travel on this path in your country within a few years of time. Your responsibility is more for my grandchildren. We all know that grandparents love grandchildren more than their children and probably the same thing may apply to me, so I may love my grandchildren more than you, provided you all work with zeal to make them true human beings. Build them up to serve not only themselves, but their brothers and sisters in their own countries. Let the heritage of yoga reach from generation to generation.

Yoga is a very intricate and fascinating subject. It develops tremendous will power and tenacity. This is the good side of the subject. The bad side of the subject is that in seeking the Truth within, we unfortunately develop a sort of pride thinking that we are better than others. This

* Swaziland, October 1976. Also published in the magazine of "The Manchester and District Institute of Iyengar Yoga", Spring 1986.

is a kind of spiritual pride. If we do not become victims of this behaviour which grows from the other end of our being, we will become the true children of yoga. It is difficult to understand pride. It is more difficult even to know at what time it achieves the potency to pull our aspirations down.

I am issuing certificates. It is the first time that I have given them out, so the honour is yours. I have still not started issuing certificates at the Mother Institute.[1]

QUALITIES OF A TEACHER

First of all you have to be strong in mind in the beginning, though you may not be knowing the subject well. You should have a positive approach within your limitations. The moment you show doubt in your teaching, it means you have sown the seed of doubt in your pupils. Do not show doubt in your teachings, nor sow the seed of doubt in them. Pupils can read your face. They will never trust you if you are doubtful in your expressions and actions.

However, do not be always sure about your teaching. If you are, it is pride. In order to confirm your knowledge, you should have a sceptical approach. "Am I going on the right path?" This gives you a chance to check with yourself and affirm. But while teaching you should not have even a tinge of doubt.

Teaching yoga is a very difficult subject, but it is one of the best services you can do for human beings. Work, not as a teacher, but as a learner in the art of teaching. Learn from looking at the pupils' body and mind as they are not the same in all individuals. As it varies, it is your duty as a teacher to bring oneness and the sense of unified feelings in their bodies and minds. As long as you cannot give this, consider that you are still a learner.

As a teacher you are gifted by Providence to learn so that you impart knowledge as your experience grows. Do not say, "I am a teacher, so there is nothing for me to learn". This is where pride enters. You have to teach affirmatively but search within and find out whether you have created doubts and confusion in your approach and study, how many loose ends were there in your expressions and feelings. Re-study your words and actions, the wrongs or rights you committed while teaching. Re-examine within and build confidence in your pupils. Rethink whatever you did, and work again on your own to find out where you went wrong in explanations or adjustments.

Before teaching, make sure that what you know is correct. Do not hide or expose your ignorance. Instead of that learn, understand and gain knowledge, confirm yourself and enhance your knowledge. Give what you know with open mindedness. Do not hide your knowledge. To

---

1 Ramāmaṇi Iyengar Memorial Yoga Institute, Pune.

hide knowledge is also hidden pride. Give both gross and subtle hints to the pupils in the art of teaching so that they gain faith and confidence.

If you commit mistakes, what would you do? Approach the students once again. Do not protect yourself or your body, but go out quicker to protect your pupils from injury. As teachers, you shun protecting yourselves, but attend to the pupils first and then think of saving yourself.

Also know that it is very rare to see a teacher strong outside but humble inside. You are my pupils and I am your teacher. For you, it seems as though there is a difference between you and me. But I see no difference between us. I consider this as a privilege that you have come to me, so I treat you as Gods inside. Treat each pupil in your heart as God but outside as a pupil. Be strong outside, but feel inside that you are serving the pupils in the form of God. This brings in you the quality of being a true teacher.

Consider this with humility. The Self is one. Your pupils' souls and your soul are the same. They might be pupils from outside but they are your friends inside. You are fellow travellers. As you serve your parents best, serve your pupils with the same attitude. Externally show the differentiation that a pupil is a pupil and you are a teacher, but not inside. This is the first quality for the development of a good teacher.

The teacher should not expect too much from the pupils, but at the same time a teacher should create and ignite interest and zeal in his or her students. You can certainly say, "I expect more from you". You have to find out new avenues for the pupils so that their enthusiasm does not die. Remember, there is no end to knowledge and understanding. Do not say that this is the minimum and that is the maximum, and this is your capacity and limitation. Rather advise them to go ahead.

There has to be duality and non-duality between a *guru* and a pupil. When children are young they are dependent on their parents and seek their guidance. But later on they become independent. The grown-up children are friends of their parents. Similarly, after you have taught well and the pupils have progressed and learnt well and matured leave them to be independent. This way the balance has to be maintained between the quality of attachment and detachment.

The subject of yoga is more important than the relationship between the teacher and student. Whether by a teacher or a pupil, the subject cannot be taken lightly. Therefore, respect the subject. If pupils go wrong, then admonishments are needed. Do not cajole the pupils all the time. Make the students know their responsibility. Be silent when one is good. The moment you praise, you are praising your own self and at the same time you are sowing the seeds of egotism in your pupils. Ego is the great enemy in the path of yoga, perhaps worse than ignorance.

ATTITUDE OF A TEACHER

These certificates are not needed from the truest point of view. Unfortunately, the world demands them. Adulteration is everywhere, in everything, whether it is material, physical or spiritual. The moment we become lax in giving away certificates to one and all, we adulterate. The demand for certification is for authenticity only. People do ask, "Where have you learned? Have you got a certificate to teach?" Therefore you need the certificate.

Often pupils come closer to the teacher. Emotionally, both get tied up. The teacher may not know the intention of the pupils. Your emotions as a teacher and their selfishness may put you in trouble. Do not get influenced. Do not show favouritism. Keep influences aside. See only that direct judgement without emotion guides for qualitative certification. If the teacher has a certificate, the pupils get confidence. Otherwise they have no confidence. The certificate is given not for misuse or to have pride that you are a teacher. Certification is not the end of the knowledge, rather it is the beginning.

Feel in your heart of hearts that the pupils are paying you the fees not as a teacher, but they are paying as a stipend for you to learn the art of imparting so that you become a good teacher. The certificates make you eligible to have stipends to become a good teacher.

Yoga undoubtedly gives tremendous inspiration, will power and confidence to help humanity with health and contentment. On the other side, it inflates the ego. This inflation of pride has to be avoided without compromises. Pay attention to the inner self.

I feel that I have done my best in enlightening you all and I hope you do good service and enlighten those who come to you. I hope that you give them the experience of satisfaction which comes through contentment in the practice of yoga in spite of the upheavals of life.

I do not expect all my pupils to be honest and faithful to me. Some may break off due to pride or inflated by knowledge. Know very well that all students who come to you do not come seeking spiritual knowledge. They come just because their health is shattered and want to get it back. Some may even come to satisfy their desires through better health for purposes of amusement or self-abuse through sensual or sexual indulgence. You have to know the natures of people who come to you. You have to guide and be ready to caution them when they are crossing the border of indulgence.[1] You need to study their psychology, you have to observe their behaviour. Caution and warn only then, when they are near the border of danger, and not in the beginning. As a teacher you have to wait for the right time to speak to the pupils with right words.

[1] In the *Rāmāyaṇa,* we come across a story on crossing the border. Sītā was attracted by the golden deer which she wanted to possess. She begged Rāma to capture and bring it to her. Though she was warned that it was not a real deer but a demon in deer form, she was adamant to have it. So Rāma went hunting for it. (continued)

Suppose, a pupil comes with a cardiac problem or any other problem to learn yoga. He comes and tells you that his doctor has told him not to smoke or drink or eat meat. You may also give the same advice, "Do not smoke. Do not eat meat". Suppose he tells you, "I have not come to seek the same advice that has been given by my doctor; I come to you for learning yoga to see how it works". There is no guarantee that he will follow your advice of not smoking and not eating meat. He may or may not listen to you. One who is addicted does not want to stop immediately.

As a teacher, without giving the clue, you have to work to stop his inner urges. You as a teacher have to see how you bring transformation in the pupils. Everybody can give advice but only a teacher can bring a real change. This is the art of teaching. As yoga acts at all levels, you have to study their physical, intellectual and emotional calibre when they come for help. Some come just for sensual satisfaction in life and they may think that yoga is the key for it. A man who is a sex maniac may come to me to learn yoga. I will not speak of his weakness, but I see whether I can convert him to yoga and keep him away from his urges prolonging the lessons as long as possible. You have to do it like this without saying, "He is no good, and therefore I do not want to teach him".

Even if you do not like a person and yet you must teach him, probably your brain will be cleansed. Sometimes you get pupils who give you the nausea. Remember they are the real *gurus* for you, because they help you to build yourself. God must have sent that person to you. Do not just say, "Sorry, I cannot teach you". It is God's test on you whether you can build up tolerance for improvement by brainwashing that pupil through yoga. If you say, "No", that means you have not shown any improvement at all as a teacher or respect towards the subject. Such crossroads are created in our approaches as yoga teachers. Be watchful and careful at these

---

(continued from 191). Knowing that Rāma was sure to hit him, the golden deer, who was demon Māricha, cried for Lakshmaṇa's help thinking that he might leave Sītā alone, so that king Rāvaṇā, who was enticed with her beauty, could carry Sītā off with ease.

Hearing the voice of Māricha which was like the voice of Rāma, Sītā asked Lakshmaṇa to go for help. But Lakshmaṇa, on the order of his brother Rāma, refused to leave the hermit. But Sītā doubted his character and abused him for not going to help Rāma. As Lakshmaṇa could not bear the harsh words of Sītā, he drew a line on the ground and told Sītā not to cross that line saying that none could harm her while she was within the limits of that line. It is called the Lakshmaṇa rekhā.

When Lakshmaṇa reluctantly left of in search of Rāma, King Rāvaṇa appeared and asked for alms disguised as a recluse. Sītā offered him alms, as is the custom of the Indian tradition, but he would not accept unless she overstepped the Lakshmaṇa rekhā. The moment she took one step outside the line, Rāvaṇa lifted her up and carried her away to Sri Lanka, keeping her in a secluded place, waiting for her consent to accept him. She not only inflicted sorrow on herself but also put Rāma and Lakshmaṇa to bear the burden of grief and had to fight in the field to vanquish Rāvaṇa. Crossing the border of indulgence may lead one into sorrow and grief. So one has to guard oneself from over-indulgence.

crossroads. Accept such situations and work. Find out whether you can take such ugly characters or personalities and ripen them for righteous living. Take this as a challenge. Never gauge a student from your standard. Gauge a student from his or her physical, emotional and intellectual standards. His or her way of talking and behaviour will guide you as to how much you can help him or her after studying their capacities. According to their standard and as per their power to grasp, use expressive words moment to moment to uplift them.

Descend to the level of the pupil to show the way. You know the path, and the pupil does not. You have to build the pupil slowly from his standard to yours.

I am happy that from 1968, the tree of yoga has grown into a huge tree in your country. Your responsibilities have increased and you have to carry a very heavy yogic weight on your backs. As the weight is great on you, you cannot neglect your practices. If you do not practise, you cannot teach at all. This is ethics in teaching. Otherwise one becomes an immoral teacher.

If a pupil comes to you with a disease, imagine that disease is within you. Think and make a self-inquiry, "What would I do if I had this problem? How can I work the affected parts? Which organs are defective?", and so forth. If you take these avenues on your own, your subjective experience will go a long way in helping those pupils who are sent to you by God to test you through them. You need your own practice to solve such problems.

Carry on your work. You and I have met through the Will of God. Through His Will we have come together and we carry on. You have to induce the next generation too to do yoga.

Do not magnify any misunderstandings between yourselves as teachers. There are three ways of not heeding to gossip: you can either forget, or forgive or be indifferent. If ill-feeling grows between yourselves, then you are not practising yoga at all. The ill-feeling is because of the inflation of your egos. "Give and take" is the only way to be friendly in yoga. If you look at a tree, some branches are straight and some are crooked; some leaves are beautiful and some are not; some are dry and some fresh. Similarly in families too there are zigzag minds. Allow a margin and teach. Find out where you and your standards meet, as you cannot ask everyone to meet at that one peak alone.

Each person has a different understanding according to the growth of his intellect. One may be mature, one may be premature, one may be in the state of maturing and one may lack maturity. We have to consider all these weaknesses and shortcomings and show the way. To show the way we cannot criticise. We can only criticise or admonish when the same mistakes are repeated several times. When a rupture takes place between teachers, it may grow later into hatred. Then it becomes the cancer of the mind. Better nip it in the bud by meeting each other, so that it does not disturb harmony within you all.

I have given freedom to one and all. I have never asked how many pupils you have or what your earnings are. When there is freedom with understanding, then there should be no room for misunderstandings.

DIFFERENCE BETWEEN PRACTICE AND TEACHING

My practices have remained untainted. Persons who called me 'Mr. Iyengar' have themselves changed later. They started calling me 'Sir' and then *'Gurujī'*, though I have not changed in my determination, approach and practice. We have to be honest within ourselves. We have to be honest in our work and we have to be honest to our pupils also. All wonderful works are done only with honesty and integrity. Carry on the work with inner humility. However, you need to show some vanity externally when you teach. When I practise, I am *sāttvic*. When I teach, I cannot be *sāttvic*. If I am *sāttvic*, my pupils are bound to become *tāmasic*. Silence is *sāttvic* in nature. Dullness and inertia are *tāmasic* in nature. I am *rājasic* in my teaching in order that pupils do not become dull. My *rājasic* teaching makes my pupils do *sāttvic* yoga. If you are *sāttvic* in your teaching, you are leading your pupils to darkness and not to light. While you are teaching, you have to be *rājasic*. When you are practising alone or with your colleagues, you should have a *sāttvic* nature. To improve your pupils you have to show a little bit of your inflated self. If you are soft, the pupil's brain gets inflated. To humble the pupil, you have to be *rājasic*. The teacher has to play a dual role. This is not dishonesty. When you practise, you are inward. You have to be within your inner body. When you are teaching, you have to forget yourself and your pupil has to become your entire self. You become a non-self, as though you are yourself entering into the pupil's body. Feel that you are in the pupil's body. To enter that body you have to make noise. In other words, what I mean to say is that since you cannot enter physically into someone's body, your explanation and the voice must be such that they penetrate the pupil's body and the pupil begins to perform.

Teaching is external. Practice is internal. If you know all these things, you can avoid the pitfalls – God also will bless you. The spiritual satisfaction of the tree is to give tasty fruits only. This happens only when it grows healthily. There are trees which never give fruit. Do not make our yoga practices barren. Do not allow only health to grow without giving mental and spiritual fruits. In order to make the spiritual fruits to grow, we have to get the whole inner organism matured and ripe, including our intelligence and consciousness, so that the self becomes ripe. I wish you all the best in your life.

THE ART OF TEACHING*

Yoga has been defined as both an art and a science. So any introduction on how to combine the art of teaching must consider both these aspects which serve as a guide to those who wish to teach. First of all, the study of the human body, of human emotional feelings, is a must. The other is to develop step by step techniques of each *āsana* and *prāṇāyāma* to increase interest in the aspirant. While doing *sādhanā*, I practised it as an art, then I learnt the theory and, combining them, used it as a science.

Teaching requires the expression of right and precise technical words that have been experienced in one's practices. The human body has an infinitely complex structural formation with so many joints, muscles and nerves and blood vessels running to thousands of miles within a structure of five or six feet in height. It has numerous organs, plexuses and glands functioning in a co-ordinated way. I have used the expression 'infinitely complex', since even now new research work in the medical field informs new findings about this mysterious body. Hence, a thorough study of experiential anatomy and physiology becomes essential to obtain a background for the physical, physiological and psychological formation of the *āsana*. Using the physiological anatomy in the practice of each *āsana*, the knowledge and experience that are gained through observation are to be translated into words later. This is how I began experimenting on myself in order to share my knowledge with others.

As life has taught me to be dispassionate, I was able to observe the moods and minds of people and I became skilled at adapting this art of yoga to suit the needs of each individual even in large classes. This combined study of human anatomy and physiology and the study of moods and modes of men helped me to transmit with the art of apt terminology and communication. I hope this illustration enhances in you the value of the art and of these essential qualities and right expressions which you need in order to grow as a talented teacher.

---

* Extracted from my book *The Art of Yoga* with kind permission of Harper Collins, London.

First of all, art requires tremendous self-discipline. One who wishes to take up yoga as a teacher should know that it demands disciplined training from the very beginning. In order to develop the art of the teaching quality, it involves the will to improve in practice and accept the pain and discomfort that follows in pursuance of this. Then one has to give up distracting activities and other interests from one's pursued goal. Yogic practice presupposes the pursuit of mental clarity and purity which are essential needs for an idealistic yogic way of life. Beauty and virtue in life create beauty and virtue in art. All art, though disciplined, is creative and the teacher must give freedom to the pupil to be creative. Undoubtedly, creativity brings joy and fulfilment. Still, the freedom for creativity should not cross the moral, mental and scientific frame. It should not divorce, diverge and dissociate from the origin which is pure and divine. Once mastery is attained the artist feels that the art is his own, his means of self-expression and his way of life. He uses his artistic frame as a vehicle towards higher and nobler aspirations and inspires men to share his vision through his talented gifts.

Art at all times is a never satisfied and exacting muse. No sooner is a goal attained, than the next one appears in view. It is a continual process of *sādhanā;* as one crosses beyond the known, the unknown moves away further into the distance. No doubt the known has a frontier, but the unknown is frontierless.

If an artist is content, then that satisfaction becomes illusory and a fall may follow. Achievement appears easy, but to maintain that which is achieved is difficult.

Art demands constant attentive practice *(nirantarābhyāsa).* For this reason, the yogi as a teacher-artist should know that he has to develop a sense of self-criticism and observation regardless of success or failure. He has to proceed in his efforts through breath control *(prāṇāyāma)* and concentration *(dhāraṇā),* to be quick in mind to observe the subtle nuances of his various movements and actions. This self-study brings in him the emotional stability and the power to discriminate. He gets himself totally absorbed in his art for its own sake as if it were his path and his goal.

Art being the goddess of knowledge, the artist must humbly wait until she chooses to grace him as she can bestow or withold favour. Without humbleness there is going to be no progress or learning, no fusion in art. The teacher too has to cultivate in his pupil a clean and clear mind so that he and his mind may be blended as one with the art. The pupil too should strive for the development of purity in art by discipline. He should take the thoughts that are good, elevating and auspicious, and learn to discard the superficially pleasant. The practitioner must learn to surmount his faults and weaknesses to rise to the heights of the art that he has undertaken. He has to impel himself to perfection by his own zeal and effort as if the art has chosen him for it to flow in him with vibrancy, vigour and purity.

In the field of yoga, the teacher guides and trains the would-be teacher by bringing to the surface his unknown hidden gifts and skills. Through these the teacher transforms him towards refinement in the work of art. He presents various means of approach and taps his pupil's intelligence with sound and brilliant techniques and instils in the pupil the energy for greater application to practise unceasingly so that he keeps constant vigilance to reach close to perfection. At this stage he becomes a dedicated artist to grasp the artistic subtleties, through which he is made to express his art with skill and grace, fineness and beauty.[1]

The teacher, by example and precept, sets the way of high standards and indicates how to bring the distant goal nearer, and the pupil accepts the teacher as his *guru* who guides him to stand well, to walk and to leap forward in the art. The teacher must have the skill to know his pupil's needs so that he can guide the pupil with love, keeping in mind the pupil's interests. He remains firm, exacting and draws the best out of his pupil.

As parents bring up their child, so the teacher with his talent corrects and uplifts the pupil in the twinkling of an eye, by surprise. The pupil should treasure these corrections, when he gets the chance to uplift his own students to acquire artistic insight and vision with which to soar towards the goal of perfection and mastery.

In the art of teaching yoga, the teacher encourages in his pupil's heart how to feel and think in order to explore the body and experiment with the *āsana* and *prāṇāyāma* along with the study of life and nature, delving deep into yoga and its philosophy. The teacher further guides and builds in his pupil the power to be an examiner not only of himself but also of his fellow practitioners, so that they are inspired to measure the sensitivity, the subtlety and the vastness of the field of yoga.

In teaching and in effort, self-discipline and right application act as the two wings of the *sādhaka* by which he rises to lofty heights. Effort is the propelling force which spurs one with the power of will and strength to start energetically to combat the short-comings of weaknesses, moods and pessimism that come in the way of learning.

---

[1] As there are grades of *sādhaka* (see *Y.S.*, I.21 & 22), there are also grades of teachers, see the article in this volume – *Anukrama Sādhanā Śreṇi*.

Effort is of two types, mechanical and dynamic. Mechanical involvement is repetitious; it is habit-forming and brings some mobility but not enlightenment. Dynamic effort is that of standing alone with a balanced state of mind *(samāhita-citta)* in the face of opposition and competition and with a sensitive and intense single-minded approach. Such intensity is essential for success.

Life has its own stumbling blocks and so does yoga. The teacher has to indicate these stumbling blocks, both in body and mind and how they influence each other, and show ways to face and overcome them.

For instance, in physical arts where the body is the base such as dance or yoga, there is a risk of physical injury bringing pain, mental dejection and depression. Any physical injury or dejection disturbs serenity and poise. If a muscle is torn through ignorance, heedlessness or over-enthusiasm, the *sādhaka* is guided by the teacher in the structure of the injured part in depth, with skilful treatment. He is shown how the affected part is to be supported and worked carefully, correctly and precisely to assist the healing force of nature in the shortest time. The pupil is made to maintain interest in the essence of his art.

Mental pains are caused by lack of inner awareness. The *Bhagavad Gītā* (XVI.21) states that desire, lust, anger and greed *(kāma, krodha, lobha)* are three things which are to be avoided as they open the gates of mental suffering. They create external and internal turmoil, stop one's artistic functioning and prevent one totally from reaching the higher aim in life through art. The teacher guides the pupil to recognise them and then to be free from them. This generates in the pupil a peace of mind which helps him to commune with his art so that he blossoms and moves with fullness of beauty, truth and purity. Then he feels he is enriched and moves to uplift man and society through the magical charm of his art.

HOW TO OBSERVE WHILE TEACHING*

When you begin teaching yoga, it is good to start with basic *āsana*. For example, take *Tāḍāsana*,[1] observe yourself how you are standing and recollect how you were standing earlier. Bring to your memory and compare the feel of understretch or overstretch by your readjustment and then judge how to explain the ways of performing it well.

The moment you look at your *āsana*, mental changes automatically take place on their own as the body adjusts. Take these sudden adjustments that take place in body and mind as techniques and teach accordingly.

While explaining to the students find out on your own body, observe and absorb yourself before you correct your students. Observe the changes that occur in your own body, which make you realise the missing links. Similarly learn to see and observe the missing links in your students and connect them up.

This way, you will come to know your students' bodies closely, and from that think of what steps in techniques have to be adapted to make them understand how to reach the state which you experience.

Learn to observe who has done well and who has not. Stop explanations till then. See the same parts of the body in all. Be quick to see and take this as a clue to explain how to act. Without calling them by name, bring evenness in their presentations by cultivating the right basic points and then proceed to build-up the next point.

Treat those who assist you as co-teachers and not as helpers. As they are co-teachers, do not show up the differences such as someone being superior or inferior. Co-teaching is just monitoring, imprinting on students of what you as themain teacher say. The co-teachers should not explain beyond what the main teacher says. They should not say things which are not connected to the main teacher's explanations and divert the students' attention. If the main

* Chicago, July 7th, 1990.

1 See plate n. 27.

teacher gets something wrong, they should remain quiet at that time and then discuss after the class and bring the attention of the main teacher to where he or she went wrong. The main teacher, who conducts the class for the pupils is the head at that time and after the session ends both co-teachers and pupils are equals.

Learn to start linking the sequential steps, but do not jump. Co-ordinate intelligence with action. Do not do and show the *āsana* faster than your words, or vice versa. It may lead the students towards confusion. Learn to adjust and synchronise your actions and words while you show and choose your words according to the student's capability of understanding and action in movement. If the student goes fast, you have to check him to follow your explanation, and if he is slow you have to control your word speed.

Both theory and practice have to go together. Theory may move like an express train, but practice may move at snail's pace. Many of you do not synchronise action with words, or the words with the movements. Words are faster than the action. The sentence gets completed but not the action. Learn to synchronise the word with motion and action. Your words should flow with action or you have to bring the word to fit into the speed and motion of action. This is the actual way of blending the intelligence of the head with the intelligence of the body and vice versa.

When you see a student to whom the *āsana* comes naturally or better than yours, then say to yourself: "Let me learn from this student's presentation, as he does not have that intelligence to know how the *āsana* has come to him." With your experience, mobility and intelligence, which have been built up through time, you will be able to grasp fast and eventually you can translate that experience and share it with students.

Teachers should not act as technocrats only; but they have to develop a humane character and mix that humaneness in their techniques. Then I am certain that he or she will grow as a real teacher.

I see many teachers teaching with their hands entwined behind their backs. If you keep your hands behind your back, can you play the violin, can you play the piano? The hands are the instruments in yoga. You have to be in touch with the instrument. But what happens is that you keep your hands behind the back and teach, and this creates distance between you and your own self as well as you and the student. You have seen how my hands are alert and active to rush forward, ready to contact, correct and help the students when they are in need. This position of readiness to act is needed to generate warmth in teacher and students' relationship. Hands behind the back means you are creating distance between you and the students. It may also create an impression that you are teaching indifferently and uninterestedly.

Often I have observed you as teachers using words at supersonic speed. Give them time to listen and adjust. Wait till they adjust and afterwards proceed. You as teacher are the first person and the students are the second person. The first person's body moves fast because you are using the word, whereas they have to listen to the word, digest and then adjust, so there is a time lapse. Hence the words have to flow in space and then enter their ears. So give time for them to listen and adjust.

First, as teachers, learn to correct the visible and perceivable parts. They are the gross parts. Then come to the less gross. First start with the visible external body and then come to the middle body, and afterwards move from middle body to the subtle body. The teachers should teach first whatever is perceivable and later teach whatever is conceivable. In the former, the students use their eyes and sensation of touch. In the latter, they use the mind and the sensitivity of intelligence.

Mind is one, but it scatters. The body is one but has many parts. So you have to use many words for attention to convey right action.

The teacher has to be subjective and objective. Subjectively you have to feel while teaching or demonstrating and objectively you have to express words to imprint on the doers. Again, when you are teaching see that you as subject and students as object become one. Also when you touch to adjust the students in their *āsana* paractice, that touch should be exact and firm.

I often said that my exact touch or hit while teaching has a psychological reaction on the students; and not on the physical level at all. It gains their quick attention and quick adjustment. The intelligence becomes alert and sharp. You as a teacher need to learn the art of touch for this purpose.

Know that the source of action begins always where the body is in touch with the ground. Make the body become one with the floor on which one is standing. Then one gets the sense of direction and understands the right action through the right and precise touch.

If the body is healthy one does not think of it. Similarly, when the soul is healthy there is no room for it to say: "I want to realise the Self."[1] So first teach how to contact the object (body) with the subject (self). Use the body as an instrument for the self to roam in the *āsana*. The body

---

1 *Tadā draṣṭuḥ svarūpe avasthānam* (*Y.S.*, I.3). Then, the seer dwells in his own true splendour.

through the *āsana* needs to be touched by the self everywhere. The self pervades the body. This is the spiritual way of practice. Though i am teaching with the body, I bring together both the body and the self as object and subject and later both as subject.

"Think before you act". You have seen that I have not kept the students inattentive either physically or mentally. If you keep the students too long in *āsana* with your explanations, their bodies rest and they lose attention and warmth in the body. So say to yourself that you will not do it again in your teaching career. This is what you should learn.

Watch while practising your own techniques that you follow and see the new movements, new awareness and new understanding coming in your bodies. Use them as a base for tomorrow's classes. Carry on this way.

While teaching, in case you lose the balance in any *āsana,* do not say: "I lost the balance". Tell them: "You lose the balance here." That is known as presence of mind. In teaching one needs presence of mind. Notice which part is giving way. How do I continue when this part gives way has to be thought out and learnt first and then taught. Presence of mind is divine. You do not need a special technique to learn divinity. When there is presence of mind you are in a state of divinity.

Learn to repeat the same instruction again and again so that they are imprinted in the students' mind. This helps the students to become more attentive to do the *āsana* better and better.

The word 'creativity' in relation to a new technique, which some teachers use, needs explanation. Know that when a person has reached exalted knowledge of the *āsana*, only then can he or she create. The immature mind cannot create. I can create, because I have tested and tasted the entire *āsana*. I have swallowed the *āsana*. You still have not chewed it, so then how can you swallow it? I have digested the *āsana* but you have not even peeled the skin off it. The pulp is inside, the flesh is inside but the skin is still gripping very hard. Can you peel an orange if the skin is too hard? If the skin is soft, it comes off easily and also can be cut easily.

While teaching we have to see the outer body, inner body, mind and awareness. Seeing their wandering minds and their lack of awareness, we instruct: "Lift this part of the body here, and extend and elongate there!" in order to bring their minds and awareness on the right track, to co-ordinate their mind and intelligence with the body while they are made to maintain and retain the *āsana*.

Patañjali says *citta prasādanam* (*Y.S.*, I.33). Levelling the *citta* in all parts of the body when one is doing and staying in the *āsana* is *citta prasādanam*. When this feeling comes, know that it is the mastery of that *āsana*. Freedom with discipline is real freedom. Freedom without discipline is libertinism.

If you build the base, the rest will follow. If you do not see and look into the base and go on doing the *āsana*, remember, not only are you injuring yourself but you become the cause for injury in others. Teach in such a way that your pupils may not get the ill effect of yoga later. Yoga declares, *heyaṁ duḥkham anāgatam* (*Y.S.*, II.16).[1] Teach in such a way that it prevents pain and suffering. Build consciously and cautiously the strength from now on so that the offensive power is not disturbed but generates zeal to grow stronger in body and mind through right practice.

[1] The pains that are yet to come can be prevented.

A WORD OF ADVICE FOR A RIGHT APPROACH IN YOGA

Yoga is a universal subject which cultures not only the physical body but also the cellular system and neurons of intelligence. Yoga acts as a bridge between the physical, mental and intellectual bodies. This bridge trims and cultures the body, the mind and intelligence for healthy, broad and universal growth of equanimity in the consciousness. As a result of this, the intelligence, the consciousness and the concept of union of man with the invisible force – known as universal consciousness or God – meet each other. Therefore, I say that yoga is the only subject existing from time immemorial that enables mankind to develop and to see the true nature of religion. Though religions vary, they all meet together at a certain point where division disappears and oneness between human beings is retained.

Teaching is a very noble profession. When it comes to yoga, there is a lot of give and take between the student and the teacher involving friendliness and compassion for the growth of qualitative teaching. The teachers and students should remain together as one family without giving any room for misunderstanding. The teachers should treat pupils like their own children and the students should respect the teacher as one respects the parents. We train our children to become healthy and happy, and as teachers we too must take the responsibility to train those who come for betterment of growth in body, intelligence and consciousness. The teachers should learn to be happy if their students surpass them in practice and teaching.

When teachers are conducting classes, the participants and the teachers have to communicate as well as commune with one another in friendliness to build up a good rapport. In the case of a personal problem, which prevents the teacher from presenting accurately as required, it is better the teacher explains his or her physical drawbacks to them and then conducts the class. The teachers can still guide them in practice, especially where they lack understanding.

The student also should appreciate the honesty of the teacher. A friendly approach will definitely increase a good relationship between them. In my life I have seen both and done both. Some explain well but cannot show; and some do well but cannot explain. Both are good tools for understanding. If one is blind to practice, the other is blind to the theory, whereas both are needed in teaching. Have confidence to bring together the theory and practice so that they are in rhythm with each other just as a blind man with legs and a lame man with eyes might help each other to move from one place to the other.

Learning yoga is a combined venture for teachers as well as students. Each student has to learn to observe the structure of his body, its movements, actions, and its contact with mind. On the other hand, the teacher has to know the capacity of each student and teach in such a way that his capacity increases. The teacher has to teach the art of connecting body with mind. The student can understand and appreciate only when he understands his limitations and the teacher uplifts him a little further.

The students should not create misunderstanding or barriers between two teachers. The teachers as well as the students should remember that they are doing *yogasādhanā* as followed by me. The branches may be separate but the root is one.

The body is not a machine which can be hammered to get the position in a day. As a student, you should take good points from the teacher and practise. Understand the teachers and accordingly listen to what they are teaching.

As teachers you have to see the good and you have to express to the participants how to do the good or at least a little better, rather than pointing out the small mistakes here or there. This way the teachers and the students probably develop a better quality of seeing and better quality of understanding. This qualitative way of seeing and understanding will be a great help to both.

Teachers should not teach something which does not come in the frame of the subject. They should not teach or talk about what has no relevance to yoga. The teachers should not misdirect the students.

As a teacher you should learn to tune the ears of every student so that they learn the art of listening. Be clear to give a good background of basic teaching to make them develop stability. Observe and ensure for yourself that what they do and what you asked them to do was synchronised. Often, you say something and the students do something else because they do not listen to you attentively.

The teachers should focus on those parts of the body where the students do not respond. See that they activate those parts. Do not proceed further unless they get the hold of them. Give an emphasis on their weak points. Let those ideas circulate in them, to be grasped.

Teach first what the students can see and feel, then proceed gradually on to points which they do not feel.

As a teacher, do the homework to analyse and practise on your own body and mind before rectifying mistakes. Decide what points are to be given to them so that they can attain what is not yet attained. Use yourself as a helping hand to help others.

The ideal relationship of master and pupil is based on a healthy way of teaching and approach to life. Yoga is about associating and putting together the objects of the self and Self. Establish proper communion, good communication and relationship. Teachers and students should proceed and progress hand in hand without giving any chance for misunderstandings. Always remember that the subject of yoga is greater than, and above, all of us. We are mortals but yoga is immortal.

A TALK TO TEACHERS*

We are meeting here today to see those teachers whom I do not get a chance to meet. I have not seen the senior teachers conducting classes for some years. After last seeing the classes almost ten years ago, I feel the standard of teaching has fallen tremendously. I do not know what has caused the standard to fall, but I was not at all happy. On this basis I would like to make some suggestions on teaching.

When you get your certificate, whether it is Introductory, Junior, Senior or Advanced, you think that you have learnt everything and you do not come in contact with senior teachers. This independent way of teaching may be one of the reasons for the low standard, because the basic background has been lost on account of want of contact and communication. After 1974, I have not watched the classes conducted by you except in medical classes where I gave some guidance on how to work on patients. The time has come for all of us to give a serious thought to this subject. A superficial way of teaching has caused sluggishness and stagnation. It may mean the death of the art. This is why I am placing some thoughts before you all.

Long ago, when the certificates were first given by me, a particular necessity was there behind it. They were demanded by the educational authorities here. The number of teachers has increased but the teachers are not proceeding step by step. The connecting links are missing and correct explanations are not being given. So we have to seriously think and work to find a way, a solution for these shortcomings. So, I suggest that levels are made in all the courses including Introductory certificate levels.

I suggest that teachers should teach only the *āsana* given in those levels. As their levels improve, then they can teach the *āsana* of that level. Elsewhere, some senior teachers moved away from the base, and I had to warn them to come back to it. Yoga is a practical matter, but what I was seeing in the classes was that the teaching went on as if one was delivering a lecture in a university. From this I gathered that the standard of teaching had gone down. You are not

* Talk given on the 17th September 1987, London.

repeating the words for students to be able to grasp the subject. If I asked the teachers what they had said a moment ago, they were not able to recall their own words. They were not connecting their words in their explanations forward and backward for students to understand. They were going on as if reading passages from a book, or they went on and on like a moving train. The teachers were not looking at the pupils, but continued with words. Is this teaching from the head or the heart? Yoga cannot be taught only from the head. Teaching has to come from the heart also. When the teacher says chest up while their own chests are sinking, how can the pupils understand and lift their chests up? You have to show with body language what you want to express. Hence, on this point we have to think very seriously. I saw a tremendous interest in the students. Hence it is our duty to see that their interest does not fade away. The teachers need to recharge their emotional and intellectual batteries. It has become a serious matter now. The teachers are lacking both the emotional and intellectual touch. They are not close to the pupils emotionally and they are not lifting the pupils intellectually. Both are lacking in their teaching.

Sometimes I saw *āsana* taught which have nothing to do with the yogic system. With this happening I do not want them to use the word "Iyengar". Yesterday I had to remind a teacher about this. Callisthenic movements were being introduced and called 'Iyengar Yoga'. Yoga is an ethical practice, where the position of the body and the breath as well as their interaction with each other are used to understand the inner mind. There should be a clear concrete presentation that shows life, the vital force and potency in the body, mind, breath and consciousness. Do not let the work be from the head. Teachers should not go on explaining with more and more words which cannot be converted into action and brought into experience. They should measure their words to make the students listen, understand and grasp. The words have to be translated into body with their meaning and feeling. Learn how to reduce this over-use of words. The senior teachers, when assessing the would-be teachers, should see that they lessen this. The teaching of yoga is not the work of the head only but the work of the head and heart.

As a teacher, we have to initially impart knowledge of techniques. Then, knowing the weaknesses of the students, we have to change the techniques to fit into the frame of their body and mind. The teacher has to see that the student, has to grasp. If they are unable to understand and do what the teacher says, then what is the point in teaching? I am worried as I am seeing you all speak of techniques without seeing their needs. Things have been moving as though in a reverse gear. One thing is that standards have to be raised. There should be a class for the teachers with the senior most experienced teachers working as monitors, and having ten teachers and ten pupils exchanging places. I did this in Boston. There, teachers were given a certain time to correct the weaknesses of the other teachers as participants. When they could not see or correct the points they explained, I pointed out that they were not yet mature for the standard they were teaching. Then I reversed the roles. This way of observation gave them a chance to see what was lacking, and then after discussion with co-teachers, I connected their words for both groups to follow. This way a uniform growth was achieved for the entire group. I conducted the group using their own points within the right frame, and used words according to the understanding of those participants.

My suggestion to them was not to go to the subtle points at once, such as which way the little toe faces, while forgetting or neglecting the gross obvious mistakes. I told them to look at gross mistakes first. When the students' bodies are toned and minds tuned, then go for minute points. When the students cannot understand the gross body, how can they understand the movements of the subtle areas like the little toe? Pointing out such minute mistakes is showing off as if one were highly qualified. This is a wrong approach for any teacher. When the gross mistakes are not rectified, students do not understand the minute ones. Only when teachers have rectified the gross mistakes should they go on to the minute ones. To go straight to the finer points like your knuckle is out, or the diaphragm is not in line, without seeing whether the arms are straight or not, or the elbows are bent or stretched, is wrong. Often the teachers themselves do not understand which knuckle is in and which is out. Similarly, the diaphragm cannot be seen from outside. Its movement is not felt either by the teacher – the seer, or the pupil – the doer. So, for the time being, keep the minute points out of your teaching. When the students mature in rectifying the gross mistakes, then build them up to see the subtler mistakes before going into the minutest points.

If a junior teacher is teaching in the presence of a senior teacher, then the senior teacher has to note the mistakes but should not intervene at once. It is not a matter of etiquette but a question of tolerance; one should not listen to wrong points alone but also good points and then guide them to correct the wrong. This builds in them confidence and courage to teach better. Often by quick remarks, confusion sets in and this may be one of the reasons why consultation is not there but the standards have fallen.

The teachers do not watch the eyes of the pupils while teaching. The most important aspect in teaching is to see the eyes of the students. If they are dull, then you should know that your explanations are not going in, hence you have to learn to change immediately to fit into their frame of mind. Do not give lectures on what you are teaching without demonstrating. Only a few demonstrated. The majority of teachers are not demonstrating but are thinking that it is their explanations that count. Because of this we have to sit together and discuss to clear the doubts of the junior teachers and rebuild them. However, this is not happening.

While teaching, one has to build up through words and expressions without forgetting the main links. First use three or four sentences and move backward and forward re-using the important words for the learner to grasp. Stop going like express trains from which you cannot see the landscape with clarity.

The "Iyengar teachers"[1] think that there is value attached to them, but the value is due to my hard work and the other early senior teachers. Do not bring a bad name to those of us who have worked very hard and built it up. For instance, take this 'A' teacher's case. If teacher 'A' does not know his/her own back movement, how can he/she teach a student with backache? If even after eight years the teacher has not found a remedy for this problem, what will be the fate of a person who comes to him/her? 'A' should go to someone 'B' who has worked it out and ask for guidance. Then the knowledge of 'A' increases and 'A' knows how to tackle such cases. The teachers feel it is below their dignity to consult the seniors and they do not work by themselves either.

Even today, an experienced student said she has sciatica, but I said that it was not sciatica since pain cannot continue for so long. Then I found out that she had an old injury. I saw her movements and the positioning of the body. I gave her many *āsana*, even *Paśchimottānāsana*.[2] Then I said, "No, it must be an old hidden pain you are getting." This *āsana* gave me the clue to come to the conclusion that it was not sciatica. I had to change the sequence to minimise the muscular pains.

Another person said that she had a burning sensation in her lumbar area and I told her what *āsana* to do but she insisted on joining the regular class. From this it appears that many do not want to follow the right advice. They want to do everything and yet follow nothing. Ambition and doing everything will not give one relief. If you do the suggested *āsana*, then you can find out how they help, then you in turn can help others. So one has to use the heart for practising yoga and not the ambition of the head.

When a teacher was teaching in a class yesterday, I saw some students whose eyeballs turned red after twenty minutes of practice. The teacher never gave a thought to this. Their red eyes indicated tension. They were all hypertensed. Then I took over and conducted the class and in two minutes the eyeballs came back to normal. So what is the use of taking an hour-and-a-half class and not observing the condition of the students' eyes? This is how the standards have fallen. You have to be careful and constantly watchful for the problems and think of solutions. Then the knowledge grows.

---

1 Certified by B.K.S. Iyengar National Association in every country.

2 See *Aṣṭadaḷa Yogamālā* vol 2, plate n. 5

When I took the classes for two days previously, the students were happy, they said that at other times it was boring. Now you have to find out why it was boring. If the majority felt the class was boring, then you have to find an answer to the question yourselves. I have shown the way. Some teachers are very good in their practice, but they teach according to their practice and not according to the groups of students who have come to learn. In teaching we have to do community work, and learn how to connect the work generally to fit into all so that all the students are benefited. All the students feel their participation. It is they who need to see the progress in themselves. The teachers have to see how the gap between them and the students is gradually lessened due to their progress.

Some may have problems like flat foot, spine trouble, hard sternum, so connect all these and then conduct the class. Observe how they receive your words, whether they have acted on what you have said or not. New students say it is good, but the criteria should be how they react when the teacher uses words or how they respond to the teacher's explanation. Do they do what the teachers expect? The teachers need self-study. Also the teachers have to watch how they react to the students' reaction. Learn to observe with a heart to heart connection.

The teaching has to be enlightening, not only for introductory levels but even in the higher levels. It is a pity that many do not even know the names of the *āsana*. In the assessments there is not enough time to do or see all the *āsana*. The assessors cannot assess asking you all the questions. It is your responsibility as a teacher to learn the names. Hence, you should learn from senior teachers. If you become a teacher, it does not mean that you are the master. There are many things yet to learn.

I stopped the partnership yoga, as it turned out more sensual than learning to make progress in the art. I introduced it with good intention so that everyone learns to help each other to progress further. But unfortunately the students received it with bad intentions. Sometimes I allow men helping men and women helping women, so that the perception in thinking is changed and attention is focused on learning the *āsana* properly.

Why should teachers laugh if the students commit mistakes? If they are unable to understand or grasp what teachers say, is it not for the teachers to understand where they lack the skill? Why do teachers not see what is lacking in them? As the teachers do not expect insult from the students, is it not their duty to see that laughing at the students is an insult to them? If the teachers laugh at the students, is it helpful to learn the art? So, correct this behaviour.

I see that the American students who started in 1973 are learning more and more while you have remained stagnant, though you all began in 1960. Therefore, either re-assess or drop your ego and correct yourselves. You the senior teachers know how I started from absolute scratch when the subject was unkown in this country. Everyone who comes to you is either new or has come with wrong imprints of yoga. Therefore correct the student to save him/her. I have done my job. When God calls me I shall go. Though I am content with what I did, now the responsibility is on you people to carry on for the best.

I saw in all the classes the teachers explaining according to their own ways of doing. They did not learn how to present an *āsana*. I do *Naṭarājāsana*;[1] but while explaining it, I shall see how their approach should be. If I can do *Naṭarājāsana*, it does not mean all can do that like me. Is there no difference between one who has mastered the *āsana* and the one who just begins to learn the *āsana?* Do you mean to say that a beginner and an advanced student are at the same level? Today I showed how to use a plank on the inner foot in order to have the weight shift for the sake of balance and the way to rotate the shoulder, standing against the wall, so that with support the student can manage. In the same *āsana*, one needs to know how to balance properly, lifting the back leg sufficiently and again rotating the shoulder.

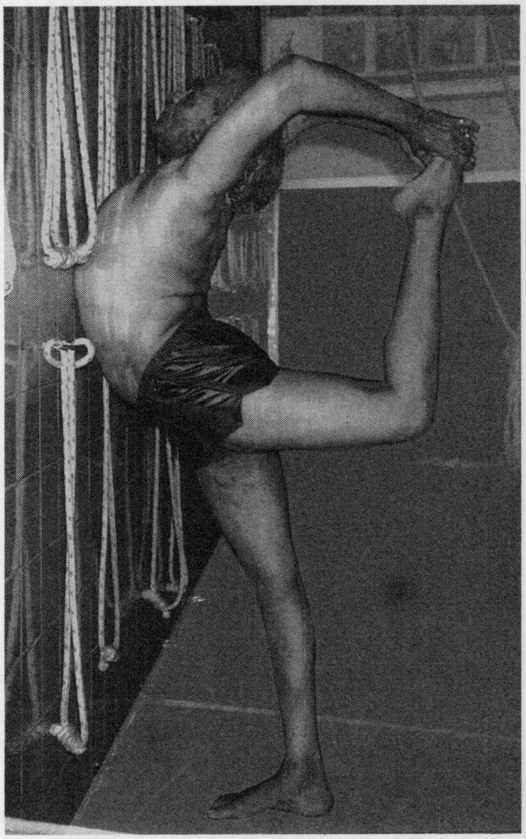

Plate n. 16 – *Naṭarājāsana* with support of a wall

There are many ways to know what is a correct movement and what is a wrong movement. One has to try various ways to find the right balance. Many teachers do not practise, saying that they have no time for it. If you do not keep up your practice, then how can you teach? Yoga is not a lecture or theory class. Definition requires the head but communication requires the heart. You have to co-ordinate these two. Most of us live in the emotions. The world cannot move for a second if the human race does not react through their emotional life with both head and heart.

In Cheltenham, I told one student that if I hit him on the shoulder blade, then he would realise his mistake there. I did hit in such a way that it started moving where it was tight. Yesterday the student told me that he had received thirty or forty letters sympathising with him when I hit

1 See *Light on Yoga*, Harper Collins, London.

him. He said that he replied to them that it was a great honour to receive a blow from me. The slanting plank was there, the plank was of the same shape as our shoulder blades. So I could exactly show how it works. He wrote an article on this expressing his joy of feeling the movement and sent it to me. As no teacher could correct him, he approached me and I corrected him in a few moments. One right hit was enough for him to know the correct action. He immediately dropped his shoulder-blade to its position! This should convey to you all what heart to heart teaching is, wherein emotion and intelligence are made to play together to bring the desired effect, in the place needed. Just saying, "Drop the shoulder blade" does not work. Often people misunderstand when I hit the students. I do not hit without a purpose. I hit for the block to release in such a way that the right required movement occurs.

I see the lack of direct communion between the teacher and the students. You talk more and you think you are communicating but you are not getting a feedback. You do not ask them what they are receiving. You do not see whether your explanation is effective. There should be a time gap between your expression and action at the receiving end. But you go on. You know I speak very fast but I still say that when I speak to a person, their movement is faster than my words. But you are not seeing the movement and still you speak fast. You have to see if what you say is translated into action or not.

The teachers should concentrate on how to improve their standard of teaching in order to convey clearly for students to understand and act rather than taking pride in expression. Students come if the teaching is good. Suppose I have shown you a new movement for the pain today. Think how that movement served to minimise the pain. Similarly, you have to think of a way of correcting on your own, before you convey to others. This way you can build up a healthy constructive growth. Otherwise knowledge gets limited, and it deteriorates. Let us understand this and let us work out to reach that meeting point on common ground.

I showed in the class how in *Utthita Trikoṇāsana* and *Utthita Pārśvakoṇāsana*[1] you do not know the movements of your heels. These things you do not observe. Learn to observe practically the weak and missing points. In each *āsana,* see your intelligence is stretched from one end of the arm or the head to the other end of the feet, like a single thread stretched evenly from the ends. Why should the heel move in these *āsana* differently while turning? When you started the *āsana* the heel was at one place and afterwards the heel was at another place. Why and how it moved there is to be thought of. In this way you check your own movements; only then can you help the movements in the students.

---

1 See plates 25 & 26.

It is my suggestion that once in a month all the teachers make it a point to meet in their areas, either London or Manchester, and exchange information. Ponder over mistakes, discuss and come to the correct conclusion with practical application. It is an opportunity to correct each other and for the exchange of good points. See how and where you miss and re-link the missing points. In Pune, Geeta and other teachers ask me what to do if they are in doubt and I immediately guide them. But here many think that they know. Why not tell each other face to face the good and the bad feelings you experience?

Let us as teachers work to exchange knowledge. Let us not come to conclusions without reconsideration. Otherwise, one has no room for observation and re-education. This is why I have called you here, to think, reason out and work in unison. As teachers, make it a point to meet once a month and work out the plans for progression in knowledge for teaching better.

Sometimes you can invite teachers and students who return fresh from Pune who could pass new information which they get there as well as in remedial classes for a number of specific problems.

What I told Geeta when she became a teacher, I would like to say the same to you all today. "Express positivity outside and always be introspective inside". You should never express doubts or confusion outside. The moment this is noticed by the students, you may end up with failure. Knowing very well you could not correct immediately, do homework on the same theme so that you find the ways to help the needs of the students. Then this self-experience and correction beams a little light in you to work with inspiration. As a teacher, if you are negative in attitude, the pupils will distance themselves from you. Even if you do not know, say to the students, "I know it, do what I say now". But speak about it the next day or when needed. Work out on yourself what you have to do for the students' queries. It is a big question which you have to work out to answer the next day or the day after. You can escape for a day, but not always. You should never teach or try anything without asking the reactions of the students. You have to get the feedback. If they say "pain", you have to scratch your head; "I don't get pain, why are they getting pain?" Do the homework. Do like the student who complained of pain and learn where he went wrong for the pain to occur and correct yourself on the pain, then guide the student to get rid of his pain.

Come together in your region to exchange all that you learn. You have a tremendous field of opportunity to grow. From now on make it a point to meet once in a while, plan constructively to do some basic things. Some senior teachers have to get together and chalk out a programme selecting two or three teachers from various areas to meet together every two or three months. In the meeting, the teachers together should make notes of their weak points, and the monitors should go through these points and tell them what is correct and what is wrong. The monitors too can make their own notes, compare, and then talk to each other. This may give tremendous confidence to budding teachers also. If confidence is lost, one loses courage. If one thinks that one is doing very well, then pride may set in. But when the problematic students come, then the required courage and confidence may not be there.

Teachers have to introduce different levels in the subject, and caution not to teach *āsana* of higher standards when they cannot perform well the given *āsana* list in their standard. So something like this is required by the Teachers' Association for checking. Otherwise the teachers may do anything and teach as they like. The efforts may go astray. The practice of yoga may end abruptly. Ethics may disappear. Remember that if you do not practise you will be a bad teacher. One should not teach from past experiences untouched by present practice.

All these years I did yoga in order to get maturity and stability. Now I am mature and with this maturity I practise to see where it leads me further. This helps me not to lose what I have learned. Even today I practise the very first *āsana, Utthita Trikoṇāsana*. Some of my senior pupils say they do backbends and are not interested in *Utthita Trikoṇāsana* or any other standing *āsana*. This is all wrong practice. I ask them if what they do in *Utthita Trikoṇāsana* and *Utthita Pārśvakoṇāsana*, can also be done in *Ūrdhva Dhanurāsana?* I can tell you exactly what works in *Utthita Trikoṇāsana* and *Utthita Pārśvakoṇāsana*, and how the same muscles work in *Ūrdhva Dhanurāsana*. I can connect one *āsana* to another. But the others are not interested in this. You feel your pelvis and sacrum in *Utthita Trikoṇāsana*. Then do *Ūrdhva Dhanurāsana* and feel the pelvis and sacrum. If they open as in *Utthita Trikoṇāsana,* the arch of the body comes well. Then decide whether *Utthita Trikoṇāsana* is necessary or not. Observe your own *Tāḍāsana*, then do *Ūrdhva Dhanurāsana* and see whether that feeling of firmness in the legs of *Tāḍāsana* is there or not in *Ūrdhva Dhanurāsana*, even with the bent knees. In *Ūrdhva Dhanurāsana* the legs remain bent. But question yourself, with the bent knees in *Ūrdhva Dhanurāsana*. Can I do *Tāḍāsana?* When the legs remain bent, can I keep my thighs and calf muscles like *Tāḍāsana?* Can I open the space behind the knees? Can I keep my arms like *Vīrabhadrāsana I?* Can I open the armpits? Find out, then you know whether various other *āsana* are essential or not for further advancement in advanced *āsana*. If your lumbar works in backbends, then you teach from the lumbar. If you have a soft sacroiliac region, you teach from the sacroiliac region. If the cervical is good, then you advise to do backbends from the cervical, by bending the neck more. How to connect the rhythm from this to that in all the movements is what you have to learn. I have often said that standing *āsana* are the base for every other *āsana*. The symmetrical, rhythmic and even movements of spine come only with the practice of standing *āsana*.

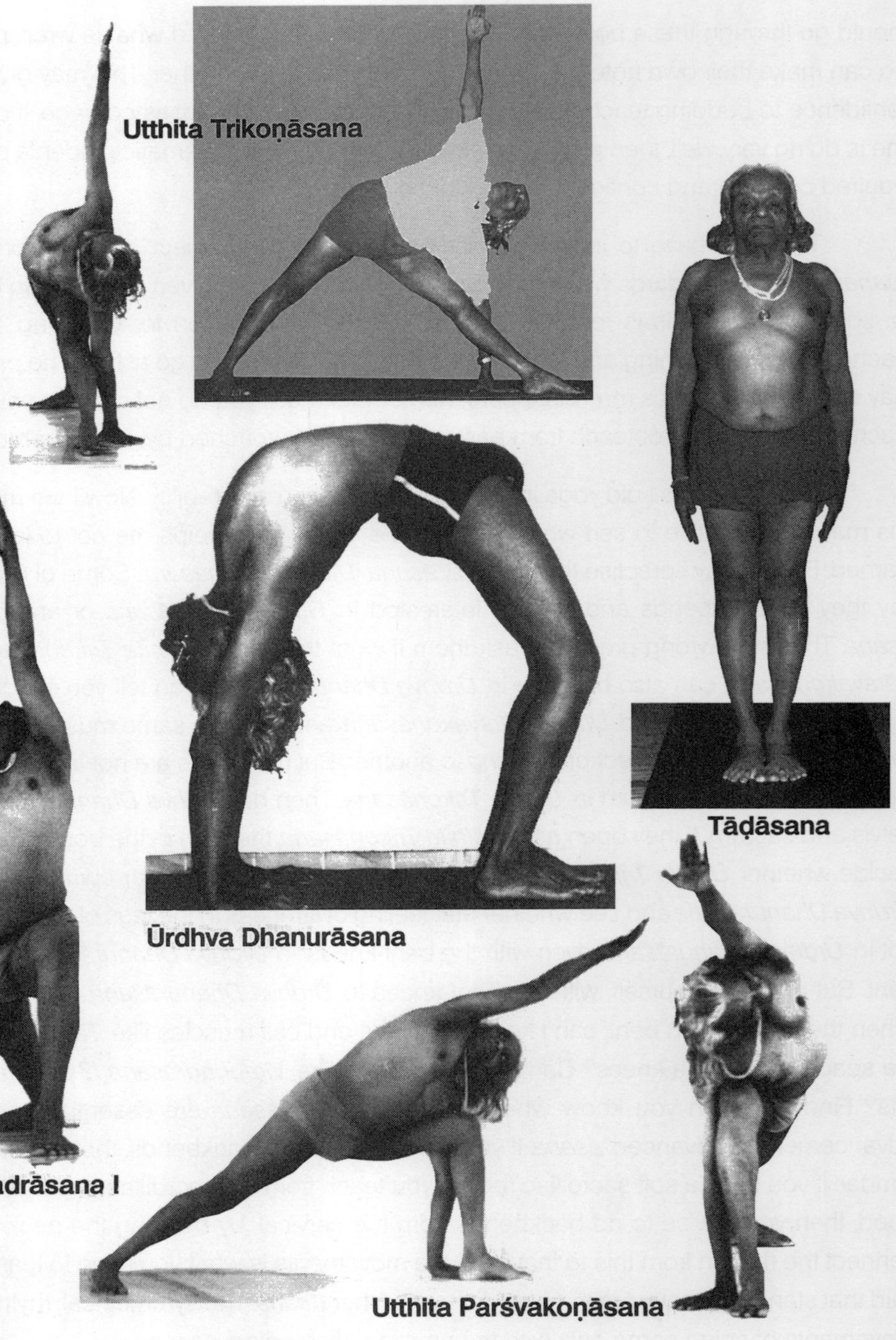

Plate n. 17 – *Ūrdhva Dhanurāsana* related to standing *āsana*.

You have to learn from Patañjali's *Yoga Sūtra*. Each joint is a *sūtra*. How to connect each joint to form the *mālā* of the body? Our joints and muscles are jewels of the body. These jewels are to be strung in various positions with a single thread, which is nothing but intelligence as one end and consciousness as the other. You see somebody doing *Ūrdhva Dhanurāsana* who bends their legs. In some the arms are overstretched and legs are understretched, in some the legs are overstretched and the arms are understretched. Some people never open the chest. Obviously the dome shape of the body disappears. What the descending or ascending order is, remains unknown. This is stagnation in practice – we have to break this stagnation. The moment you learn that nothing is coming, know that you have lost something in the practice.

Some teachers think they have progressed. If some parts of their cells are active, they think that they are improving, but in their heart of hearts they have to feel where the cells show deterioration in action. Where the cells do not work, know that there is the death of the cells. Think of all these, then I admit that you are improving. Often our cells, our body, will not allow us to master the *āsana*. Though we use our intelligence, we do not use our discriminative intelligence. We may think that we are doing well because there is no pain. But where is the equilibrium? Where is the evenness? Where is the understanding? Where is the distribution of energy? All such practices end up with *viparyaya* and *vikalpa* in *āsana*. The *āsana* remains misconceived, illusory and a fanciful idea without any substance in it.

Hence, I want my teachers to refine what they know. Not refine but "re-fine" your fine *āsana*. Each pose has to be reposed. Reposing is meditation. Posing is action. Then you have to reflect; what has come, what has not come; where have I turned more, where have I turned less. Where have I done, where have I not done; where have I attended, where have I not? With this knowledge, you reach a higher level and you can become an able teacher.

Remember, yoga requires tremendous subjective awareness as well as subjective criticism. Music and dance are objectively criticised. Others can criticise easily the other arts. But in yoga others cannot criticise, only the person who does can criticise. That is the beauty of yoga.

So get together and re-fine your practices. Teach well. Go from the gross to the subtle points. Observe the pupils, their positioning, their movements. Learn to unlearn in order to re-learn. Do not teach only to please the students. Teach so that they open their eyes. The imprints of wrong practice remain stronger than those of correct practice. Therefore your efforts should be to teach correctly. Bear this in your mind. You, as a teacher, are doing *saṁskāra* on students. Let them carry the correct and auspicious imprints with correct and auspicious practice. May God bless you all.

GUIDELINES ON *ĀSANA* FOR TEACHERS*

First of all let me make it clear that I have come here to guide you teachers and pupils. Earlier I have conducted several classes, intensive courses and attended conventions. I have taught *āsana, prāṇāyāma* and *dhyāna* during all these gatherings. Now, it is time for me to see what you do, how you conduct the classes, how you proceed. Of course, if there is any problem or lack of understanding, then you can certainly ask me.

But the way you are demanding and commanding is surprising to me. Remember you have come here to study and learn and not to dictate to me to teach what you want to learn. Learn to follow what the teacher teaches and study with reflection, but do not demand from me and do not try to command me. First behave like a pupil and not as my colleague. You are all at the bottom rung of the ladder of yoga. Perhaps some of you are seeing me for the first time. So all of you should be humble from inside to earn knowledge. Be humble and modest while learning.

Some being beginners and some being senior students, do not demand from me but ask that what is relevant, basic and simple for all of you to grasp. But your arrogance is such that you are asking what has not been tried or started by you.

As pupils, when you cannot do the basic, simple *āsana*, why should you jump for backbends? Your own teachers may say: "Never mind, I will teach you". Teaching yoga is not a business. It does not run on the principle of "supply and demand". Unfortunately, it has been used by some as a business. The teachers who supply according to the demands of the pupils, treating them as customers and consumers, may become popular teachers, but not ethical or religious teachers.

If one teaches according to the whims of the pupils, then it is purely selfish with commercial gain at heart. I do not want that type of teaching from my teachers. The teacher's job is to build up that which evolves the pupil from the physical level towards mental and spiritual growth. The teachers should aim at bringing about a transformation in the pupils.

* San Diego, USA, June 27, 1990.

When you ask for back bends, first find out whether you know your own body. You are not going to get this body-knowledge by looking at an anatomical map. Anatomy is taught and learnt on a dead body, skeleton, or from drawings in the books. The practice of yoga teaches you the subjective anatomy – the live and functional anatomy. It makes one a subjective anatomist. Medical science gives an objective knowledge of anatomy. If the latter is acquired knowledge, the former is an understanding knowledge.

The back bends, which are called *pūrva pratana āsana*, are no doubt attractive and fascinating. The pupils want to do them. That is why you asked me to teach backward bendings – the *āsana* such as *Uṣṭrāsana, Ūrdhva Dhanurāsana, Viparīta Daṇḍāsana, Kapotāsana,*[1] so on.

Though you want to do back bends, there is always a psychological fear from within. The fear is on account of not knowing the function of the posterior trunk. This not knowing the back of the body acts as an enemy that pounces and seizes the body. That is why when there is fear one tenses the fibres, resists the tendons or the ligaments and gets injured while practising. It is not fair to attribute your invited injury to a teacher. Listen attentively to the words of the teacher and then go to the *āsana* with understanding. The resistance of the body and mind acts as an enemy due to the instinctive fear in one's practices. Both overstretching with overenthusiasm and overconfidence and understretching due to fear, are injurious. Know your capacity and try to extend a little more than is possible. By this you learn the art of balancing not only the effort you put in but also the fear and courage.

This is advice to the pupils. Let me advise teachers too. The psychology of most of the teachers is that they look to the stronger side and never on the weaker side of their pupils. It requires special eyes for the teacher to look at the weaker side. Always you explain to those who do things easily. But you do not address their weaker side to correct for them. The teachers need to learn the art of looking. It is easy to appreciate when one does well, when one is good at presentation. But it is very difficult to see the defects which remain hidden underneath the good performance and showmanship. The pupil expresses this by saying, "I can do the *āsana* but it is painful". The pain and defect remain hidden under the garment of pride. Often one side or one part of the body remains stronger and aggressive, and one obviously attempts the *āsana* with efforts from the stronger side. The weaker side gets neglected and it hides itself without participation. The pupils will not be knowing what they are doing and how they are doing, but the teachers cannot neglect this important and vital point. They need to develop the eye to look at these hidden and dormant defects. The skill of the teacher lies in this visualisation and correction. The teacher may demand a workout from the pupils and be satisfied with what the pupils have done. This is a kind of pride or heedlessness in the teacher. But remember that the responsibility

[1] See *Light on Yoga*, Harper Collins, London.

does not cease. On the contrary, the responsibility begins here. After teaching or making the pupils perform, the teacher needs observation and introspection and recollection of how the pupils fared, where the defect was, what happens when mistakes are made, what is correct and what is incorrect.

Why should there be complaints regarding *Sālamba Śīrṣāsana?* Without seeing the weaknesses in students bodies, the teachers teach *Sālamba Śīrṣāsana*[1] and I get letters to solve their problems. The one who taught becomes free but not me! Such things should not happen. In case you do not know how to correct, feel free to approach the senior Iyengar Certified teachers. You all belong to one Iyengar Yoga community. Tell the pupils that there is an experienced Iyengar Yoga teacher very near us to whom they will take you for advice so that you and I can work with confidence and clarity. In the case that the one you come across has not had the experience of the problem you are facing, then find out others who had undergone training with me for a long period. This way you may find somebody who can help you the right way to teach or ask me for guidance. This kind of approach is found even in Vedic times. The *Upaniṣad*[2] says that when the solution was not found, the teacher along with pupils went to the masters. But they did not teach something when they were not sure about it. Similarly, you as a teacher should not play upon the pupil's body and mind when you cannot handle them correctly. This becomes unethical teaching.

As a teacher when you teach a new *āsana*, or as a pupil you do a new *āsana*, both have to know their responsibilities. As a teacher, you have to see that you do not teach wrongly. Your teaching, though limited, should be a correct and positive one. Similarly, the pupils should listen to the teacher's explanation properly, watching the teacher's presentation carefully. The teachers should be precise in showing the actions and adjustments, emphasising key points. They should use apt words so that the pupils do not misunderstand or misinterpret. They should not be misguided. The pupils on the other hand should see, watch and listen so that they absorb the instructions properly in order to translate them on the body.

If you as a teacher or a pupil remain irresponsible, then wrong habits will be formed. Habit does not break easily. In order to become a yogi or a yogini, one has to have a flexible and mobile intelligence. Habit makes the intelligence rigid. Rigid intelligence does not take us to the level of understanding the finer points. Break that rigidity and make the intelligence become pliable. Pliability and expansion of intelligence alone help to build up the policy of give and take. Rigidity cannot take nor give. The body and mind will not accept the good and correct method, or reject the bad and incorrect method. You really need to be careful.

1 See plate n. 28.

2 *Chāndogya Upaniṣad,* V.5.1.

You do not know how to teach the healthy person *Sālamba Śīrṣāsana*.[1] Now you ask how to teach when there is an injury to the brain. When there is an injury you have to be doubly careful.

As regards a person with brain injury, one has to get feedback from him before advising *Sālamba Śīrṣāsana*. One has to begin by introducing the *āsana* where the flow of blood does not rush towards the brain cells but is made to percolate or seep through them, before attempting *Sālamba Śīrṣāsana*. Build up courage in them by resting their heads; in (b) *Uttānāsana,* on a stool; in (c)*Prasārita Pādottānāsana,* with support for the head; in (a) *Adho Mukha Śvānāsana* with support; and legs resting on a stool in (d)*Halāsana* which makes the brain get aclimatised to the blood flow. Then they can attempt (e) *Sālamba Śīrṣāsana* first by resting the head on the blankets, with legs bent and then straight with feet on the floor so they are made to get used to the head-down position before taking them into *Sālamba Śīrṣāsana*. Give the sequence in such a way that it protects them from harms and injuries and build up confidence physically, physiologically and psychologically.

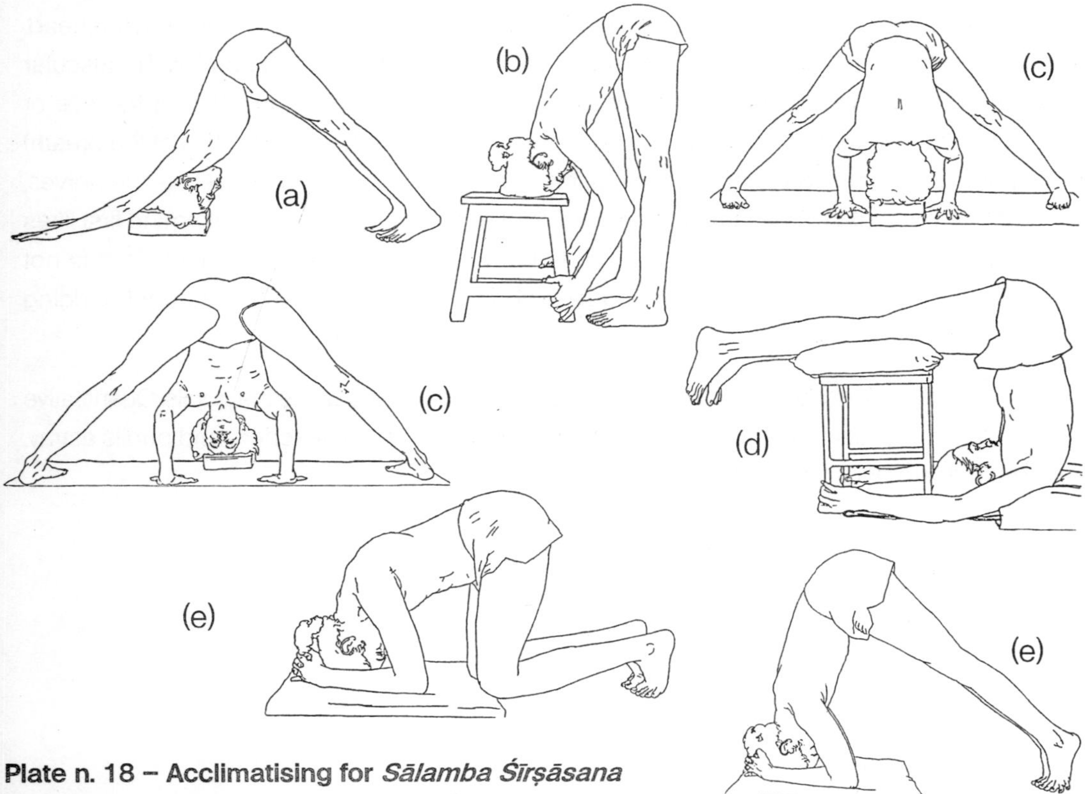

Plate n. 18 – Acclimatising for *Sālamba Śīrṣāsana*

1 See plate n. 28.

I have taught many who have come to me with brain injury. There was a woman who was injured when her house was robbed. She got up in the middle of the night as she heard a sound and the robber hit her on the head with an iron rod and she fell unconscious. Later, she was hospitalised for treatment. The head-ache and blackout persisted for years. Finally, somebody suggested my name to her. It took six months for her to get rid of dizziness and blackouts. While teaching, I had to be careful throughout since she was having these during *āsana*. Later she did *Sālamba Śīrṣāsana* with comfort and began driving a scooter after a break of years.

Let me explain about *prāṇāyāma*. Someone asked me to teach *antara kumbhaka*. See how your demands are. They are not only irrational and illogical but also destructive. As the butterfly goes from one flower to other, your minds flit to anything. Somebody asks for back bending, somebody asks for *Sālamba Śīrṣāsana*. Somebody asks suddenly for treatment of injury in the head and someone for *antara kumbhaka prāṇāyāma*.

For each *āsana* and each *prāṇāyāma* there is a sequential approach. You cannot pick up anything that you want when your body, mind, awareness and understanding of intelligence are unprepared. Whoever does *kumbhaka* egotistically, feels irritation and heaviness in the head. If one feels irritated after *prāṇāyāma*, one has done inhalation retention not only with muscular tension for a longer period, but also forcefully. If one has a headache, irritation in the eye or itching in the ear, know that it is a sign that you have done *kumbhaka* (the holding of the breath) without paying any attention to the position of the spine, chest and head, as well as the nerves, brain and the very breath. You cannot force *kumbhaka* on the body or mind. Your mind first likes to concentrate on the duration of holding of the breath – "Can I hold on longer?" That is not breath control, rather it is violence on the body, mind and breath. Duration is quantity but doing it properly and rightly is quality.

The teacher's responsibility is to teach qualitatively in order to guide the pupils. Quantitative teaching may prove futile. Quantity without quality may lead both the teachers and pupils astray. Quantity builds up pride and ego. Quality brings humility.

ADVICE FOR PRACTITIONERS*

Today is *Patañjali Jayanti.* Tomorrow will be *Naraka Chaturdashi,* which we all celebrate as *Diwāli* or *Dīpāvali.*

Dīpāvali is the festival of lights. That conveys us many things. It is the festival which expresses the conquest of evil and the path towards the light of knowledge. It is a festival of enjoyment, and on this day we meet and greet our near and dear ones as well as our friends and well-wishers.

Though the human being is a beautiful and wonderful creation of God, yet man has invited moral and mental weaknesses by his way of thinking and working. Lord Krishna, in *Bhagavad Gītā,* gives the list of *asura saṁpad* – the demonic qualities. Narakāsura was a demon in whom the demonic qualities had reached such an intensity that people under his regime were experiencing nothing but the hell of suffering. *Narak* means hell. On *Naraka Chaturdashi* Lord Krishna killed Narakāsura and brought freedom to the suffering.

Our *cittavṛtti* is somewhat the same as *naraka.* The *vṛtti* of man are neither trained, nor tamed nor cultured. The *vṛtti* shape the mental faculty of man. His mind *(citta)* is nourished and nurtured on *vṛtti.* The five *vṛtti,* namely correct knowledge, illusive knowledge, delusion, sleep and memory, construct our mental faculty. However, these indisciplined *vṛtti* get mixed, overlapped and multiplied in our vast chamber of *citta,* oscillating our thinking process and actions. Often *vṛtti* mislead our thinking processes and actions. Patañjali calls these *vṛtti, vitarka vṛtti* – the defective thinking process which leads towards dubious knowledge. The reason behind dubious, illogical and unethical knowledge is basically because of *lobha* – desire or greed, *krodha* – anger, and *moha* – delusion, infatuation. The thinking of man is based on these weaknesses of the mind. The crop will be according to the quality of the field. When the field of man, i.e. the mind is itself of a poor quality with desire, anger, greed, delusion, pride and jealousy, the action based on it would be pain, sorrow, grief and ignorance.

---

* From *Yogadoot,* nº 2. May 1993.

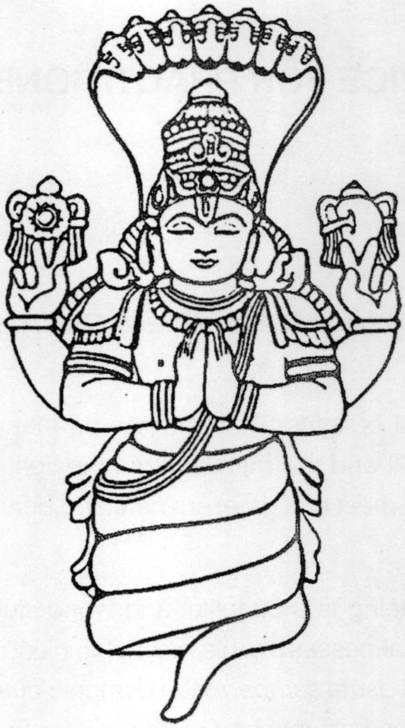

Plate n. 19 – Patañjali

Our thoughts and actions sprout from *ahaṁkāra* and *buddhi* and often a clash between these two would be there. *Ahaṁkāra* on its part misdirects and misleads due to lack of discrimination. One needs to develop the quality of discrimination *(vicāra śakti)* and the power of deliberative thinking. When the thoughts and actions are provoked by *ahaṁkāra, buddhi* has to intervene to advocate and administer the power of discriminative thinking.

Dubious knowledge creates *naraka* in us. The crop of demonic qualities grows abundantly faster. We need the crop of divine qualities – *daivī saṁpad.* We need to sow the seed of discriminative thinking so that the *vṛtti* are disciplined and channelled in the right way. The misguided and misleading *vṛtti* bring distress. These are tormenting and painful *vṛtti – kliṣṭa vṛtti,* whereas unstressing, untormenting *vṛtti* are *akliṣṭa vṛtti.* We have to vanquish this *kliṣṭa vṛtti,* the *Narakāsura* within us which creates dubious thinking and then leads towards inauspicious actions.

See the icon of Patañjali (above) with folded hands in the hall. His folded palms (the *ātmānjali mudrā*) are the symbol of humbleness. This is same of the *daivī saṁpad.*

By this what has to be learned is to submit yourself to the cosmic force (God) and drop the *naraka* caused by *ahaṁkāra*. The moment you drop the *ahaṁkāra*, the facets of wisdom surface.

Patañjali is an incarnation of a dignified gloriousness. He says, develop friendliness *(maitrī)* towards those who are happy, compassion *(karuṇā)* towards those who are in sorrow, gladness *(muditā)* towards those who are virtuous and neutrality *(upekṣā)* towards those who have vices. If somebody is happy and well placed in life, we may develop malice and hate. If someone is in sorrow we may remain indifferent, heedless and selfish. When somebody is virtuous having divine qualities, we may land up in sorrow because we feel we lack such qualities, and when somebody has vices we may be friendly with them. Know that *Narakāsura* will be born out of all these qualities feeding the ego *(ahaṁkāra)*.

Patañjali does not talk about non-friendliness, animosity, non-compassion, hate or unasked involvements but on positive qualities like friendliness, compassion, gladness and indifference or rather neutrality. Learn to develop such qualities and find out yourselves what happens. All these qualities are hidden in us. We only have to bring them up in action.

Today being *Patañjali Jayanti* and *Dhana Trayodashi*, we have to adopt and assimilate the meaning of this *sūtra*, *maitrī karuṇā muditā upekṣāṇāṁ sukha duḥkha puṇya apuṇya viṣayāṇāṁ bhāvanātaḥ cittaprasādanam* (*Y.S.*, I.33). It is through cultivation of friendliness, compassion, joy and indifference to pleasure and pain, virtue and vice, that the consciousness becomes favourably disposed, serene and benevolent.

These four facets cultivate character in us which lead us to knowledge in the form of *vitarka*, *vicāra*, *ānanda* and *asmitā*. *Vitarka* means analysis, *vicāra* means synthesis. With this two sided blade comes clarity. This leads to joy or *ānanda*, and *asmitā* then leads one towards the study of 'I', or me or mine. By this *tamas* and *rajas* are conquered and the *sāttvic* level of *ānanda* rises up and tells you that you can now understand "me". This may take a life or even lives for us to experience and understand its hidden meaning.

In one single *sūtra* he has brought the *daivī saṁpad* and wants the yoga *sādhaka* to drop his *kliṣṭa vṛtti* in order to move towards *akliṣṭa vṛtti*. In short, it means the education of our *vṛtti*. He wants our *citta-bhumi* not to be a hell *(naraka)* but to be a heaven. Let us cultivate these four aspects of human character so that we become cultured.

So in the beginning, Patañjali gives us *citta vṛtti nirodha* by which we may understand the quality of demonic nature and be able to still it.

Patañjali has given us a method to eradicate dubious knowledge – *vitarka* or *viparīta tarka*[1] – into *viśeṣa tarka*.

Patañjali gives us a methodology to think so that our thinking process remains on a proper track. If *maitrī, karuṇā, muditā* and *upekṣā* are four pillars to build up the human character, then *vitarka, vicāra, ānanda* and *asmitā* are four pillars to build up the human intelligence.

Patañjali introduces these four pillars of *prajñā* to cleanse our thoughts so that we come in close proximity of *saṁprajñāta samādhi* with right knowledge. We as aspirants of yoga have to develop this methodology from the very beginning of our *sādhanā*. *Vitarka* means analytical thinking from which to infer. It is the process of analysis. *Vicāra* is proper reasoning in order to reach a result after a complete logical deliberation. Logically, certain things might be correct but they may be impractical. *Vicāra* in this sense is synthesis. With *vitarka* and *vicāra* clarity comes. This clarity in intelligence leads one towards *ānanda*. This is a state of elation or bliss. *Ānanda* is a pure state of untainted happiness. When the thinking process and deliberation are cleansed, the weeds of *viparīta tarka* are eradicated: with the absence of *viparīta tarka* of *krodha, lobha, moha* (anger, greed, delusion), the *sādhaka* gets free from doubts and dubiousness and enjoys pure and true happiness.

Now, let us study *asmitā*. The I-consciousness *(asmitā)* in its grossest form manifests as pride and ego, leading towards selfishness. But in its subtle form it is very close to Self. The words "I am" indicate our existence, our presence. In Sanskrit, *aham* means 'I' – the very pure existence of one, and *asmi* means 'am'. *Asmi-tā* is "am-ness" and not I-ness or I-consciousness. It stands for *ātman*. This 'Universal I' is the *ātman* in you, in me and in everyone.

We need to go to this pure form of am-ness where there is no pride and no attachment. This *asmitā* is the cultured self on the verge of pure Self. For this we need to build up these four pillars of *prajñā* in order to eradicate the defects *(doṣakṣaya)* in us.

Teachers especially should develop or raise the level of their intelligence and be humble at the same time. While teaching have a *maitrī-bhāva, karuṇā-bhāva, muditā-bhāva* and *upekṣā-bhāva* towards the students as each one belongs to different categories. Some may be doing better than you, some may be suffering, some may achieve quicker than you and some might be a hard nut to break.

---

[1] See the footnote on pages 152-153, in the article "Parallelism Between Yoga and *Āyurveda*".

While teaching, do not teach in a way which may mislead the students. See that your teaching, explanation and presentation is logical, practical, reasonable, and brings happiness to the students first and then leads them towards Self-realisation.

On this *Dhana Trayodashi* and *Dīpāvali* festival, let us receive the message of Patañjali in a positive and practical manner. Let us worship and acquire the wealth *(saṁpad)* of divine qualities. On *Naraka Chaturdashi* day, one applies oil to the whole body and takes a head-bath *(abhyanga snāna* or *gangā snāna)* for one's own purification and sanctification. It is a religious ceremony in everybody's house. Let us have a bath which purifies our intelligence through the four states of *saṁprajñāta samādhi*. So let us have this *jñāna-gangā snānam* – consecrating bath, for the intelligence to shine brightly for one to face the Self.

Then it is a *Diwāli* day for all of us. Let us light the lamp of *ātmajñāna*. Let us live in bliss *(ānanda)*. Let us have the fire-works of *buddhi* (intelligence) by which to see the grandeur and splendour of soul.

GURU – BEACON OF LIGHT AND WISDOM*

Guru is one who is full of knowledge, full of light. *Pūrṇimā* is a full moon day. The sun throws the light and the moon receives it. *Guru* too who is full of knowledge pours that knowledge for his disciples to receive it. Therefore, this day is called *Guru Pūrṇimā*. It is a very significant full moon day on which to celebrate the *guru-śiṣya* relationship.

MY *GURU*

You heard that my book *Light on Prāṇāyāma*[1] received a national award. I am very happy that I received the *prasāda*, in the form of a national award on this very *Guru Pūrṇimā* day. This award, I received through the blessings of my *guru* and yoga. Yoga is my *guru*. Yoga alone taught me yoga.

My *paramparā* is traced back to God. This yoga is presented to us by Patañjali, who is also my *guru*. Patañjali says that God is the first, foremost and absolute *guru* unconditioned by time and ever present, who guides us from within. He is also my *guru*. This *guru* is nearest and dearest to me. He dwells in my heart and speaks to my heart, and I salute Him who is within me.

When I look back myself, I feel surprised how the Lord residing within guided me! In 1935 I simultaneously started practising and teaching yoga. I never thought that the tree of yoga would grow like the banyan tree. I never thought that the hidden knowledge will sprout in such a gigantic manner. I am grateful to my *guru*, who sowed the seed of interest in me in his own rough and tough way. But the seed survived and grew into a tree giving me a magnanimous fruit. It was my fate that I had to go to my teacher at Mysore for domestic help. But through fate I was fortunate enough to receive this knowledge. I got converted to yoga; and the faith in it uplifted me to this level.

---

* Talk on *Gurupūrṇimā*.

1 Harper Collins, London.

In those days I was like a person possessed. I was possessed by yoga. There was nothing but a single thought "yoga" in my wakeful or sleepy or dreamy, or aware or unaware states. I was haunted by yoga consciously, unconsciously, subconsciously and perhaps even supraconsciously.

I am also thankful to you, my students of yoga, who indirectly acted as my teachers. But for you I would not have communicated this art. You all committed mistakes. The more you committed mistakes, the more homework I had to do to correct myself as well as you. Your differing natures taught me how to communicate and impart this knowledge. At that time yoga was not an accepted art as it is today. People were looking at it with an indifferent attitude. I first worked to make them accept it as an art. I made them understand it as a science, and then made them absorb it as philosophy or as a way of life.

QUALITIES OF A TEACHER

Yoga is a subject which has to be taught with full love, devotion and proper communication. When you make me sit on a platform and you sit down to listen to me, there is little communion. Often in the classes, while teaching, my harsh voice and intensity in teaching are mistaken for intemperate behaviour. This is because of the often quoted and misplaced notion that a teacher has to talk sweetly.

I grasp the mistakes fast. I read your mind faster than yourselves. My body and mind vibrate while teaching. Therefore, my adjustments are quick. The mistakes that you commit may take years for you to realise. One does not know how deep the mistakes penetrate within. By the time you realise this, you are lost; so I show my quickness in correction. This is mistaken as harshness. My eyes move faster than yours. I catch the mistakes instinctually and instantaneously even if thousands of people are in front of me. I am not a person of the type who say "go slow and learn". If I can catch the mistakes and correct you, why should I go slow? How can you go slow? Do you know, when the toast is hot, you can butter it quickly, smoothly, evenly and more nicely than when cold. Similarly, I too toast you so that the impurities are burnt faster. You can do your own buttering.

Secondly, while practising or teaching, I am not Iyengar. Something inside kindles me to forget myself and makes me an impersonal entity.

Another meaning of *guru* is weight or heaviness. It is a weight of knowledge that the *guru* puts on you. Those *gurus* who are light as far as knowledge is concerned pretend that they are sweet and serene and appreciative of your work. Ask your mind honestly whether it is true or not. If you are afraid to touch someone while teaching and correcting, you may break or tear something; that is why you are slow. One who has a fear complex will never be able to communicate properly or totally. His so-called merciful look is nothing but fear. I have no fear because I have clarity when I teach.[1] It is my dedication which brought this clarity. Can you stop the brain-work of a mathematician who is quick in calculation? You cannot. For you, it may be very fast because you are slow. But you cannot ask a mathematician to be slow. So also, if I am fast in correction, if I am quick in my approach, if my answer is ready before yours, you cannot ask me to be slow.

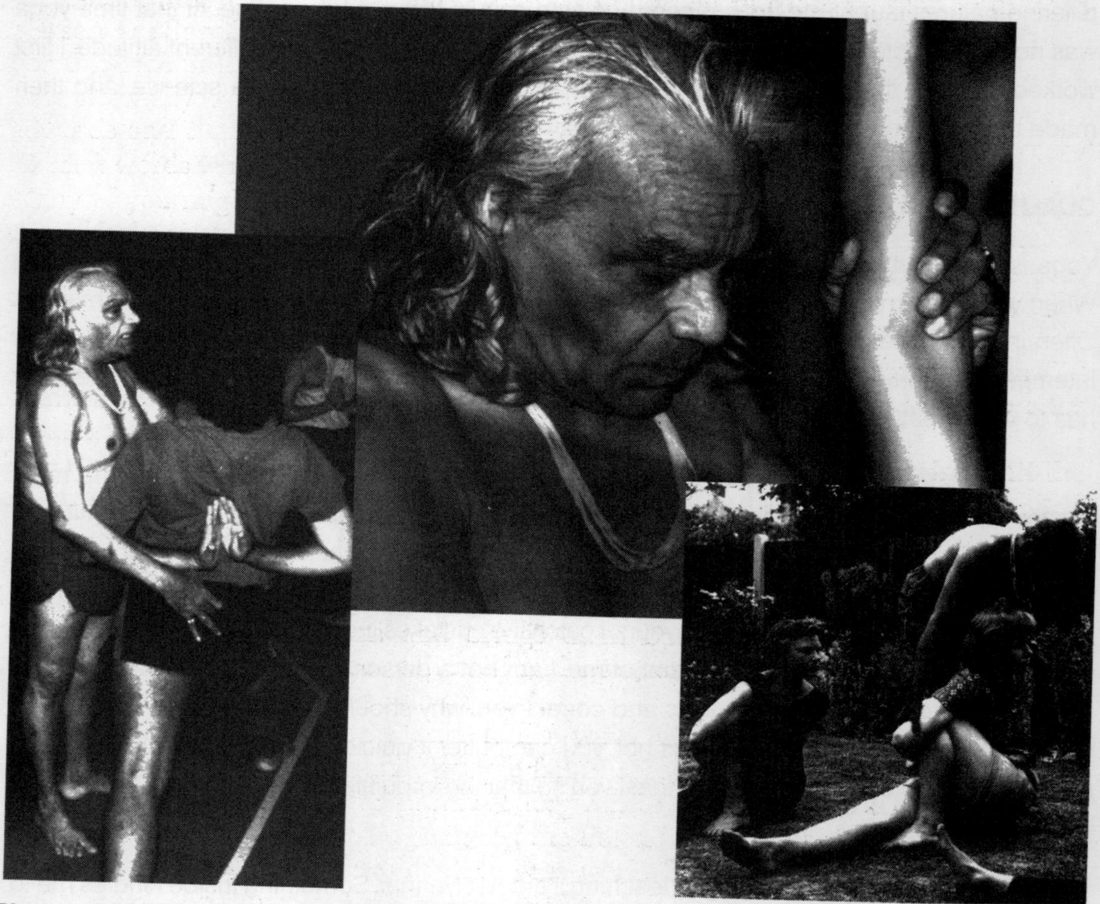

Plate n. 20 – Teaching, guiding, correcting

---

[1] Often the teaching of *āsana* and *prāṇāyāma* is done sitting or standing away from the students. *Gurujī* helps the pupils directly with his touch in order to place the body in proper state in *āsana*. He supports, lifts, extends, moves or turns the body of the person in an exact way and exact place so that the student does the *āsana* and derives the expected result.

If I point out mistakes one after the other, why should you feel insulted? A scientist comes to a conclusion after repeated proofs of his experiments. Then he is accepted because he has already experimented and proved. In the same way, if I have already experimented and have already suffered by committing wrong and ask you to correct yourself so that you do not suffer, do you call it mercilessness? Tell me, should I bring life in you, or allow you to have a merciless death, when I know how to revive your life and restore your health? What is mercy? Should I allow you to go slow knowing well what cannot be avoided without corrections. Is it mercy? Correcting at once in a way you may find hard to grasp but whereby you can make progress, is this approach non-merciful? Search in your hearts for an answer.

Remember, dedication is a very sweet word. It is an enchanting word. At the same time, dedication is a harsh truth. We have the mythological story of king Hariṣcandra, who lost the kingdom, his wife and his son and became a guard at the funeral place – cremation ground. For the sake of holding on to truth, he had to refuse his son Rohitāśva's cremation because he could not collect money from his wife and he could not allow her to the pyre without payment. Then Gods appeared and blessed them all to their previous glory.

VANISHING OF THE EGO

Loving or loveable talks always have some selfish ends. Loving talks do not hurt. However, any hurt or any injury or any loss is recoverable. But an "ego-hurt" is such that you are at a total loss. All your struggle is to see how you save your ego and how you preserve it. You have reserved the place for ego in the head and preserved it in your heart. Then where is the place for God there? Have you tried any day to reserve the place for God in your consciousness? Ego and God cannot both stay at the same place.

Guru pūrṇimā is a day of dedication where the pupil surrenders himself to the *guru*. He follows the words and works of the *guru*. He works selflessly and gains self-respect. As a pupil, if you do so, you need not preserve your ego.

You, being students, are *tapasvin*. One who does *tapas* is a *tapasvin*. A *tapasvin* is a self-disciplined student who practises devotedly. A *tapasvin* practises with full inspiration giving his whole and soul to the practice, bearing all onslaughts. Are you all inspired to become a *tapasvin?* Are you ready to bear any amount of difficulties with full patience? Have you a burning desire to know? Have you the passion for knowledge?

If you are a *tapasvin*, then I am a *svādhyāyin*. *Sva* means self and *adhyāyin* is one who studies. *Svādhyāyin* is one who studies "self". *Sva* stands for the vehicles of the self. As a teacher and a *svādhyāyin*, I lead *sva* (the vehicles of the self), which includes body, mind, I-ness, intelligence and consciousness, towards the self. You think that as a yoga teacher I have to rectify only your *āsana*. No, then it will not be yoga. Rectifying merely the *āsana* will be at a physical and physiological level, whereas in the process of teaching, I touch you at the psychological level; even if I touch your mind and intelligence they do not hurt you much but if I touch your ego, it hurts you. Ego reflects your real nature. Ego is a replica of yourself which reflects exactly what you are and therefore you feel hurt.

As a *svādhyāyin* I rectify your *sva*. When you yourself begin to rectify your *sva*, then you are an *Īśvara praṇidhānin* – or a devotee, a *bhaktan*. A *tapasvin* has to become a *svādhyāyin* essentially, and a *svādhyāyin* essentially has to become a *bhaktan*.

You may be a scholar, you may be an intellectual person, and you may gain a great amount of knowledge. But the soul does not shine as long as the quality of the *sāttvic* nature is not acquired. As long as ego or *ahaṁkāra* is there, the *sattvaguṇa* of *asmitā* cannot shine. Ego, or *ahaṁkāra* is a greater enemy than *avidyā*. The *sva* has a shape. It recognises itself as a pronoun 'I' or capital 'I'. The body, mind, ego, intelligence and consciousness all come under this *sva* or 'I'. This 'I' is just I-ness and not a real 'I'. When this I-ness or seeming 'I' comes in contact with the real 'I' in you, there is a clash and that is *ahaṁkāra*. It is this mistaken identity between 'I' and I-ness which separates one from real 'I' – the soul – and causes the ego to flourish. This ego or I-ness has a shape, whereas the Self is shapeless. I-ness has *ākāra* (shape). The Self has no shape. It is *nirākāra* (shapeless). Therefore, it should be very clear in our mind not to get cheated and misled by identifying I-ness as Self. Therefore, we need to conquer *asmitā*.

For the sake of conquering *asmitā*, not only have you to be a *tapasvin*, but also a *svādhyāyin*. *Asmitā* is a word which expresses *aham asmi*, i.e. I am. *Aham* is 'I' and *asmi* is 'am'. It indicates the existence of 'I' in us. This 'I' which is away from soul expresses I-ness, ego. When it is near the soul, it expresses itself as self. Transform this 'I' which is in contact with *sva* – the seen – so that it reaches nearer to *svāmi*, the Seer. *Tapas* is meant to conquer *ahaṁkāra* and *svādhyāya* is meant to conquer *avidyā*. A *tapas* without *svādhyāya* is fruitless and aimless. *Tapas* has to be done intensively with full inspiration and *svādhyāya* has to be done with full attention. *Tapas* needs intensive inspiration and *svādhyāya* needs intensive attention. Attention balances the inspiration. Overinspiration is harmful. *Tapas* without *svādhyāya* inflates the ego, whereas *svādhyāya* (self-study) imparts the knowledge to understand the real 'I' – the soul in you. Wisdom comes when this I-ness is known as a separate entity from the soul. The *sādhaka* moves from this wisdom towards *Īśvara praṇidhāna*. He surrenders his I-ness to the supreme Universal Soul. The finite self *(jīvātmā)* surrenders and dissolves in the infinite Self. *Īśvara* is God and *praṇidhāna* means surrender or profound religious meditation. So, *ahaṁkāra* has to surrender. Then *avidyā* vanishes and *vidyā* (knowledge), sets in. God being Infinite, the Infinite surfaces. It is like going from one horizon to the other. The more you realise the truth and you surrender yourself, the more the *tapas* is intensified.

Tapas, svādhyāya and *Īśvara praṇidhāna* open new horizons to lead you towards *vairāgya* (renunciation). *Vairāgya* does not come by wearing saffron robes. *Vairāgya* is a quality. *Vairāgya* is to surrender the ego. *Rāga* means attachment. *Vi* indicates negation. *Virāga* means negating attachment. When the ego is surrendered, it is the culmination of detachment – a total desirelessness. *Tapas* is meant to conquer *tamōguṇa, svādhyāya* to conquer *rajōguṇa*, and *Īśvara praṇidhāna,* the *sattvaguṇa.*

PURITY IN YOGA

One needs education in yoga too. It is the way and reality of living. One has to bring the right vision in one self to discriminate between right and wrong and then discard the wrong to stick to the right.

When there is an uninterrupted flow of intelligence passing through you, that is called *vidyā*. This *vidyā* is not the acquired worldly knowledge. It is *parāvidyā*. It transcends worldly knowledge.

Guru and *śiṣya*, the teacher and the pupil, come on one level when both of them drop the ego and they lose their identities. This is called maturity. Until maturity comes, there is a difference. From today onwards follow *tapas* and *svādhyāya* in such a way that the *sādhanā* ends up in *Īśvara praṇidhāna*. *Īśvara praṇidhāna* is *bhakti*, the path of devotion. In *bhakti* there is no differentiation. All are one. All are devoted. All are the servants of the Lord.

Do not practise yoga at a commercial level. Do not commercialise it. Do it with love. Touch with love. Teach with love. It is a subject of dignity. Unfortunately these days, yoga has been commercialised. It is in your hands to maintain its purity. These days anything can be sold in the name of yoga. But I do not want my pupils to follow that track. My directness in teaching, though it may look a bit harsh, is for this purpose. Do yoga as *tapas*, accept yoga as *svādhyāya* and offer it to others as *Īśvara praṇidhāna*.

We are all *sādhaka*, practitioners of yoga. Yoga is the practice and yoga is the soul. When *sādhaka, sādhanā* and *sādhya* (aim) become one, it is union, it is yoga – the goal. You are yoga and yoga is you. Kindle the light of yoga, so that yoga enlightens you to become a wise man.

God bless you!

REFLECTIONS AND EXPERIENTIAL WISDOM IN *ĀSANA* AND *PRĀṆĀYĀMA*[*]

Today being Patañjali Day, this recitation has been a very auspicious start. You heard all the four chapters of Patañjali's *Yoga Sūtra*. I think it is the first time I have heard your pronunciation of the Sanskrit words which was very, very good. That is the way to catch the words and the language. When you repeatedly say and hear, it expresses the meaning of the words without even going through the text to understand them.

We are celebrating the *jayanti* not for the sake of fun, as other birthdays are celebrated, but to review each year and feel to what degree we are victorious in our practices. That is why we are celebrating Patañjali Day, to find out how far the progress has been achieved by ourselves through the grace of Patañjali. We are celebrating this as victory-day in our *abhyāsa* (practices). As yoga *sādhaka*, we have to reflect on what we have done, what needs to be done and how far we have gone and to some extent what we achieved in our *sādhanā*. So, it may seem to be a selfish programme, yet it is essential. The festival of lights also begins today. It is a very big festival in India. For the practitioner of yoga it is more important since he has to keep the light of yoga burning. Once in a while we need to look back on what condition we were in and in what condition we are now. To look back is a lion's eye-view which gives a chance to see what we achieved and where we failed. It is also a bird's eye-view to see what impediments or hitches are in our way, what we neglected and where the fissures have appeared.

We have often heard the exposition of the four chapters of Patañjali.[1] The first chapter offers the whole range of how to reach the end of the *sādhanā* with various views on the subject.

For us, even the very first *sūtra* has a high and significant meaning. *Anuśāsanam* in the first *sūtra* conveys disciplined and devoted practice. So, what is yoga? It is a devoted and disciplined practice to reach the very core of our being. Why do we have to practise devotedly? So that the mind, which moves, fluctuates second to second, is quietened and silenced. How does it happen? Only by discipline.

---

[*] Talk on *Patañjali Jayanti*, 1998.

[1] See *Aṣṭadaḷa Yogamālā*, vol. 1, section III.

Well! All this seems to be easy. Yoga is disciplining the *citta*. Patañjali says, *yogaḥ citta vṛtti nirodhaḥ*. Yoga is restraining the movements of *citta* in order to bring their cessation. The mental current tends to go with the crowd of thoughts. This is the movement of *citta*. As mass psychology has to do with a crowd, the *citta* too follows the crowd of thoughts. Yoga asks the *citta* to discipline itself. So it does not follow the crowd, but it follows its leader – the soul.

In order to reverse the journey of *citta*, a support is required since it is all alone on the reverse journey. This support is called *ālambana* by Patañjali. For instance, there are two types of *samādhi – sabīja* or *ālaṁbana* and *nirbīja* or *nirālaṁbana*. *Sabīja* is with support whereas *nirbīja* is without support.

I am not speaking of the support in *samādhi* now. I am speaking of the support which is needed in order to develop devotion and discipline of consciousness which are essential for spiritual growth. Patañjali speaks of the fluctuations of mind, ego, intelligence and consciousness. All these change second to second. Hence, he wants us to follow a discipline with support, as the quietening of fluctuations depends on support.

In order to diminish the fluctuations of *citta*, Patañjali gives various alternative methods, one after the other. Though I am not going into detail with each method, I would like to invite your attention on a beautiful, educative and scholarly *sūtra: viṣayavatī vā pravṛttiḥ utpannā manasaḥ sthiti nibandhanī*[1] (*Y.S.*, I.35). *Viṣaya* means thought waves or objects. He wants us to find out whether the thought wave or the object illumine us or not. He suggests we take the object as a focal point, which will illumine us. If we go with that one thought, our mind automatically comes to a state of steadiness. When it comes to a state of steadiness, then the consciousness, which is closer to the mind, appears. This consciousness expresses itself when the mind is quiet. Particularly when you are doing the practice of *āsana*, I have given you the experience of understanding this *sūtra*. When you are doing *Sālamba Śīrṣāsana*, *Sālamba Sarvāṅgāsana*, *Setu-bandha Sarvāṅgāsana* or *Halāsana*,[2] the senses of perception are drawn inwards. When you are awake but not doing yoga external objects create ripples in the mind which take you outside. When you are doing yoga, you are awake without the influence of external objects and hence there is no room for ripples in the mind. Especially, in the above mentioned *āsana*, you experience this state.

---

1 The consciousness becomes also composed, serene and benevolent) by contemplating an object that helps to maintain steadiness of mind and consciousness.

2 See *Aṣṭadaḷa Yogamālā* vol 2, plate n. 5.

While you are doing these *āsana,* the senses of perception, namely eyes, ears, nose, skin and tongue, which often go out to acquire objective knowledge, are reversed and turned inwards, so that you feel that you are moving towards the core. You are cut off several times from outside thoughts, though it is not a continuous process because you are all still beginners. Therefore, it is "interrupted quietness". As you have all experienced this, I say this is an achievement for you. What I am indicating is that when you are doing these *āsana,* your senses of knowledge are completely quiet and silent and there is no chance for thirst for outside objects.

When you are inhaling, you take in the breath, and say we have filled the lungs. Do you not? But while the breath is going in, something springs up and expresses itself. Have you ever noted that? You can try, with slow inhalation. As you are inhaling, the breath goes in, but something which is dormant, which is hidden, slowly surfaces and makes room for the inbreath to be engulfed in your lungs. This is what you have neither noticed nor studied. As you are inhaling, as the breath goes in, your very core gives room for the breath to enter in and at the same time makes the mind remain non-existent. This conveys the feel of *viṣayavatī vā pravṛttiḥ utpannā manasaḥ sthiti nibandhanī* (*Y.S.,* I.35). Here the mind is stable, but you realise there is something higher than the mind which moves through your inhalation. This is the hidden dormant life-force which we call self, surfacing in your existence.

Similarly there is one more attractive *sūtra* which draws your attention. While you are doing the *āsana,* often you feel the meaning of *svapna nidrā jñāna ālambanaṁ vā* (*Y.S.,* I.38), and experience their states of consciousness. Here Patañjali wants the *sādhaka* to study and recognise the different levels of consciousness to that of the wakeful state of consciousness, so that the stable knowledge *(sthirajñāna)* is built up in the *sādhanā.*

For example, in sleep your mind is in *abhāva pratyaya* state. The *citta* experiences absence of thought waves. There is no fluctuation in the *citta* in sleep. Not knowing anything is the modification of mind in sleep. Fluctuation in sleep is a dream. In the wakeful state often the mind behaves as if you are dreaming. In sleep, we recognise the fluctuation of *citta* as dreams, while in a waking state we recognise it as the wandering of *citta.* The knowledge from the sleep is that the mind is in a steady quiet state. So in the *sādhanā;* simulate the quality of sleep, without allowing the mind to wander. Sometimes your mind will be wandering while doing *āsana.* That is why I used the words "interrupted quietness". You learn consciously with the support of the knowledge of sound sleep, not to have fluctuations while doing *āsana* or *prāṇāyāma.* Then there will be no fluctuations in your senses of perception, as the mind has moved inside. When it is withdrawn, it traces something new which keeps you alive and active. This new feeling, new experience, takes you near, closer to the experience spoken of by Patañjali, *viśokā vā jyotiṣmatī*[1] (*Y.S.,* I.36). Let me give you a glimpse of it.

At certain times when you are doing *āsana*, you feel exhilarated; you are full of joy. At that time, what is it which brings the feeling of exhilaration? For a while you feel that you are free from *rāga* (lust). You are free from lust and at the same time you experience exhilaration in the practice of *āsana*. You feel as though you have no burden on your shoulders, as though you have nothing to gain and nothing to lose. You remain unattached to past experiences. Have you experienced it or not? This experience is the seed in us, a support to continue our practice further and further in order to reach a state of complete fullness in the entire machine of the body where the acumen is encaved. When there is this feeling, there is no oscillation, your intelligence becomes more sensitive. You put an end to the use of words like "stretch your arm, stretch your leg, stretch your back," and so forth. You remain in *āsana*. You are in *āsana*, you are just merged in *āsana*. You feel the state of *vītarāga viṣayaṁ vā cittam*[2] (*Y.S.,* I.37). You are free from lust, a *vītarāgin,* while practising *āsana* or *prāṇāyāma*. Now your understanding in *āsana* would be the use of your own self-energising force, the very core of the being.

Though this self-energising force exists in the entire human body, mind and intelligence, yet it may be dormant a little here or it may be active elsewhere. Even our intelligence is dormant in certain parts, active-passive in certain parts or shifting from place to place every now and then, or sensitive with a single stretch of the intelligence and the self-energising force in the entire human system as if the body is not charging, but you are charging the body. How many of you have tried to look into yourself in this way when you do the *āsana, prāṇāyāma* or *dhyāna?* Have you ever thought of it this way? Patañjali says that when the consciousness is clear and ready to gravitate towards emancipation, heedlessness or carelessness on the part of the *sādhaka,* fissures in consciousness may appear and distort the consciousness. If this happens to a *sādhaka* who is on a high pedestal, then what about the *sādhaka* who is on a lower pedestal? Therefore, while practising, do not show poverty of consciousness. Feel the flow of sensitivity, touch and spread of consciousness remaining evenly.

Today, I want you to know how to bring these noble feelings to the surface. Let us all observe where our intelligence has been purified and sensitised in our practices. For example, when you are asked to do *Uttānāsana*,[3] have you ever studied the movement of energy? You

---

[1] Or inner stability is gained by contemplating a luminous, sorrowless, effulgent light.

[2] Or, by contemplating on enlightened sages who are free from desires and attachments, calm and tranquil, or by contemplating divine objects.

[3] See *Aṣṭadaḷa Yogamālā* vol 2, plate n. 5.

only know that you are bending forward and your hands are going down. But how do the energy and consciousness spread in the body? Patañjali uses the word *citta prasādanam.* Do you bring this aspect in your practices? When you do *Uttānāsana*, do you ever observe whether your consciousness expands from the back towards the sides, or do you only observe the vertical downward movement? When every *āsana* is multi-petaled, why do you make it single-petaled? In *Tāḍāsana*,[1] have you ever observed that you have to do *Tāḍāsana* with the inner mounds of the feet? Probably you have to think. For some the inner mounds touch the floor, for many the middle mounds touch, for some the outer mounds touch. If there is no equanimity of the petals of mounds of the bottom of the feet, which means they are drying and disfunctions may take place in the other parts of the body. Similarly, is it not so in a flower? These indications of your drying feet will one day say that you have no sensation. Do not lose *Tāḍāsana* action when you do *Uttānāsana*. If the tree is healthy, the flower is healthy. If the flower is healthy, the petals are healthy. As the petals are connected to the stem, so are the petals in the form of anatomical or physiological terminologies connected to the core.

We do not know which part of the mound of the foot touches the floor in *Tāḍāsana*, in order to understand how the changes have to take place in *Uttānāsana*. Actually the imprints of *Tāḍāsana* vanish in a split second in *Uttānāsana*. When you do the *āsana*, you do not watch the feeling of *Tāḍāsana* on the mounds and study the expansion of the consciousness in your side legs, in your back legs and in your front legs. Basically, this expansion of the consciousness comes through the practice of yoga. Withe the practise of yoga you cultivate the intelligence to a state of sensitive alertness that direts and expands the consciousness simultaneously in each and every part of the pose. Without the cultivated intelligence to expand and direct, the consciousness cannot spread. If the cloth is dirty, one spreads it out to be cleaned. In the same way, through the expansion of consciousness, the dirt has to be cleansed. This is what *Pātañjala yoga* teaches us, to develop that sensitivity so that you electrify your practices.

You may be doing *Ūrdhva Dhanurāsana*.[2] How many of you are aware of the upper arm and the exact middle portion of the trunk? Is there a rhythm? Does the energy flow from the back of the wrist to the back of the heel without any division? If there is a division, what have you to do to avoid it? If there is no supply for the stem of the flower, the petals dry out. Similarly you have to know in this *aṣṭadaḷa yoga*, how you handle the petals, namely the muscles, the joints, the tendons, the cartilages and so on, carefully and attentively. Do we look into that? We do not. Because consciously you do not spread awareness.

---

1 See plate n. 27.
2 See *Aṣṭadaḷa Yogamālā*, vol 2, plate n. 12.

Hence, my message to you is that what is cognisable often remains in an uncognisable state. Begin to practise by recognising the cognisable parts regularly, then the parts which remain uncognisable begin to surface. For example, when you place your palms on the floor in *Adho Mukha Śvānāsana*[1] you have to find where your life energy is present and where it is absent, where the life force is active, or overactive, and where passive and inactive.

Use your *prajñā* (awareness) and intelligence so that the feel of the consciousness flows all over in the *āsana*. This is the state of *saṁprajñāta* or self-awareness in *āsana*. Observe that what challenges the body flashes on your intelligence and how it tests you with your own awareness. Bring this co-ordination with the rhythmic action of the body in your practices so that the mind feels and corrects the right flow of energy. Then through this interaction of mind and body, observe whether the consciousness touches the body evenly. So from now on make the flow of energy steady and study the movement of consciousness and find out in your daily practice of yoga how the ingredients of nature *(prakṛti)*, through this given instrument, the body, guide us to evolve and be involved.

With this awareness in the *āsana*, try to spread the Self also. Do the *āsana*, *prāṇāyāma* and *dhyāna*, not compartmentally but totally using the power of intelligence and movement in body, rhythmically. Commune with the energy of the self to mingle with the consciousness, and the consciousness with the flow of energy. This is the message which you all have to strive for to gain *jaya* or success. Then it becomes *jayanti* (celebration).

Now experience what the *Bhagavad Gītā* says, "Do the duty well and do not think of the fruit". At the same time if you read the *Bhagavad Gītā* carefully, it says, "Correct *karma* brings right fruit". Even Patañjali finishes his aphorisms establishing that the aim of the yogi is *kaivalya-avasthā*. Let me explain this with *āsana*. Do the *āsana* with accurate motion and action with a measured breathing, and adjust in such a way that you feel the presence of the soul everywhere. Then learn to come out from the *āsana* with this feel of soul to that position from which you went into the *āsana*. Do them with this dynamic sensitive approach like water that percolates gradually. To reach towards the *āsana* is evolution, and to come out of the *āsana* is involution. This method of evolution and involution is not only by the body, but also from the sensitive intelligence. When that develops, the union with consciousness takes place. Then both intelligence and consciousness merge in the Self. This is *kaivalya-avasthā*. This is the elixir of *sādhanā*. This is the ambrosia of yoga. I hope you savour the ambrosia of yoga throughout your life.

See *Light on Yoga*, Harper Collins, London.

DIRECTION FOR EVOLUTION*

This is the silver jubilee year of our Institute, and the response to this first important function here is so unbelievably great that I am in a dilemma. I am in a dilemma because of the frame of mind in which you have come. Your thought waves are different from mine. This course is not an intensive course like the ones I used to take. Your mind is probably feeling inclined for an intensive class from B.K.S. Iyengar and you may be disappointed that these classes will not be like the ones I used to conduct regularly. This is purely a guiding session for teachers to know their good points as well as bad ones. The idea of this special session is not only a re-learning process, but further consolidation to obtain maturity in the subject.

I think that many of you who received the information about the objective of the course have probably not read the information accurately. When we asked for questions regarding your difficulties in your practices and in your teaching, I received more than 180 questions but not a single one about the obstacles in your practices. All were on health problems. Seventy to eighty percent of the questions were repetitions from different people. Many of these questions have been answered many a time by me during my teachings over the years. This means that the senior teachers who have learnt directly from me and taken up the teaching have their own frame of mind. Therefore the teaching goes not according to the subject but according to their frame of mind. Some questions have been repeatedly answered for the last 60 years!!

This session was meant to solve the difficulties you have in practice and in the art of teaching *āsana* and *prāṇāyāma*. However the questions were more personal, "It pains me now and then." Why is there so much confusion in the minds of teachers to raise their own personal questions again and again? Either you do not communicate with senior teachers or you may be proud in yourselves. Or have I to take it that the senior teachers are not conveying the subject in the right perspective for misinformation and doubts to arise every now and then?

---

* Talk at the beginning of the course for teachers on the occasion of the 25th anniversary of Ramāmaṇi Iyengar Memorial Yoga Institute, 16-22 January 2000.

I started yoga from scratch. You have all seen me, what my practices are and my way of teaching. I have not deviated from the subject though I have moved from the gross to the subtle and from the subtle to the finest. Having taught from the gross towards the subtle, why is there so much confusion in carrying the message to others? That is my dilemma. It is something which you and I have to sit together and give a serious thought to, to work out and find the means through words and actions, in order to move from the bank of doubt and confusion towards confidence and clarity. Let us work together to cross over to the other bank of spiritual contentment, satisfaction and unison in our practice and teaching.

The coming generation will be an unhappy generation as unknown diseases are going to be increasing. Even medical science may have to think, study and understand the symptoms of the coming diseases. Exactly for this reason yoga comes into the picture, as it is a holistic, preventive and a curative system. Yoga will have a big role to play for this generation, as well as for posterity, so that one lives and lets others also live in peace and contentment. Let yoga act as a good seed of health, happiness and contentment.

Yoga is the best means for you to learn, understand and use that defensive strength which co-exists with disturbing forces. If you get confused without giving any thought to trace the cause of confusion, then you are not only the losers, but the coming generations will also be losers. Therefore, pay full attention to what is going to be said and shown in these sessions as they are meant to remove the misgivings, misunderstandings or non-understandings and misconceptions.

Again, I will show and explain from the base, as if you and I have not met before, as if we are facing for the first time to hear fresh words – as if the subject is new and fresh. I will do my best to help you to study yoga afresh so that you learn to become critics of your own practices, sayings, behaviour and teachings. Let us keep aside our human nature of finding faults and criticising others in such quick succession. Let us be quick enough to understand our own differences and weaknesses, and to learn to criticise ourselves and our own shortcomings, so that the study of the subject, as well as of our own mental egoistic behaviour brings us to know our own true state of being. Let us keep our egoistic self aside.

Yoga is self-study. Your mind, which plays a dual role, has to be tested by you. You need to have an extraordinarily sensitive mind to find out your weakness and work on your own, by various ways of thinking and action, so that you become a human being in its true sense. Our aim is always to find faults in others. This habit of finding faults in others is not an achievement. But to find faults in our own selves is a great achievement. This is the reason why and how this session is going to be held.

Hence, I am planning to make you understand the basics of *āsana* and *prāṇāyāma*. You have to grasp these and work on yourselves from moment to moment. Your mind may be stable, your intelligence may be stable but your cells may not be. Or, your cells may be stable but your mind may not be. This differentiation goes on, and you may not have even thought about this. You do not question why you are careful in certain parts and not in others. You only find excuses but not the real fact. Find out how and why does your mind flow in particular spots and not in the entire body. This is what I want to guide you in and to show you how the mind and energy should move harmoniously in your practices. If you can grasp what I show and explain, which I shall show repeatedly, then I say that your doubts and confusions will fade out and good luck will dawn on you all. If you cannot grasp them, then I say it is your bad luck. But with your bad luck do not carry a wrong message! If you have not understood it, then it is your duty to tell me that you have not understood so that I show and explain once again, and later ask your teachers for guidance so that they will be able to explain if they have understood.

No doubt, evolution is not easy. You have to elevate yourself from what you are and what you were. This session will show you what you should be looking for and learning. You cannot say from your mind that this is what I want to be, or this is what I like to do. You have to keep your mind fluid and mobile to accept new constructive thoughts and things. If you cannot keep your eyes, ears and mind open, then you cannot reach the stage of the right foundation at all. If you know the present, then the future takes care of itself. This is the philosophy of yoga where you keep yourself attentive on the rays of your own thoughts from second to second, from moment to moment. There are ways in yoga to minimise or to be free from affectations or prejudices and to take the mind away from these bindings and attachments. Knowingly or unknowingly you change your thoughts and direction of thinking and you must learn to bring them back to a state of awareness in your yogic discipline. Like the charioteer who holds the reins of ten or twelve horses and controls all of them, similarly you should know which rein is loose in your body and which is strong. The strong one may pull in one direction and the loose one may not react at all. If the horses run in different directions when they are gripped wrongly, you fall to the ground. Only if you grip the horses i.e., your capillaries, your muscles, your fibres, evenly as a single unit, will there be no accidents. Both you as a charioteer and the horses (your senses), ride smoothly with the chariot (body).

The other dilemma is that the hall cannot hold more than 300 participants. But, the Indian mind wants to be very hospitable especially if their prestige goes up *(laughs)*. Having accepted their hospitality, I hope that you also accept by extending your own hospitality to accommodate all with a friendly gesture.

This can be possible if you all recollect the *Yoga Sūtra* of Patañjali, *maitrī karuṇā muditā upekṣāṇāṁ sukha duhkḥa puṇya, apuṇya viṣayāṇaṁ bhāvanātaḥ cittaprasādanam* (*Y.S.*, I.33).

We need to learn this *sūtra* from a different angle. I am going to divide it into two parts. *Maitrī, karuṇā, muditā* as the first and *upekṣā* as the second. *Maitrī, karuṇā* and *muditā* are the three qualities meant for you to show to your neighbours. However, the *upekṣā* has to be shown to yourself. If you have to accommodate one and all, keep your *sukha, duḥkha, puṇya* and *apuṇya* aside. Do not be selfish and seek pleasures. In this guiding session I definitely show *maitrī, karuṇā* and *muditā* with love and affection for you all. However, I will be indifferent to myself as far as my health, my pain and my discomforts are concerned.

I hope that when the session is over, this will open a new path and a renewed hope in you and your practices of yoga. With this message let us be friendly to one and all, let us be co-operative, let us co-ordinate with one and all and cultivate a constructive touch in the art so that all of you grow in harmony and concord with no doubts and dilemmas and go back with renewed confidence.

May the session bless you all in this new vision of yogic discipline.

HOW TO SEE THE *ĀSANA**

BE A RECEIVER

You have learned from your teachers various words, various expressions and ways of explanation. Though they may change a little here and a little there, the basic idea must be to get the right and precise *āsana* by co-mingling the various parts of the body and then co-ordinating these various explanations and expressions with the aim of accuracy.

While listening to the teacher, the students should not calculate. Keep your brain as a receiving instrument and leave your problems to the teacher. The teacher is the thinker while teaching, and not you. Follow what the teacher says and incorporate them in your body.

ADVICE TO TEACHERS

The teachers study the students calibre and capacity to introduce the techniques of correct deep breathing. This should be thought of only when the teacher knows that the students are not making mistakes in performing the *āsana*. The one who has perfected himself knows the mastery of the *āsana* and does deep breathing without oscillating the body. Many move and disturb the body when they do deep inhalation and exhalation. If inhalation is inflation, exhalation is deflation. Do not introduce oscillation, inflation or deflation in the body while teaching deep breathing in the *āsana*. Study carefully and then you realise that your deep breathing in *āsana* is like those who breathe when they do physical exercises. Learn and then teach *prāṇāyāmic* breathing without jerks in the body. Better to teach first forward or backward *āsana* with normal breathing.

Disciplined and conditioned normal breathing acts as an organic exercise. Do not say that you are introducing *prāṇāyāmic* technique in *āsana* as Iyengar does not teach this aspect of breathing. It is you who have not given a thought as to why I do not teach deep breathing in the beginning. You boast that you have created something just to earn favours. I have tried all these

---

* July 1, 1990.

long, long ago, and as a teacher. I dropped what is not good for the students. Some follow my teaching, knowing that the breathing techniques emphasised unnecessarily do not help the students to master the *āsana*.

If one says that he is following me, then why deviation under the mask of creation, and that too, which is harmful?

To teach the inverted *āsana* is more difficult than teaching backbends. Beginners do yoga compartmentally, not totally. Therefore, as teachers you have to notice what comes in your practice of *Halāsana* to introduce in *Sālamba Sarvāṅgāsana* and what is coming in *Sālamba Sarvāṅgāsana* to introduce in *Halāsana*.[1] The teacher has to give the understanding regarding the balance, and the spinal work required for the balance of the inverted *āsana* so that students gain confidence.

PRACTICE SHOULD BE AUSPICIOUS

When you are practising, do not just do that for the sake of doing. Learn to reflect while you are practising. Make your mind and brain observe and re-learn what you are doing. Doing is mechanical; learning is dynamic.

Patañjali's *tasya vācakaḥ praṇavaḥ*, and *tajjapaḥ tadarthabhāvanam* is a guide. The Lord is identified with the sacred word *ĀUṀ* known as *praṇava mantra*. Reverential repetition of the *praṇava mantra* with contemplation on its meaning and feeling (Y.S., I.27,28) is real *japa*. Repetition of *āsana* is *japa*. You have to repeat the *āsana* with reverence. There should be devotion in your practice. Then you have to know the meaning of the *āsana* in order to do it effectively with its meaning. Then you have to learn to feel the *āsana*. If you do not know its feel, you oscillate. By feeling, you develop stability and poise. Feel in order to live in it. Convert the *āsana* into a cave for you to penetrate within to be closer to the soul.

Good *āsana* practice develops in involuting the senses, the mind and consciousness. If you are not totally involved, then you become an exhibitionist. Involution is meditation. Meditators say take your senses in. This is what we do while practising or teaching the *āsana*. I hope you understand the meditative value of *āuṁ* in *āsana*. As you are inter-penetrating while doing the *āsana*, your senses go inwards. That is *pratyāhāra* in *āsana*. One should use this *pratyāhāra* in the *āsana* as a springboard for spiritual growth. One does not practise *āsana* or *prāṇāyāma* for the health of the body throughout *sādhanā*. It may be in the beginning but not later.

---

[1] To see these *āsana* see *Aṣṭadaḷa Yogamālā* vol 2, plate n. 5.

SALIENT POINTS ABOUT PRACTICE AND TEACHING

ĀSANA

I. FOR RAW STUDENTS: In the beginning, teach the students the basic techniques, like left foot in, right foot out, in standing *āsana*. Do not go details. Introduce the details when they have learned the basic form.

II. DISTRIBUTION OF ENERGY: Distribution of weight in body while in the *āsana* implies distribution of energy on physical, emotional, intellectual and conscious levels. Just as we have to learn about distributing our weight correctly in the *āsana*, we have to learn about distributing our emotional, intellectual and physical energy.

The students have two different ways of working in *āsana:* some students work from muscular power, as they are inclined to develop the muscles, but their inner movements and refinements are not there because they strain their muscles with too much effort; and some students have less strength due to poor muscular development, but they have the enduring power to bring subtle actions and subtle adjustments involving balanced distribution of weight, effort and energy.

III. CENTRALISATION AND DECENTRALISATION. Each *āsana* is a balance between centralisation and decentralisation. If some *āsana* are done with a centralised focal attention, with no room for freedom and expansion, others need vastness of space in the body for extension and expansion.

One teacher spoke of using certain terms with reference to *Bakāsana*.[1] She said that while teaching beginners, it is better to have the arms kept apart (decentralisation). It may be easy to get the *āsana* with hands apart, but to bring the hands closer and closer together (centralisation) develops lightness and endurance. However, within this centralised tight movement, you also have to create room for decentralisation so that no contraction, contortion or constriction

---

1 See *Light on Yoga*, Harper Collins, London, plates n. 409 and 410 are showing this *āsana* performed as centralised and decentralised respectively.

takes place. The body should not remain untidy in such *āsana*. The chest has to expand and open up. Every cell in the body has to find the intra-cellular space.

IV. FEEL OF HOLDING AND NOT HOLDING: An *āsana* should have both a gripping action, where there is a certain amount of fixity and yet holding nowhere, and also the flowing energy which involves total freedom of movement. Thus, each *āsana* is made up of action of fixity and flow of energy.

V. CENTRE OF GRAVITY: In sitting *āsana (Upaviṣṭha Sthiti)* or in forward extension *(Paśchima Pratana Sthiti)* such as *Padmāsana* or *Paschimottanāsana*, find out the centre of gravity so that one does not lose the balance. Especially in *Jānu Śīrṣāsana*,[1] once you find that centre of gravity, there is a certain weightlessness. Since the weight gets distributed properly, the energy too spreads and flows evenly.

It is much more difficult to discover the centre of gravity in backbends, because often you get excited with movement. Motion and movement are enjoyed by all. However, in order to find the centre of gravity you need to be attentive and steady. In backbends, the breathing remains rhythmic if one finds the centre of gravity in the body.

Patañjali says that the *citta* is drawn strongly like a gravitational force towards emancipation due to the exalted position of the intelligence (IV.26).[2]

The practice of *āsana* should be such that you not only find the centre of gravity on the physical body, but of your whole existence. The *āsana* has to be performed in such a way that the action, movement, adjustment, the energysing process of every bone, muscle, cell, is in touch with the core of the being.

VI. FOR THE TEACHERS: For your own practice, learn how to go deep into the *āsana* instead of doing many *āsana* at a stretch. Learn how to balance the *āsana* with ease and rhythm though the condition and constitution may differ from one to another.

PRĀṆĀYĀMA

I. *PRĀṆĀYĀMA* IN *ŚAVĀSANA*: Beginners should not be taught *prāṇāyāma* in the sitting position *(Upaviṣtha Sthiti)*. They should practise *prāṇāyāma* only in *Śavāsana*. Again, they should choose only *Ujjāyi prāṇāyāma* and learn to work with the inhalations, retentions and exhalations.

---

1 See *Light on Yoga*, Harper Collins, London.

2 *Tadā vivekanimnaṁ kaivalya prāgbhāraṁ cittam.* Then consciousness is drawn strongly towards the seer or the soul due to the gravitational force of its exalted intelligence.

II. THE APPROPRIATE TIME FOR PRĀṆĀYĀMA: It is better for beginners to practise in the evening instead of the morning. Though one is fresh in the morning, one does not understand whether one is doing the movement right or not as the body wisdom is not alert. If one feels nice, then it is a different matter. The evening time is better for the beginner to understand and get the right method of breathing. However, when one is able to practise *prāṇāyāma* in the mornings in a right manner, then alone is the spiritual contentment felt.

III. THREE STEPS IN THE PREPARATION FOR *PRĀṆĀYĀMA*: 1) It is important to be relaxed in the brain and passive in the nerves. Therefore, in the beginning of the practice of *prāṇāyāma* pupils are made to do fifteen to twenty minutes of *Śavāsana*.[1]

Even if one is doing *Sālamba Śīrṣāsana* and *Sālamba Sarvāṅgāsana*[2] before *prāṇāyāma*, *Śavāsana* for fifteen minutes before the *prāṇāyāma* is essential. One should follow the same principle of doing *Śavāsana* after the *prāṇāyāma*.

2) The beginners have to open the chest physically, particularly the sternum and the ribs. There are various ways of working with the pillows placed underneath the trunk to open different parts of the torso. For example, lying over a horizontal pillow makes the abdomen soft and lying over

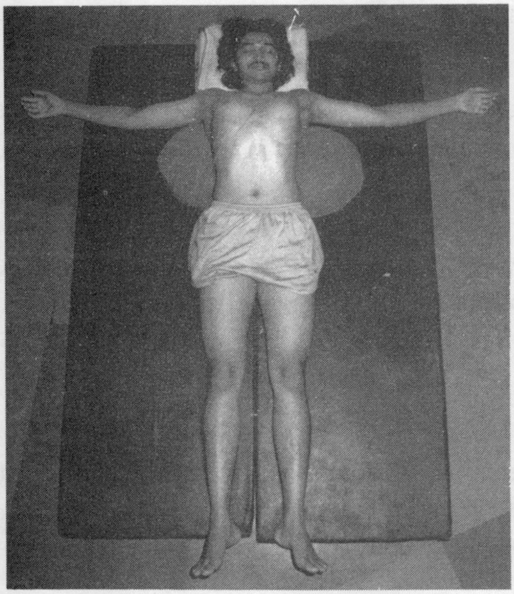

Plate n. 21 – *Śāvāsana* – horizontal pillow

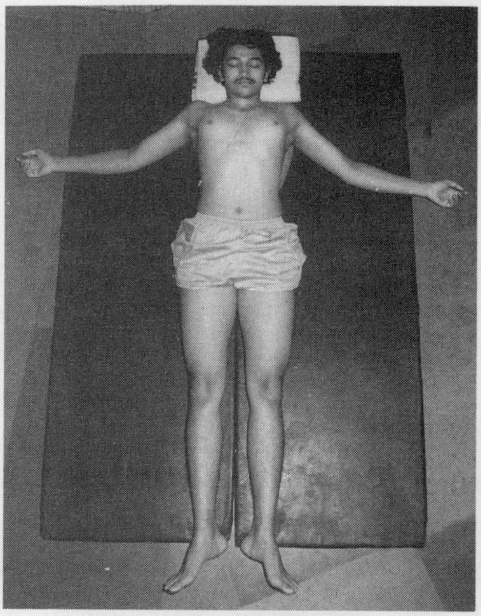

Plate n. 22 – *Śāvāsana* – longitudinal pillow

1 See *Aṣṭadaḷa Yogamālā* vol 2, plate n. 3.
2 See *Aṣṭadaḷa Yogamālā* vol 2, plate n. 5.

a longitudinal pillow helps the sternum and chest to spread and open well. This way one can learn to adjust pillows to get the right feel, which enhances not only the physiological body, but the mental body too.

3) The beginners have to be emotionally prepared in order to maintain stability in the practice of *prāṇāyāma*. They need to get maturity in their minds to go into the depth of *prāṇāyāma*. This implies serious devotion in the practice as well.

V. GUIDANCE FOR BEGINNERS:

1) Observe the exhalation: When you begin practice, it is important to observe first the flow of exhalation. The exhalation leads towards quiet relaxation. Here, you experience the neutral state of body and mind. Know that proper exhalation leads towards proper inhalation.

For some, exhalation is more difficult than inhalation and for others the reverse. In exhalation you have to meet the one who resides inside. You are made conscious of your existence. In inhalation, you get to know yourself. This way you may not have to face fear in exhalation. *Ujjāyi* with attention on inhalation builds confidence and strength.

2) If one does the *prāṇāyāma* hurriedly or hastily, one will find that the flow of the breath gets disturbed. The direction of avenues inside changes. This way one disturbs the channel of the breath. As one gets better one can reduce normal breathing between *prāṇāyāma*, as the channels get opened.

First do a couple of cycles of normal breathing in between the *prāṇāyāmic* cycles, whether *Ujjāyī* or *Viloma*. Then, limit by decreasing the normal breathing cycles by increasing more *prāṇāyāmic* cycles. The mind has to stay fresh with each breath. When the breathing becomes mechanical the mind loses its purpose and begins to wander. You have to bring the mind and *prāṇa* together. It is easy to reach any city on this globe, but the inner journey towards the soul is difficult. *Prāṇāyāma* helps the inner journey.

VI. GUIDANCE TO TEACHERS:

1) Intermediary normal breaths: In the beginning the teacher should make students do normal inhalation and normal exhalation between a few cycles of each *prāṇāyāma*. They should train the spine, the chest, the intercostal muscles, the lungs and the diaphragm. This relaxes the organs of perception and the brain and gives time to 'understand and catch the breath' with care.

2) Unknown tensions arise in the beginning for any beginner. So teach the students to do each movement of breath, carefully preparing the brain to remain fresh. Prepare awareness in normal breathing in order to understand the depth in deep breathing. It is important to cultivate awareness

and passivity in the students when they are learning *prāṇāyāma*. Through the intervals of normal breathing, they gather energy for awareness and prepare the body and mind for a good *prāṇāyāmic* cycle of breathing.

Whether teachers or students, while teaching and learning, both share equal responsibilities. Both the teaching as well as the learning should be done with open eyes – with total awareness.

SECTION VI

YOGA IN SCHOOLS

THE NEED FOR YOGA EDUCATION IN SCHOOLS AND COLLEGES*

Whether one wants to follow the science of duty, earn a livelihood, enjoy life or seek liberation, health is a must, as health is the wealth of everyone. The *Upaniṣad*[1] proclaims that a weakling cannot enjoy the pleasures of the world nor become a master of the self.

Before I deal with yoga and its need in educational institutions, let me define yoga and education as I see them.

For me yoga is character building. Each one develops habits and behaviours without giving a thought to them or to whether they are integrative or disintegrative. Yoga is the reconditioning of the behaviour pattern in each of us ensuring unity and harmony in each and every cell of our body, poise and calmness in the mind and serenity in the self. This is the best personality one likes to possess wherein one not only lives within oneself in perfect maturity, clarity and peace but also with society.

What is education?

The word "education" is derived from the Latin "educare" meaning "to educe", "draw forth", "lead out" or "unfold" the latent or potential, i.e. to develop the talents and gifts of an individual. In short, it is the drawing out of the best qualities of a person. Though the approaches of both are identical, education views objectively and yoga subjectively, hence, the need of yoga in educational institutions.

We are all endowed, in our individual ways, with innate capacities which need to be unfolded. Some of us have a keen sense of truth or justice, of beauty or loyalty. Some, on the other hand, may be extremely intelligent but lazy, indifferent or pleasure-loving; others may lie, cheat and remain selfish.

---

* First published in *Bhavans Journal,* June 11th, 1972; completed in Pune, 6th September 1982.

1 *Muṇḍaka Upaniṣad* 2:4

It is the task of a good educationist to help his students to realise their strength as well as overcome their weaknesses; to contribute to their growth and development on the one hand and to help them to eradicate their weaknesses on the other. Yogic discipline is an excellent aid in such an education for it attempts to remedy the defects and to cultivate the good in oneself. It brings discipline into the life of the student, be it at the physical, mental or spiritual levels, and make him aware of his strength as well as his weakness.

Nowadays, instructions are given in educational institutions to enable a student to pass an examination. They are often confused with the term "education", which is mistaken for a licence to obtain employment and to earn one's livelihood. Of course, one cannot underestimate the need to earn a living, but does man live by bread alone? Is it not his duty to cultivate his own personality too? He must learn to understand his own physical and mental well-being so as to be perfectly conscious of his words, thoughts and actions.

Does yoga help one to build up such qualities?

With my vast experience in daily practice and teaching of yoga, I say without the slightest hesitation that yoga plays a positive role in the development of an individual as an integrated person. The daily practice of yoga helps one to achieve a perfect understanding of the intelligence of the body, for the body has its own intelligence. This knowledge of the working of one's own body is based on direct experience.

For example, the brain may be sure of being able to perform *Sālaṃba Śīrṣāsana*. By this I mean that we may know the technique of doing *Sālamba Śīrṣāsana*[1] to such an extent that we feel confident that we will be able to do it. But when it comes to the actual performance of the *āsana*, one realises that one has to understand the use of the arms, the neck, the correct position of the spine and how it supports the legs, how the legs are to be stretched, where exactly the weight should be and how one should balance by distributing the weight on to the various parts of the body, without putting a strain on the arms or the neck and especially the head. In this way one gradually masters the art of keeping the body energy in a "zero" position, i.e. observing that the energy within the body touches evenly all its frontiers.

By this training one learns what the body intelligence is and what direct perception means. This is the factual knowledge, as the intelligence of the body brings to the attention of the brain a new light, a new experience, and teaches it to adjust or adapt itself.

---

1 See plate n. 28.

This pliability of the intelligence and its capacity to learn from new experience leads one to true education as distinct from an education which depends upon information gleaned from books and lecture notes.

Yoga is a subject that has to be practised and experienced, not merely discussed or argued about. Even if one wants to discuss it or argue about it, one has to experience it. What one experiences is the direct imprint of understanding, and it is the imprint left by this direct knowledge which makes discussion possible. If the experience does not co-ordinate with the mental image or the thinking process does not co-ordinate with experience, then either the experience is insufficient or the thinking process may not be precise. The experience and thinking process, should both tally. Yoga teaches to verify this aspect. This is real education.

Through the practice of yoga one attains not only physical well-being or toning of the body, but emotional stability and clarity in the intelligence. Hence yoga is an educational art which disciplines and develops the body, the emotions and the intellectual faculties, its purpose being to refine man.

Yoga is a science, since it is a systematic study based on the principles so pithily expressed in the aphorisms of Patañjali, and also in other books on yoga such as the *Yoga Upaniṣads*.

It is a philosophy, as it studies the principles of right conduct and shows thereby the road to right living which has a backing of centuries of experience.

The path of right living is paved with eight stages: *yama, niyama, āsana, prāṇāyāma, pratyāhāra, dhāraṇā, dhyāna* and *samādhi*. All these are integral parts of yoga, building the physical, ethical, vital, emotional, intellectual and spiritual needs of all of us to make us really human beings.

As we guide children what to do and what not to do, yoga too insists what not to do through *yama* and what to observe through *niyama*. When children grow, we insist they go and play, so it is the same with *āsana*. Afterwards we send them to school to study and learn. In the same way, *prāṇāyāma* is taught for the study of the mind. This helps to channel the energy and control one's own behaviour and learn about one's own self. From school, the youths go for graduation. Similarly the four aspects of yoga are dealt with in depth to make the students eligible for graduation. After graduation, when they go for jobs or social service, the *pratyāhāra* of yoga guides them to use their lives fruitfully for their good as well with their neighbours. Then comes *dhāraṇā, dhyāna* and *samādhi* to reach the highest summit in one's life, i.e. from Self-realisation *(ātma sākṣātkāra)* to God realisation *(paramātma sākṣātkāra)*. Thus yoga starts with the growth of the body and ends with the fruit of the vision of the soul.

I have taught yoga in educational, cultural, military and other institutions with beneficial effects and I cannot overemphasise the need for yoga among the young today. We live in an era of speed, stress and strain. Such a life makes heavy demands on our nerves, which are but invisible branches of the brain. When the nerves collapse, anxieties and neuroses of one kind or another set in. The individual becomes a nervous wreck. "Prevention is better than cure", and yoga is the "preventive system". It ensures strong yet elastic nerves that can take in a good deal of hectic activity with equanimity and poise. It is the only system, as far as I know, which develops harmoniously both brawn and brain. It can be taught without heavy financial investment and without equipment. It can be done at any time, according to one's convenience and can even be adapted to the needs of the undernourished or the over-fed! Yoga is meant for one and all since it is beyond gender, caste, class and creed.

In countries like the United States and England, Educational authorities, for whom I provided syllabi for *āsana* and *prāṇāyāma*, introduced yoga in 1968 under my supervision.

When yoga has become so popular all over the world, I fail to understand why we in India are still feeling shy to take a bold step. Is it because it is associated in our minds with a recluse who renounces life, runs away from society and isolates himself on some remote mountain top? Yoga is life abundant and not life negation.

Now in Japan, people are going back with a vengeance to the old traditions of its past glory in order to revive their country. They want to free themselves from modern influence. Then why should we not accept yoga, which is as beneficial as it was centuries back? One cannot stress enough the need of yoga for our students. So let us introduce yoga as a drill up to IXth standard, anatomically and physiologically from the Xth to XIIth standard, as mind culture in colleges, and as spiritual culture in Universities. This is the way to form a syllabus in yoga.

In fact, after forty-five years of teaching yoga I feel so strongly on the subject that I would insist on witholding the award of a degree to a student unless he is found fit not only intellectually but physically too.

What I wish to emphasise is a harmonious all-round development of the student in body, mind and intelligence as well as a well-rounded personality with a strong character. Only such students can build a healthy, just, honest and self-reliant character. Therefore education in yoga is a must for a healthy and a happy world for the younger generation.

The beauty of yoga is that it will not necessarily change the world for you, but it will change you for good to face the changing world.

SUGGESTION TO INTRODUCE YOGA FOR SCHOOL CHILDREN*

CURRICULUM IN YOGA FOR SCHOOL CHILDREN

In the absence of a background note, theme paper or draft proposal, I find it difficult to articulate my views. However, I am setting forth my comments and suggestions in the hope that this exercise will lead to serious and fruitful discussions. I need hardly add that a great responsibility rests on the group of esteemed experts and teachers who have been entrusted with the task of framing a graded curriculum for teaching yoga in schools.

OBJECTIVES

We should be clear in ourselves about our purpose in introducing yoga in schools; for, in the final analysis, the curriculum will reflect the pupils' physical and mental growth. Vague or idealistic objectives will result in vague or idealistic syllabi. Vagueness will lead to confusion and idealism will make impossible demands on the teachers and lead the students to frustration. The objectives should be concrete, visible, approachable and practicable. They should begin with the body, the envelope of the soul, and then proceed to guide the content in the body for the realisation of the soul. These objectives can be considered on the following lines:

a) The first and foremost objective should be to improve the health of the students. The word health is being used in a comprehensive sense. It should be *sarvāṅga-sādhanā* wherein body, mind, intelligence and self are involved and yet it should be dynamic, attractive, igniting keen interest in the students to further the yogic practices. The present day curricula train a part of the body at the cost of other parts or without inner penetration of intelligence, from the skin towards the self, or the outer penetration, from the self towards the skin which can be termed *aṅgabhāga-sādhanā* (partial movements of the limbs) ending in *aṅgabhanga* (body in pieces).

---

* Text submitted to the Government of India (National Council of Educational Research and Training) when they had asked my views about the subject. The Hindi translation of this text was published by the N.C.E.R.T. in its *Indian Modern Education,* vol. 7-1, July 1989.

b) The philosophical content at this level should be NIL, as the students have neither the inclination nor the maturity to grasp it. Often, at a tender age, philosophical education makes the students negative. Our first responsibility is to make them positive.

c) The teaching should be universal and free from bias without bringing in any sectarian religious dogmas. It should draw upon physical, biological, physiological and psychological sciences and should have a spiritual base. What is spiritual is universal. Patañjali calls yoga *sārvabhauma* and therefore, yoga is universal. India being a multi-religious society, the syllabus has to eschew emphasis on any particular religion.

Today we can say that discipline is religion and indiscipline is irreligion. Right conduct, right living, is religion and a life of a libertine is irreligion. This does not mean that religious education should not be imparted in schools. It can be explained so as to fit in all religious frames of thought. However, sectarian religious ideas should not be mixed up with yoga as it may create room for suspicion in the eyes of the students who belong to other religions.

d) Psychologically, it should make the students active and alert, sharpen their mental faculties and provide them with a positive outlook on life.

e) The curriculum should be designed keeping in mind the capacity of the average students.

f) It should be flexible enough to be applicable to pupils in diverse situations and conditions in any part of India and the globe.

CONTENT OF YOGA

The word yoga is one of the most tortured terms in use in India. There are so many interpretations of the concept and theory. According to the authoritative text, *Yoga Sūtra* of Patañjali, there are eight aspects of yoga. Of these, the ideas contained in *yama* (abstinences) and *niyama* (rules or observances) can be imparted in other courses which deal with ethics and moral science. Some of the ideas can be introduced during practical training. It is undesirable to offer weighty discourses to children on these matters. Similarly, *prāṇāyāma* should not be taught at the school level. It is a subtler teaching demanding maturity on the part of the practitioner. If introduced at an early age, it may lead to a prematurely aged appearance. *Pratyāhāra, dhāraṇā, dhyāna* and *samādhi* are higher techniques and children should not be exposed to these.

We submit that *āsana* alone of the eight aspects should be imparted to school children. Properly imparted and practised, *āsana* will provide both physical and mental health and lead to balanced growth. Being active physical movements, the children will readily take to them and the practice of *āsana* can be easily corrected. However, the following points should be noted as regards *āsana:*

a) The *āsana* should not be static ones. Anything repeated mechanically will be boring to children. The *āsana* should be dynamic and full of speedy movements. These will attract the children who are likely to be distracted otherwise.

b) Variety should be introduced. Variety not only makes *āsana* interesting but it also makes them purify and strengthen various parts and organs of the body. Changes in variation develop good memory.

c) It should be borne in mind that children are less prone to injuries and they recover more quickly. At present callisthenic methods (P.T. Drill) are taught in schools. The change from callisthenics to yoga should be effected smoothly. We should take care not to cause disturbance during this period of transition.

d) In the initial stages, since the *āsana* are to be taught on a mass scale, they may be done in the pattern of a drill by numbers.

PUPILS

The secondary school covers students from standard V to standard X, i.e. children between the age groups ten to sixteen. There should be graded *āsana* from simple to complex, for students of different classes. Broadly from standard V to standard VIII the emphasis should be purely on the physical level. For standard IX and X the emphasis should be on anatomical and organic aspects of *āsana*. In junior colleges and undergraduate classes the emphasis should be on mind culture. Only in postgraduate classes should emphasis be on the philosophical and spiritual dimensions.

TEACHERS

Any educational experiment or programme will succeed only if teachers have the necessary training and commitment. A few comments are made:

a) It may not be possible to substitute the present teachers imparting physical training, but these teachers may be trained in two or three months' time to take up teaching yoga instead of callisthenics. Or the P.T. teachers may be trained in yoga during their diploma courses.

b) The syllabi for training the teachers will naturally be more advanced.

c) Ramāmaṇi Iyengar Memorial Yoga Institute, Pune, will help to train teachers' provided boarding and lodging arrangements are made by the Government or the schools themselves.

d) It is necessary to offer refresher courses to teachers on a continuing basis so that the teachers themselves will be fit to impart subtler explanations of the same and remain alert and updated.

SCHOOL

Communities in India have been divided into four categories: villages, towns, cities and metropolitan centres. The schools in these areas show wide differences as regards facilities and standards. The syllabus should be flexible enough to be workable under different conditions; e.g. some schools may lack suitable buildings, compelling yoga to be done in the open, or they may have uneven walls or there may be non-availability of blankets for inverted *āsana*.

KRIYĀ

Many in India are very much enamoured of *saṭ-kriyā* such as *dhauti* and *neti*. I may be pardoned for my candid remarks. They are aesthetically repulsive for performing in public and are very messy. These *kriyā* should not be taught on a mass scale. When drinking water is not available in villages, how they can use water for *neti* and *dhauti* and how they will keep the cloth clean, have to be considered. Before introducing *kriyā*, if deep breathing methods are taught, will they not serve the purpose?

PILOT PROJECTS

To introduce on a large scale any programme without testing it on a small scale is fraught with dangers. It is necessary to have certain pilot programmes and on the basis of the experience gained modify the syllabi to be taught on a wider scale. In fact it will be worthwhile to select a few schools and impart different systems of yoga there. This would enable one to compare later and evaluate the technique and approach of different persons and institutions.

EVALUATION

It is necessary to have an inbuilt system of evaluation so that the progress and problems can be constantly monitored.

RECOGNISED TEACHERS

The present policy appears to consider those who have secured some kind of diploma or degree from certain institutions in these courses. This eliminates those teachers who have great proficiency and experience and who belong to institutions which do not offer such courses. Ways and means should be found to draw upon the knowledge and experience of such teachers. So some established institutions of reputation may be asked to recommend their candidates.

SPORTS

Yogāsana should not be considered a substitute for sports at this level. They should be viewed as complementing each other. It is necessary to emphasise Indian sports as they require minimum expenditure and facilities.

It is necessary that we should go about implementing the above programme carefully. A hasty step may create a negative attitude in the minds of the children and eventually yoga training will be considered by most children as an evil to be avoided or suffered under compulsion. While teaching, the subject should not become a mechanical, soulless practice without creating interest amongst the children. Much depends upon the yoga teachers who by their example and enthusiasm can create the necessary favourable disposition in the minds of the pupils. There is a tendency in mass psychology to belittle or berate yoga and make its teaching a thankless job.

I may mention here that I started teaching yoga in 1936 and taught yoga in schools and colleges of Pune as early as 1937 and in National Defence Academy for the cadets and officers since 1955, which is continuing till now. From 1968, the Inner London School authorities introduced my system of yoga which has become a permanent feature of the curriculum. One reason for the spread of yoga was the benefits gained by the parents who consequently encouraged their children.[1]

---

1 I am happy to let the readers know that yoga and *yogāsana* have been taught on a regular basis since a few years ago in Doon School for boys, Welham School for girls and Ann Mary's School in Dehra Dun, Uttaranchal, as a regular subject (both in theory and practice) like other academic subjects. Even examinations have been held and certificates issued, as per their level in *Ārambhik, Prāthamik, Dvaitik, Traitik* and *Pramāṇapatra* so that, if they choose to become teachers of yoga in schools, they can teach with comfort. - May 2001.

YOGA AND PHYSICAL EDUCATION

Physical education means the training of the body for perfect health and harmony. Let me see how the subject of yoga fits in regarding this aspect.

Before dealing with the subject of yoga it is only natural to know what health stands for.

Health is a state of perfect equilibrium where one forgets one's own body and lives in a state of poise without feeling the sense of duality between the outer body and inner body. This feeling of well-being is felt when all the systems of man work harmoniously.

In the present age, science has advanced very rapidly and equally diseases are on the increase too. Pharmaceutical shops are evident everywhere and each shop is crowded with people asking for medicines to gain health, strength and vitality. Though these things are necessary in some cases, it is a folly to run to shops for health. They are not going to eradicate or prevent diseases completely. They may help to some extent but nature alone has to play the role of putting such disturbances in the right order.

Here comes the necessity of *yogāsana*. If one has to live a healthy, harmonious and long life, the training of body and mind is essential. *Yogāsana* not only works as a preventive method but also helps in curing diseases. It is akin to nature. In yogic *āsana*, the quality of blood and its proper flow is maintained throughout the body. Yogic *āsana* do not end only with physical well-being but also work in keeping the body agile and the mind alert and light. The practice of *yogāsana* brings physical, moral, mental and intellectual well-being.

The science of yoga has a broad vision regarding health. While analysing health, yoga explains the impediments which come in the way of health. Normally, we think that when the body and mind are diseased, it is unhealthiness. But the science of yoga elaborates the disease further since it affects one's body, nerves, breath, mind, ego, intelligence and consciousness. For instance, languor and laziness are great impedimennts which make both the body and mind dull, slow and stupid. Similarly, when one doubts each and every thing, it becomes the disease of the mind. Heedlessness and carelessness make every action of ours faulty as we lack proper thinking and a proper plan. It is a failure of intelligence. Having intelligence and the capacity to organise the efforts by which to achieve the expected goal, one may nevertheless remain engaged in sensual pleasures, which we can compare to bad habits or mis-conduct such as smoking, drinking, drugging and incontinence or sexual indulgence. Fickle-mindedness and lack of sensitivity may lead towards failure, since one does not recognise or identify the real aim. Illusion misleads such people. One misses the bus. Some people dream and remain in an illusory world and do not come out of that dreamland and fail practically to face reality. Some strive and put in effort. But in spite of that, they fail which may bring about a sense of inferiority. Some may reach the goal, achieve everything what they want but fail to maintain themselves in that state. Their success culminates and terminates in failure because of their own ego, behaviour, nature, character, misplanning and discontinuity in efforts. Often all these happen because of an unhealthy mind. Weak nerves make one nervous. The body cannot face emotional upheavals. One experiences shakiness in the body because of fear as well as anger. The breathlessness and hyperventilation may seem to be the physical problem but its root cause is in the stress factor and the anxiety of the mind. The weak mind cannot face the onslaught of sorrows and pains. When a person is in misery, the body, breath and mind suffer. The mind, being weak, becomes negative, desperate and dejected.

This analysis of impediments is not only applicable but apt, since everyone experiences these problems in life. We come across people who develop such defects if not in childhood, but later in life.

Each one keeps his house clean and surroundings tidy for a happy dwelling. This body is the kingdom. The intelligence acts as a king and commands the mind to act as a chief. The senses of perception and the organs of action are soldiers. Soldiers need regular discipline to keep vigil on the frontiers so that aggressors are not allowed to step into the territory. Similarly, if this body is not taken care of, disease enters and creates ill-health, unhappiness, misery and so forth. The practice of yoga is needed to keep our inner army ready to fight against the above described impediments so that, by proper attention on the systems of the body, health and harmony are enjoyed in abundance.

Yogāsana can be adapted to the young or old, man or woman, valid or invalid, diseased or healthy without any barrier.

With all these reasons, I affirm that the practice of yoga is the best physical education and it should be introduced to children of school level, so that they could become stronger physically, mentally, morally, intellectually and spiritually to face the unknown future.

SECTION VII

YOGA FOR SPORTS PERSONS AND ATHLETES

YOGA FOR ATHLETES*

Yoga has become a word much bandied about and has been linked with several esoteric groups and popularised by all kinds of pop groups as the Beatles. In the frantic search for spiritual and transcendental experience through yoga akin to psychedelic and hallucinatory experience induced by drugs, the strong physical foundation of yoga has been ignored. For this reason the immense advantages of the *yogic āsana* or postures for athletes and sportsmen have been very largely forgotten.

The Olympic Games being held at fairly high altitude as in Mexico City demand from both the athlete and the sportsperson a degree of acclimatisation if they are to give their best. Various countries have come up with solutions, such as training at high altitudes. Perhaps India with its experience of thousands of years in the practice of yoga can give the most perfect solution to the problem.

Athletics and all sports demand vigourous physical discipline to develop speed, strength, endurance, precision and agility. While the muscular portion of the body is developed, very often the inner organs remain weak or stifled and the mind may actually be dulled. Athletes are unable to maintain supremacy in their fields for very long; while consumption of energy is at a maximum, the recuperative powers are hardly developed. Here it is that yoga can assist athletes and sportsmen.

YOGA AIDS

It is here that the art of yoga can assist athletes and sportspersons. The yogi's understanding and mastery of the body is far more intricate than that of the athlete. It recognises five layers of the human body: the anatomical body, consisting of bones and muscles, the physiological layer, made up of the respiratory, nervous, circulatory and alimentary systems, the psychological or emotional layer, the mental or intellectual inner layer, and finally the blissful state of being. No other system has mapped out with such precision the development of these various layers of the human being.

---

* From *Poona Herald*, Diwāli Special Supplement, 21st October 1968.

The usual repertoire of exercises for the athlete includes exercises for contracting and expanding the muscles. Weight-lifting, running, swimming and playing games develop the anatomical structure of the body, but at the physiological or organic levels attention is nil. We often have a huge bulk hung onto small, poorly developed internal organs. Yoga is not simply content with the external development of the muscles. It believes in the proper communion of the internal organs and the anatomical structure of the body. Freedom and strength are given to the spleen, pancreas, liver, heart, kidneys and all other organs by the same process of contraction and expansion that is normally used for the development of the muscles.

One of the characteristics of *yogāsana* is precisely that it never works only at the muscular level, but muscular action stimulates the circulatory system and inner organs in a particular way, not only by contraction and expansion, but also by twisting and relaxing them.

Also the anti-gravitational positioning of the inner organs in the inverted *āsana* such as standing on the head or on the shoulders revitalises the organs as the blood circulation is improved due to the change of the gravitational pull.

Finally, the attention given to the absence of tension in the organs and to their response to the action of the muscles makes it much easier for those organs to go quickly to a state of relaxation and therefore to be quickly recharged by the energy generated by the practice of *āsana*.

Also, elasticity is given to the intercostal muscles, rib joints and spine as well as the lungs, and the breathing capacity is enhanced by the techniques known as *prāṇāyāma*.

The basic *prāṇāyāmic* technique employs inhalation, retention and exhalation. With inhalation there is an intake of energy. Retention distributes this energy throughout the body, while exhalation expands this energy.

BODY ACIDITY

Sportspersons expend more energy in a short time than they take in. This generates a great deal of acid in the body which results in fatigue and stiffness, making the body heavy and dull. Yogic techniques teach fast recovery from stiffness, heaviness, dullness and fatigue.

Prāṇāyāma also is not just forceful deep breathing by simply pulling the intercostal muscles of the chest box. It is more than that. Each and every remote part of the lungs is made to absorb the energy slowly and rhythmically through the drawn in breath from the pelvic diaphragm to the top of the lungs, so that the topmost ribs feel the full extension and expansion of the lungs. The frontal ribs should move up and forward, while the side ribs should move horizontally. The fullest possible expansion of the lungs is given by these horizontal and vertical stretches.

A heavy shower runs off the ground, whereas a gentle drizzle soaks into the earth benefitting the crops. So also sharp forceful inhalation will not be as beneficial as a quiet steady intake of breath. Retention of breath increases the circulation of blood and keeps the body warm and clean: whereas the athlete uses the upper portion of the lungs while active and the intercostal muscles while resting. With smooth, rhythmic, slow movement of inhalation, the lungs are fully utilised. Similarly the exhalation too is made to move rhythmically and slowly, to reabsorb held in energy as much as possible.

The learning of yogic techniques of breathing is beneficial to athletes and sportsmen and helps them to withstand strain at any altitude. The *āsana* together with *prāṇāyāma* tone the nerves so that acclimatisation is soon realised. The warming-up process in cold countries is helped by the inverted poses such as *Sālamba Śīrṣāsana* and *Sālamba Sarvāṅgāsana*.[1] Yoga also helps in gaining emotional stability and many of the ugly scenes at sport and track meets can be avoided if athletes learn through yoga to keep their tempers under control.

Emotional stability leads automatically to clarity of mind and greater energy output.

Some sportsmen who underwent training at the Institute[2] soon realised the beneficial effects of yoga. Though they spoke to their colleagues about this, their is lethargy in the officials concerning yoga. In 1960 I gave a yogic course to many pre-Wimbledon tennis players at Lady Crossfield's house. Lady Crossfield was herself at one time a tennis champion and pioneered modern tennis kit for girls. Our own Professor D.B. Deodhar practised yoga for several months at the Deccan Gymkhana Club in 1937 and played better cricket after yoga practices. Even today many cricketers, athletes, runners and sprinters are undergoing training at our Institute.

Our hockey team has been challenged for its supremacy. As India is already in touch with Pakistan and several Western European teams, they would do well to learn a few basic *yogic* techniques before proceeding to the Olympics. Recently, we taught hockey players in Pune before they left for Tokyo and the Asian Games. The result was startling. India won. Let us impart yoga on a full time basis to bring laurels to our motherland.

---

1 See *Aṣṭadaḷa Yogamālā* vol 2, plate n. 5.

2 Ramāmaṇi Iyengar Memorial Yoga Institute, Pune.

YOGA AND SPORTS

Yogāsana have a long way to go as "demonstration sports" for the Olympics. But yoga has entered not only the sports field in a big way but also the Olympic consciousness.

At the Barcelona Olympics, according to the media, a pressman was asked to wait as Dr. Samaranch, the Olympic Committee Chairman, happened to be doing his personal yoga practice when the pressman called on him. The great basketball player Kareem Abdul Jabbar says that it kept him in position well past his 40th birthday. Yoga has a profound ability to combat stress in moments of tension when the sportsmen want to put the last ounce of vigour in the final burst of energy to reach the tape, because the intelligence of the body develops quick relaxation before the mind can intervene.

Many athletes have of late discovered that yoga is a tremendous boost to their training because it stretches and relaxes muscles and ligaments. This improves the range of motion and helps prevent injury. It offers the athletes precision in the way of the various positions and emphasises the development of stamina, balance, strength and flexibility as well as meticulous anatomical alignment.

Early this year one of my foreign students wrote to me that coaches of two New Zealand rugby and cricket teams have asked for assistance in the training programme for their players. They are hoping yoga will prevent the increase of "bad knee" and lower back injuries their players suffered over the last year's playing season. On my advice, my student started with the standing *āsana* to cover various aspects of knee and lower back injuries and I am told that they all felt better.

I recall some accounts that came to me over the low key performance of our hockey team in Mexico. The team was advised to do *Śavāsana*[1] before play to gain total energy. Their bodies became cold and they were nowhere in the matches. I do not know from where they got

---

1 See *Aṣṭadaḷa Yogamālā* vol 2, plate n. 3.

this advice. Anybody with an elementary sense of yoga would have said that it would be counterproductive. When the team had to be ready to go into battle a few minutes later, it was asked to lie down. When the opponents made them prostrate, the defeated team and their coach blamed "yoga" for their inglorious defeat instead of investigating if their foot work, team work, running and stick work matched those of the opponents.

Nearer home take the instance of Kiran More, who worked under my guidance. The first impression was that he had grown taller, added a few inches. This was hardly the matter. He looked taller because most of the time the wicket-keeper has to work bending over and watching the ball.

Kiran was asked: The wicket-keeper is the only player in the field who has to be alert every moment. How do you keep yourself that fit?

Kiran: "Plenty of exercise and net-practice. Besides I take guidance at the feet of *Gurujī* (B.K.S. Iyengar). I am well-poised, maintain my mental calm and concentration. Yoga has tremendously helped me to combine quick reflexes with a very high degree of concentration and anticipation about which ball will have flight in what direction and how agile I must be within my reach to get to the ball. Concentration is enhanced by yoga and when there is nothing much happening around in the game I used to get bored and lethargic. Yoga has taught me to be alert even when there is no action under way for a spell."

Do not think that sportsmen have no problems. Azhar sought instant relief and sought my advice. So did many other cricketers and their coaches. Even the English cricket players approached me for help. It's not fair to mention names. I am told that the New Zealand cricket teams did yoga of sports before they plunged into the battle.

I feel that Indians who are endowed with high skills and technique lack the resolve and the "killer instinct" in international competitions. It's a question of morale. If the martial arts combining Zen have helped root the Japanese deep to their tradition, to blaze a new trail in sports and athletics, why cannot our sportsmen and players draw from our ancient goldmine of yoga and its traditions to gain glory for our country? Low profile Indian cricket manager Ajit Wadekar once asked me what he could do about his protruding belly. "Work", I quipped and added: "I mean workout". Yoga is action, every moment, there is no respite from its mill because relaxation too is an action – active relaxation, not the passive lying down. Turning to yoga for reducing stress is one aspect, and we should seek creative interaction with the given basis of life – a fundamental transformation.

Brian Wilkinson, who gave up cycling races, has this to say: "I had needed precise body control and a close interaction of body and mind to survive in the tight situations of hard track and grass-track racing and yet these were challenged as never before by *Tāḍāsana*.[1] Surprisingly it wasn't long before I observed beneficial effects outside my practices".

One of my pupils says that she used breathing exercises, yoga posture relaxation techniques and meditation when working with athletes.

"By using the Iyengar Yoga system, I am able to offer a method of structural and functional fitness and a way of dealing with physical and mental stress".

Sportspersons around the world have found in yoga what was lacking in their training. I feel that our Indian athletes should benefit of this art which is so close to them. As an ardent patriot who wants India to retain its glory at national and international meets, my advice is freely available for those who want to compete.

Sport is one aspect of life. Life is far larger and "whole". While the sportsperson and athletes should strive in their areas of application, my advice to them is outlined in Patañjali's *Yoga Sūtra* (III.47): "They should acquire the wealth of the body so that he or she has perfect formation in the body, possessing beauty, grace, strength and a complexion which is as lustrous as a diamond. And last but not the least, the body should be endowed with firmness and compactness".

---

[1] See plate n. 27.

IMPORTANCE OF YOGA FOR SPORTS AND GAMES

It is a great pity that when we are in this new millennium, sports persons and the administrators of sports have no idea of what Indian yoga can do for the benefit of sports.

Yoga is a direct human science that deals with the upkeep of the whole of man, in physical fitness and for a mentally alert condition.

Lots of misconceptions are in the minds of sports authorities that if sportspersons take to yoga practice, then there must be something wrong with them. What a pity that such educational authorities have no sense to peep into the subject to understand what yoga is or the value it offers to make better sports persons.

Is yoga a pathology – the science of diseases – according to them? Do they believe that yoga is meant only for invalids? Without knowing the value of yoga, why assume that those who come to learn yoga must have some physical diseases or problems? Why not see how yoga cultures each and every part of man's body from the tendons, fibres, ligaments, sinews, muscles, joints, the vascular, the cellular, respiratory, circulatory and digestive systems, mind, intelligence and will power?

If yoga is a science of diseases or therapy, is that why the authorities reject it? If so then why are the so-called physiotherapists engaged? Are they not part of a certain therapeutic science? For me they are more of physical therapists, whereas yoga is not only physico-physiological, but also a neuro-physiological, physio-psychological and physico-intellectual art and science. If the physical body of man is considered as the structured body, the physiological body as the organic body that supplies life's elixir to the entire body, then do the physiotherapists pay attention to the health of the organic body? It is yoga alone that makes all the sheaths of man, woman, boy or girl work and build up to an optimum level of dynamic health, from the skin to the self and from the self to the skin. So yoga is not merely a pathological or therapeutic science but it is an all-round health scheme.

In yoga there are strenuous *āsana* to challenge the stamina and endurance. There are several methods of performance to develop speed and strength,[1] recuperative *āsana* to recover from physical and mental fatigue and at the same time there are several *āsana* which help to keep the needed part of the body rested and rejuvenated. Also, various positions are invented, discovered and re-discovered to get immediate relief. One can provide practice programmes before the game to have alertness, quickness, sharpness, readiness and freshness and practice programmes after the game for relaxation, recuperation and restoration of mental balance and poise. The major importance of yoga, concerning sports and competition, is the re-generation of energy and the re-oxygenation of the body in the shortest period of time and at the same time to be fit and fresh for the next day or the next event. When yoga can give so much, it is a pity that the decision-makers who wield power know nothing of yoga and its benefits. The athletes and sportspersons who practise yoga, have to learn and practise secretly, since they are afraid to express the good that it has done to them, merely because yoga is not recognised by the authorities.

Athletes, sportspersons and players of other games are expected to be sharp, agile and quick in their movements such as running, turning, bending and picking up. For them to achieve this, the mind too has to be trained along with the body. Hence they demand vigourous and rigourous physical training, mental discipline, will power and determination to develop speed, strength, agility, stamina, endurance and precision.

They should also understand that the aches, pains and injuries are part and parcel of all games, be it athletics or sports. Unfortunately today's athletes and sportspersons have the illusion that they can do well at the given time without perspiration or inspiration, without paying any attention and respect to the needs of the body and mind to be successful in games. How do they meet the challenges without training the muscles, the tendons, the ligaments, the joints and the organic body as well as the mind which has to be firm, steady and swift as well, is beyond my comprehension.

It is a fact that one has to use different parts of the body according to the needs of particular games. But it does not mean that they should not pay any attention to the other parts of the body. The body along with the mind needs to have a total approach. How can they claim to be dedicated athletes when they are heedless regarding the body and mind? Their unattended parts of the body develop weakness, mind becomes petty, negative, and they become a drag on other players. If the body movements are swift, intelligence develops freedom to see beyond and reach vastness to achieve the goal with comfort.

---

[1] See *Aṣṭadaḷa Yogamālā*, vol. 2, *Vinyāsa Yoga*, pp. 245-256.

This is why wise men of yore differentiated between *aṅgabhāga-sādhanā* (part body actions) and *sarvāṅga-sādhanā* (whole body training with attention and alignment). On account of the partial development, sportspersons remain under strain and therefore the concentration and agility fail at the crucial time.

To understand the body as a whole, athletes should know that man is made of physical, physiological, emotional, intellectual and the blissful sheaths. Accordingly exercises are connative, cognitive, mental, discriminative and exhilarating. When all these are attained, then only does one become a full athlete or a sportsperson. Otherwise, they succumb to failure and dejection.

Also, they should be made to understand the value of good health. It is not a commodity that is to be bought in a pharmacy. It has to be earned by inspiration and perspiration, attention and devotion.

As life force is dynamic, health is dynamic.

If one observes, one can feel that each muscle of the body moves in different directions with actions and counter-actions, pressures and counter-pressures, firmness and agility. In order not to reach the wrong multifaceted actions, one has to build up the challenges and counter-challenges accurately. Daily workout is essential to build the needed qualities and stamina in the body. Hence culturing of the body and mind is a must in all sports, so that they support, sustain and uphold for the needed action of the game at the right time.

To achieve this, body and mind have to act together, understand and co-ordinate with each other. They have to be made to realise the intelligent and unintelligent parts or sensitive and insensitive parts, so that equi-wisdom is built up through body language, recharged with right action and motion along with quick and sharp reflexes. The soma and psyche need to work in unison.

Here comes yoga, which plays a great role in helping athletes and sportspersons to improve from the gross body to the subtle body, then mind, intelligence, energy and consciousness. First, the practice of yoga makes the eyes become sharp as they are closer to the brain. The sharpness in the eyes and brain create confidence.

Yogāsana help in bringing to our attention the weak parts of the body. They help in mobilising the joints, increase the range of movements, bring efficiency in action and sharpness, correct the faults that occur in games and keep one always fit and in a state of efficiency with minimum strain. They also lubricate the joints and keep movements and dynamics of the body at the optimum level.

Athletes and sportspersons consume more energy than normal in a very short time. This burning out of energy generates acids in the joints and muscles bringing stiffness and fatigue. Yoga practices supply fresh blood for circulation keeping the joints free from accumulation of acid and muscles free from fatigue.

With the practice of *āsana,* the sportspersons begin to understand how to co-ordinate each and every action with the movement of the breath. Yogic breathing generates enormous energy, which is stored in the store house of energy, to be used at the time of need with full force, known to players as the 'killer instinct'. *Prāṇāyāma* techniques generate energy, organise storage and release only toxic air. It keeps the body warmer and helps to withstand strain with comfort.

Thus, this way, yoga helps to build up accurate movements with alignment, flexibility, firmness, co-ordination in motion and action. Yoga helps all, be they a swimmer, a runner, a body builder, a weight lifter, a cricketer, a footballer, a hockey, badminton, tennis or rugby player, as it covers all the hundreds of muscles and joints to work in harmony.

For example recently an opportunity was offered to one of my students, Shri S.N. Motivala, through the good office of Shri Ashok Mankad to conduct yoga classes for fourteen state cricket players in Mumbai.

When standing *āsana* were taught, the cricketers realised how inadequate their hamstrings, abductors and thigh muscles were. By doing the inverted poses, they could feel the coolness in the brain and body, while in backbends, they felt the enormous expansion of the chest cage. They also experienced freedom in the lateral movements of the spinal muscles in the twistings, a strengthening and stretching of the arms by arm balances, and an auto massage effect in *Vīrāsana* and *Baddhakoṇāsana.*[1]

At the same time, they could realise that with the practice of yoga injuries were minimised as the body could absorb the faulty action as with shock absorbers. Even if injuries occur, they were able to bring immediate relief or at least could minimise or keep them in check. The body resistance to such problems could be seen easily. They could easily face them. This is an unknown fact or unknown effect of the practice of yoga which very few people know. Yoga teaches a self-recovery and self-healing process. It brings the body intelligence to the surface so that one begins to understand the method of using the muscles, bones, joints and whole of the body in such a way that the injured area is not further injured. However, this is understood only after a long run of practice. It cannot be taught in a two or three day course. The yoga training needs to go synchronously with the sports training.

---

[1] See *Light on Yoga*, Harper Collins, London.

Thus the cricketers realised that yoga not only builds up power, endurance, agility and swiftness in body, quick reflexes in mind and a determined will. I am also happy to hear that the national cricket centre at Bangalore under the guidance of Brijesh Patel has made yoga a necessary subject for national players and others.

Yoga associates the body with the mind and mind with the self. It makes one understand a sound mind in a sound body and a sound body in a sound mind. This is the essential need for all athletes, sportspersons and players.

Therefore, I feel that the introduction of yoga to athletes and sportspersons all over India must become a part of their daily routine, so that they become better athletes and better sports persons and build up national prestige and honour.

SECTION VIII

ON YOGA AND SOCIAL LIFE

STAGES AND AIMS IN MAN'S LIFE*

It is assumed that the life span of man is one hundred years. We in India pray with sincerity and devotion to the Sun God, who is regarded as the manifestation of Brahman – the Creator – in visible form, to bless us with clear eyes to see, ears to hear, tongue to speak well, virility, firmness and steadiness, in order to enjoy life with purity, happiness and contentment for a full one hundred years.

We believe in continuous refinement and perfection. Likewise, we should accept that life has a continuity beyond death, in other words, rebirth. As old thoughts die out and new ones crop up, so also life and death follow alternatingly like seed and plant. Unfulfilled cravings, actions and aspirations go into the new life according to one's *karma* and quality *(guṇa)* entwined with one's past life *(pūrva-janma)*.

Let us look at an example. In the breeding of dogs and horses one sees to the pedigree. The quality of seed is verified when one sows the seeds. Agricultural technology has advanced to produce hybrid wheat, paddy, maize and fruits. To reach the pinnacle of one's life and living, purity and distinguished qualities of mood and behaviour *(guṇa-karma)* are essential. The life that takes birth will imbibe the qualities of thoughts and feelings of the parents at the time of union. The sperm and ovum that form into a nucleus bear their characteristics. Think for instance of a pot which contains odiferous and stinking materials. The pot when emptied continues to give out the same smell as the former contents. Even when earthen pots are broken, the pieces bear the smell of the respective pot to which they belonged. The imprint of smell is left behind very strongly. Similarly, human beings carry on the imprints of *vāsanā*.

The present life is the result of past actions. The conditions and qualities of the coming birth are decided from the very moment of conception. There are instances of worthy children born to impious parents and dull children to very high intellectuals. Yoga has a solution for this, though one in a million may rise to lofty heights of Absolute Aloneness. Despondency should not be allowed to hinder making attempts in the pursuit of yoga.

---

* From *Bhavan's Journal*.

Though the caste or class system is waning because of wrong interpretations and misuse, the stages of life enumerated by our great sages remain eternal as they are a part and parcel of each one's life. The stages of life *(āśrama)* are divided into four groups. They are: (1) *brahmacarya* – stage of learning, (2) *gṛhastha* – stage of a house-holder, (3) *vānaprastha* – where man guides his children to maintain the family, at the same time learning to detach himself from worldly matters. He lives aloof from life's ups and downs and frees himself from desires, which is the foundation for the last stage, (4) *sannyāsa* – wherein he renounces completely all pleasures and devotes his time and energy to attaching himself in thoughts of Almighty God.

These four stages of life exist even today though they may not be seen in their pristine forms and duration. It may not be possible for all to live one hundred years. Therefore, it is better that one considers to adopt yoga early in whatever the stage one is living in.

The life span of a person is evenly divided into the above four stages. A person has to learn, earn, maintain and establish himself and his family and at last reach freedom from wants and ambitions. His noble, majestic and peaceful life should be remembered even after death. As the stages of life are four, the aims *(puruṣārtha)* thereof are also four. They are *dharma, artha, kāma* and *mokṣa,* and they coincide with the four stages of life.

Dharma is that which teaches the essence of right thinking, living and acting. An individual undergoes training in acquiring knowledge of the world and of God to distinguish between what is merely pleasant and what is good, the ephemeral and the real under the guidance of an able teacher.

A *brahmacārin* is one who, while maintaining celibacy (called *brahman*) and studying *veda* and *vedāṅga* (also called *brahman*), moves in the thoughts of Brahman – thus befitting fully the term *brahmacārin. Brahma* is Universal Supreme Soul, *car* means to move, so *brahmacārin* is one who moves in the thoughts of *brahma.*

The observance of *dharma* and study of *brahman* go hand in hand. When the teacher is satisfied that his pupil has absorbed the teaching, the teacher blesses him and asks him to get married and live a pure life as taught by him. Here begins the second aim of life, *artha.* This is the beginning of earning honestly and living independently. When he finds financial security, he marries and during this stage he acquires wealth so that he is not dependent on others for maintaining his family. His *kāma* (desires and pleasures) is supposed to be fulfilled on entering the second stage – the wedded life. *Gṛha* means house. *Stha* means to establish. One who has established himself in the house (family) is *gṛhastha.* Here he experiences the turmoils of pleasure and pain, joy and sorrow. Then he arrives at the third stage, *vānaprastha* and assumes the role of an adviser or a guide to his family. He behaves as if he is one with them but inwardly he develops non-attachment. *Vana* means garden or forest. *Prastha* means to march towards. One who leaves the house and marches towards the forest is a *vānaprasthin*. This prepares him for the further stage of *sannyāsa*, where he renounces worldly bonds tending to the last aim of his life, *mokṣa*. When he finds himself mature physically, emotionally and intellectually, he wishes 'good-bye' to the family and lives alone within himself, serene and quiet, giving all his belongings in the service of God. *Sannyāsa* comes from the root *sam-ny* which means throw down together. Throwing down or abandoning is *sannyāsa*.

Just as the stages and aims are categorised, persons are assessed according to their mental development. The stages of mental development are: 1) *mūḍha* – dull, 2) *kṣipta* – a state of neglect, mentally scattered without a base, 3) *vikṣipta* – a state of agitation and distraction, 4) *ekāgra* – steady mind, and 5) *niruddha* – a state where one loses one's identity and becomes one with the Maker. Only a person in the *niruddha* state is fit to become *sannyāsin*.

In the stage of *brahmacarya*, the person may have any one state or combined states of mind. If he is *mūḍha*, he is taught *yama* and *niyama*, so that he understands the commands of *yama* and the disciplines of *niyama*. When he becomes *kṣipta* or *vikṣipta*, he is taught *yama, niyama, āsana* and *prāṇāyāma* so that he develops concentration, and the oscillation of his intelligence is checked. In the *ekāgra* state, he may develop arrogance which may inflate his ego as he is able to concentrate. For him, besides the first four aspects, *pratyāhāra, dhāraṇā* and *dhyāna* are taught to maintain purity in his concentration and develop humility. *Samādhi* is an experience, depending upon the qualitative development and progress of the person. *Samādhi* is like the fruit of a tree which may bear fruits in one season and may not blossom again for years. The tree of *samādhi* is nurtured through continuous *sādhanā*. In the practice of yoga, all cannot reach *samādhi*, since it is not a life-time achievement. One has to get matured in *sādhanā* so that *sādhanā* is fructified into *samādhi*.

The *sādhanā* of the aspirant varies according to his prevailing state of mind or *guṇa*. It may have to be changed according to the situation prevailing for the day. This point should be borne in mind as no link in the chain of yoga can be neglected, though each aspect has a tremendous bearing in building up one's character and personality. In all the eight petals of yoga, the journey of the *sādhaka* is from *dharma* to *mokṣa, brahmacārya* to *sannyāsa* and *tamōguṇa* to *guṇaśreṣṭam* (pre-eminent in virtues).

The discipline of yoga is given according to the state of mind. It is also taught according to the four stages of life. *Yama, niyama* and *āsana* are taught to a *brahmacārin*. Emphasis on *prāṇāyāma* is advocated for a *gṛhastha* or a family man, so that he may regain his dissipated energy and remain virile. At the same time he is trained in the art of controlling his desires and senses by practising *pratyāhāra*. This gradual development in *pratyāhāra* makes him fit for the third stage of life, *vānaprastha*. Here he learns, in addition to the five earlier stages of yoga, *dhāraṇā* or contemplation. Then in the last stage of *sannyāsa*, he is ripe to perform meditation *(dhyāna)* where he becomes one with God. This makes him a perfect Divine man and he shines like a light unto all!

YOGA: A TRUE CULT FOR PEACE AND HAPPINESS*

What is yoga?

Yoga means union. Union of the individual self with the Universal Self.

There is a lot of misconception in the minds of people when they hear of yoga. Many seem to think that swallowing nails, drinking acid, walking on water and fire, reading fortunes and so on is the end and aim of yoga. This is the most misunderstood, misrepresented art and science and yet it is the most popular. There are many living examples to prove the efficacy of yoga.

Yoga is a perfect practical science of its own, as its practice is a real necessity in our daily lives.

The aim of yoga is to achieve harmony between the body and the mind and between the mind and the soul – enjoying the unalloyed peace from within. No doubt, there are several paths to reach the peak of the mountain as there are several means to realise unalloyed peace. They are *rāja yoga, haṭha yoga, bhakti yoga, karma yoga, jñāna yoga* and so on. But the fountain of all paths are *haṭha yoga* and *rāja yoga.*

DISCIPLINE IS NECESSARY

The practitioner of yoga begins in training himself with moral, physical and mental disciplines.

Moral discipline involves both social and individual ethics. They are the commandments enumerated by Sage Patañjali. They are non-violence in words, thought and deed, truthfulness, non-covetousness, non-stealing, continence, prayers, contentment, practice, perseverance, kindness and surrender to the ONE who is the source of all sources. But the most important basis of all the ethics, which we have to remember, is the body. The body has been bestowed to us as a great capital to start to show our discipline and creativity. This instrument is given to us

---

* 1974.

by unknown hands to protect and to live not only for ourselves but for future generations as well. If we abuse the body, we are breaking the very first moral discipline. When the body or the temple of the soul is kept in a perfect state of health, then the mind is freed from the body and reflects on the self. This is the aim and end of yoga.

THE HINDRANCES WHICH DISTURB HARMONY

The disharmony in our body and mind is caused by various psychosomatic factors such as shakiness in the body and fear in the mind that shatters the very art of living.

To eradicate these psychosomatic factors, sage Patañjali codified the great science of yoga with its eight constituents namely, *yama, niyama, āsana, prāṇāyāma, pratyāhāra, dhāraṇā, dhyāna* and *samādhi.*

If *yama* and *niyama* are the moral commandments of yoga, *āsana* is positioning of the body which trains its various limbs to remain as assets for a sound perfect health. *Āsana* and *prāṇāyāma* not only purify the nerves, regulate the secretions of the endocrine glands, strengthen the digestive organs, improve the circulation of blood and help in evacuating toxic matters, but also keep one always young and agile to withstand the dualities of cold and heat, pleasure and pain patiently and cheerfully.

YOGA IS FOR ALL

This art can be practised by young or old, weak or strong, firm or infirm, irrespective of gender and under any climatic conditions. However, the practice must be done according to the requirements of the individual, the circumstances and temperament.

It is no doubt a great achievement that our present generation pays greater importance to the development of the brain but unfortunately it pays very little attention to the brawn. Both are essential. If neglected, one becomes physically weak and emotionally unstable. The attention and effort to the development of the body and brain need to be equally balanced. If one of these is neglected, one becomes a burden not only to oneself or to one's parents but to society as well. If proper care is taken, happiness, peace and love will be in abundance.

Primarily yoga aims at discipline and results in health and emotional stability, mental control ending in Self-realisation.

It is my experience that without physical, moral and mental discipline, spiritual discipline is an impossibility. As the gardener takes care of the sapling to enable it to grow into a gigantic tree by manuring and watering it regularly and then enjoys the flowers and the fruits, so also *āsana* and *prāṇāyāma* develop one's physique to perfection and lead one to that spiritual perfume – Self-realisation or *ātma-jñāna*.

YOGA: A PATH TO PEACE AND HARMONY*

Consciousness is close to the body as well as the Self. As long as there is no communication from the inner self to the body and as long as there is no understanding between the external self – the body – and the inner self, there is no poise within or peace outside.

Peace and harmony are wonderful words. Harmony is the language of the heart and not that of the head. Being the language of the heart, it is very difficult to express the experiences of inner quietness. Yoga is the means to attain it. As long as the means are not perfect, realisation in the form of peace and harmony cannot be achieved.

Mr. M.P. Pandit of Aurobindo's *ashram,* has made the suggestion that we should have a physical focus for our sanctuary. No doubt, we should have one for the sake of the community. But the place – the body – as well as the force – intelligence –, has already been given to us by God. Let us use that intelligence to experience poise and peace.

We have had in our times three great men – Mahatma Gandhi, Sri Aurobindo and Sri Ramana Maharshi. Mahatma Gandhi was static inside and dynamic outside. He met everyone, his means *(karma)* were very superior, very divine. Sri Aurobindo's approach was love, which is *bhakti*. It was a great help to all people like us. Ramana Maharshi always said, "Find out who you are, so that you may be freed from the state of *avidyā* and *asmitā*". With even a bit of the *jñāna* of Ramana, the *bhakti* of Aurobindo and the *karma* of Gandhi, we should be able to see peace – not only within ourselves, but all around us. These three great men are the examples for us to follow in our day to day practice. Without *jñāna* there is no *bhakti*, and without *bhakti* there is no *karma*. They are all intermingled.

In the *Rāmāyana*, there are three types of *Īśvara bhaktas* – Rāvaṇa, Kumbhakarṇa and Vibhīṣaṇa.[1] The devotion of Rāvaṇa was *ahaṁkārik* – egoistic, *rājasic* to fulfil his selfish ends. Therefore, the *jñāna* and *karma* took a back seat. He lost poise and the balance of mind. The

---

* Speech of the Chief Guest (The Sanctuary of Peace and Harmony), October 1977.

1 See the illustration in *Aṣṭadaḷa Yogamālā*, vol. 2, p. 239.

devotion of Kumbhakarṇa was *tāmasic* and inert, which made him lazy and sleepy. With a strong body, he remained empty within. The devotion of Vibhīṣaṇa was *sāttvic* and had pure intention. It is important for us to learn from these three devotees. We need to drop ego and become humble. We need to drop laziness and learn like Vibhīṣaṇa to surrender ourselves totally to *Paramātmā*. He had the physical firmness, emotional stability and intellectual clarity to experience *sāttvic dhyāna*. In *sāttvic dhyāna* alone harmony and peace come to us. Today many people jump to meditation and end up with Kumbhakarṇa's *tāmasic*, inert state of emptiness, or become egoistic or take pride in saying that they are meditating. They ignore the body, they ignore the mind and think that they know the Self. Vibhīṣaṇa never declared his devotion and meditation. He surrendered to Rāma – *Paramātmā*, giving up all ties. To have peace and harmony one needs to have a proper approach.

I am confident that those who work for peace and joy will pay attention to yogic discipline. I, being one of the members, know that it is also my duty to carry on at least with my pupils, trying to know what inner peace is.

NOW AND BEYOND*

Though man is born free, nature's heritage, consisting of three qualities – illumination, activity and inertia, entwines him. Like the earthen pot which carries its contents (good or foul), the wheel of time moulds and remoulds man according to his own makings and behaviour. He will have a body with either a dull and stupid mind, an agitated or distracted mind, a controlled and marshalled mind or a divine saintly mind.

Due to technical and scientific progress, man has to move at a supersonic speed in whatever state of mind he is in. This supersonic speed in thinking and action diminishes the physical frame, tenses the nerves and tautens the intellect. If he cannot release these tensions and relax, he falls prey to sleepless nights, which in turn affect his thinking. His anxieties multiply; doubts and incapabilities set in; attitudes of jealousy and malice develop. Then he becomes negative in his approach to life. He is evasive, reserved, indifferent, depressed, lazy, ill at ease and creates his own philosophy of illusion, seclusion and isolation. From these he switches to artificial ways of living. In order to find peace and happiness, he gets addicted to tranquillisers, sleeping pills, alcohol and various other psychedelic drugs. These may allow him to forget his anxieties and worries for a short time, but the cause remains unresolved and taunts him unabated.

Yoga is based on morality, physical discipline, mental alertness and spiritual awakening. We have been endowed with a body to express the Self that lies within. It is the duty of each of us to treat the body with the respect which is its due. Here begins the ethical discipline. The *yogis* of yore never thought that the body should be treated as something to be neglected or left unnoticed. On the contrary, they observed that the body's energy should be transformed and sublimated to the level of the intelligence and then of the Self. The moment negligence is shown to the body, it is contempt towards the Self. It lies in our hands to transform and sublimate the energy of the body through the process of *sādhanā* or to show carelessness to it. The continuance of the *sādhanā* is morality and neglecting it is immorality.

---

* *Yoga Journal*, issue no. 30, January-February, 1980. Symposium: *The Oracles of New Age*

No part of yoga can be practised without total involvement of body, mind and self, though in the beginning the divisions of the external and the internal are taught for sake of convenience. With thoroughness in the *sādhanā*, each movement in body and mind becomes the quest of the Self. When one practises either *āsana* or *prāṇāyāma* or *dhyāna*, there is a certain ethics demanded by each posture, each movement of inspiration or expiration and each adjustment required of the intelligence in the art of meditation. Each movement has to be observed, and the adjustments to be made precisely and immediately. For instance, in meditation, the body should be as firm as a diamond, as alert as a hooded cobra and as sharp as a razor. The brain, which is situated in the skull, has to be kept passive, as gentle as the thin end of a leaf which moves even at the most gentle touch of the breeze. The passivity of the brain helps to register each and every movement of the senses of knowledge, mind, intelligence and consciousness, which takes place at the time of meditation. When the brain is completely passive and alert, the mind situated at the centre of the heart reveals itself, being nothing but the outer layer of the soul. The conscious energy tosses between the intelligence of the head and the heart. By effort, the brain is made to remain silent and purged of its load so that the *yogi* is poised within himself, or he reaches the state of impersonality where he is face to face with his own self. Again, if the *āsana* is done for the mind to be alert, the brain is made a mere receiving instrument with which to see the faults in the movements and to help the senses in making adjustments. Then one realises that yoga does not simply deal with physical discipline but demands a greater mental discipline. Accurate performance of *āsana* reveals a total awareness of every pore of the skin and firmness of the unwavering intelligence. The energy of the body is thus gradually raised to the level of the intelligence.

Now let us consider the aspects of *prāṇāyāma*. Philosophically, inhalation means drawing in of cosmic energy, whereby the cosmic force comes in contact with the individual soul *(jīvātmā)*. In exhalation, the individual goes out to come in contact with the Universal Soul *(Paramātmā)*. In the inhalation-retention – *antara-kumbhaka*, the cosmic consciousness is held by the *sādhaka* to mingle *jīvātmā* with *Paramātmā*. In this state one experiences the cosmic force as all pervasive. *Bāhya kumbhaka* implies that the individual self in the form of breath is released to meet the Universal Self with humbleness. *Prāṇāyāma* process makes the body, the brain and the mind fit vehicles for meditation, since they are made humble by this process. *Prāṇāyāma* teaches us not only to be firm and still in the body, nerves and mind, but also engrosses us in the Universal Breath and surrender of our breath to the source of all – the *Paramātmā*.

In normal awareness the sense of 'I' functions in the brain; in the state of sleep the energy of the brain and the sense of 'I' do not function, but descend to the seat of the conscience.

In meditation, the body and spine have to be held straight like a firm pillar. The cells of the brain, along with the sense of knowledge, are released from the load of stress and strain. Then the energy of the brain is made to descend towards the seat of conscience *(dharmendriya),* and at the same time the energy of the consciousness and conscience *(antaḥkaraṇa)* is raised up to receive the descending energy of the intellect. This simultaneous action stops the thinking processes and brooding thoughts. The intellect does not waver, but dissolves in conscience, leading to a composed peace, calm and motionless mind. This, according to Sri Aurobindo, is "the opening out of mortal limitation into the unlimited immortality of the Soul".

Hence, practice of yoga is the only art and science which helps to eradicate these afflictions and brings back hope, confidence, courage and life free from prejudices of the past or the future, wherein we are able to face the present constructively and usefully with poise and peace.

Could we not conclude that it is not only knowing the known, that is the very body, the mind, the intelligence and consciousness, but moving beyond the known, to the Self which resides in us.

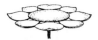

YOGA MAKES ONE THE MASTER OF CIRCUMSTANCES*

Yoga is an infinite art as are all other arts. Words are finite. It is very hard to convey the infinite greatness of the art of yoga through finite words in the limited time of a few minutes.

When God created man, He created also the qualities of *sattva*, *rajas* and *tamas*. Man, caught in the web of these *guṇa*, became a prey to the polarities of pleasure and pain, good and evil, love and hatred, the permanent and the transient. In seeking unalloyed bliss, he found out yoga and God. He defined God as a generating force, organising force and destroying force and yoga became the instrument to reach Him.

Yoga is one but it is called by such various names as *rāja yoga*, *haṭha yoga* , *laya yoga*, *jñāna yoga*, *bhakti yoga*, *karma yoga*, *mantra yoga*, *tāraka yoga*, *kuṇḍalini yoga*, *śakti-pāt yoga* and so on.

I am concerned with yoga. Though Patañjali nowhere mentions that he is dealing with *rāja yoga*, modern commentators labelled it as *rāja yoga* as it speaks of stilling the thoughts and branded *haṭha yoga* as physical yoga. Both *rāja yoga* and *haṭha yoga* are inseparable. United they lead towards *mokṣa* since they help to experience the state of liberation or aloneness.

Yoga is a psycho-physiological and psycho-spiritual subject. Nobody knows when and where the body ends and the mind begins and when and where the mind ends and the self begins. The sages divided our body into gross, subtle and causal. *Haṭha yoga* starts from the body and ends with the soul whereas *rāja yoga* starts from the mind, climbs down to the body and again lifts one towards the soul. Hence for me both are the same, being a psycho-spiritual subject.

Yoga is mainly a spiritual subject, but its by-product of health has assumed a major role and has almost come to the level of a therapy. Due to stress, strain and speed, its utility to conquer these three has gained momentum.

---

* From *Pune Service Wheel*, vol. 45, nº 18 – 2.11.81. Talk given on 12th October, Rotary Club.

Health is a conscious state of freedom from all shackles of suffering such as one experiences in deep sleep. Yoga works not only on the muscles, but also on the organs and the systems of the body along with mind and intelligence.

The body is like fallow land – uncultivated. Like a farmer who ploughs the land, removes the weeds, waters it, sows the best of seeds, tends the crops to get the best of the harvest, man ploughs the body with yogic practices. He removes the toxins and impurities accumulated due to wrong thinking, wrong behaviour and food; he irrigates bio-plasma or bio-energy, which is called *prāṇic* energy in yoga, and cultivates right logic and reasoning to free the mind from the pastures of worldly desires by sowing the seed of *ĀUṀ* as prayer, tending the mind as a crop from which to harvest peace and harmony. Thus he learns to live in peace within himself and with his neighbours and becomes a master of his circumstances.

SECTION IX

MULTIPLE ASPECTS OF YOGA

A THING WHICH WAS IMPOSSIBLE EVEN TO DREAM BECAME A FACT OF LIFE*

A few years ago it would have been a mad man's crazy idea. But now it is the pride of the people of his village, a school for his village's children.

When I was ten years of age, I remember that I was imitating Mahatma Gandhi wearing clothes like him and in my mind thinking of living like him to serve the people. I was sickly, weak but very hot headed even at that tender age. I lost my father and the responsibility of my up-bringing fell on my brothers. They had their own worries and difficulties and we the younger brothers were neglected. The future was very bleak and there was little hope even of survival. Often it occurred to me that the remedy for all unfortunate ones was – suicide. I even went to tanks with the intention of drowning myself. But last minute fear of becoming a ghost kept me away from this ghastly action.

When I was a boy of fifteen I casually agreed to follow the advice of my brother-in-law[1] to learn yoga to improve my health which was affected by various ailments. I went to Mysore and stayed there for two years. But my lot of misfortune was with me. I failed in the Secondary School Certificate examination of 1936. I was allowed for Public Service and not for entry to the college as I failed by three marks in English. I was thinking in my mind that I was only fit to work as a servant in a hotel or as an attendant. This was not for me as my temperament was to seek freedom from domination.

As I knew a few yogic *āsana* I thought in June 1936 that I should go from place to place and give demonstrations in the Educational Institutions of the State then known as Mysore. It was not as easy as I thought at first. The heads of the institutions used to ridicule my request and I had to go without food and shelter to other places to try my luck. It was a great joy when I gave a demonstration in a Middle School in Chikkaballapur and the head master handed me the sum of twelve *annas* (seventy-five *paisa*) for my demonstration which he had raised from the students, contributions ranging from 1 to 3 *paisa*. Then I went from place to place. I was helped at certain places and at other places I had to be content with nothing.

---

* 1967.

1 *Guru* T. Krishnamacharya.

How on earth was a boy like me ever to live a decent life – leave alone the philanthropic ideas which I was visualising thanks to the example of Mahatma Gandhi.

It was in the same year 1936 that the Maharaja of Mysore asked my brother-in-law (now my Guru) to go on a tour of North Karnataka to propagate yoga. At that time he asked me to follow him. Fortune was favouring yoga as my source of inspiration. There, some professors and others wanted to learn yoga. Their family members wanted to learn too. I being the youngest of the lot was placed in charge of the women's yoga class. Thus the seed of my career was instilled in me by the hands of destiny. Though I was destined to be a teacher of yoga, I had to face hurdle after hurdle to make a living out of it I faced opposition and hunger with calmness year after year with but one motive – to live and die for yoga only.

In August 1937, I was invited to Pune to train the college students in yoga for six months and since then with ups and downs in life I have stuck to my practices and now I say that sincerity and tenacity alone were my key to success. Though I started teaching, I had no more than ten pupils then. Now they are countless.

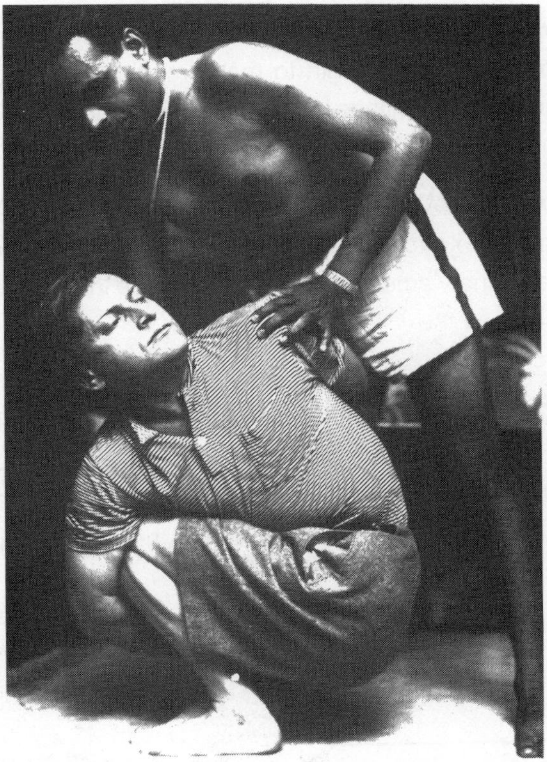

Plate n. 23 – Teaching Yehudi Menuhin

MY CONTACT WITH THE WEST

I was introduced to the famous violinist Yehudi Menuhin in 1952 by a pupil of mine, Smt. Mehra Malegumwalla of Bombay. He was keen to learn yoga not only for his health but also to improve his violin playing. This had been affected by overstrain and his nerves were in a state of exhaustion. Though he was introduced to several yogis, destiny brought us together. Our friendship has remained firm even to this day. He derived much benefit through yoga which prompted him to invite me to Europe and America as his guest in 1954 and 1956.

Though I had been visiting Europe since 1954, it was only in 1961 that I could impart my knowledge to the ordinary public in England by conducting regular classes in various parts of the city and suburbs. The classes were also conducted in cities of Europe. Now many of my senior pupils are conducting classes and call themselves B.K.S. Iyengar Associations, Institutes and Centres.

ADOPTION OF THE VILLAGE

It was in 1963 that some of my pupils wanted to help me financially. I told them that God had favoured me with a noble art and strength to make my living. Still if they want to help me I suggested that they could help any village in India by approaching the Bharat Sarvodaya Mandal to give them a village.

The *Bhoodan* Movement[1] gave them a village called Ramagiri in Mahbubnagar of Andhra Pradesh. My pupils soon set out to give a token of their boundless gratitude by adopting this village which lacked the ordinary amenities of life, through the international organisation 'War on Want'.

Through artistic and cultural events and by collecting jumble house to house and then selling these at a bazaar, they fetched the required sum of pounds 450, then the equivalent of Rs 6000/ – demanded by the *Sarvodaya*.[1] This sum was raised to provide facilities like drinking water, pump sets for irrigation, agricultural implements and so on. Out of this sum only Rs 2000/ - has been made use of and the rest of the amount is not yet utilised or accounted for. It is strange but true.

---

[1] *Sarvodaya* and the *Bhoodan* Movements, launched by Acharya Vinoba Bhave

ADOPTION OF BELLUR VILLAGE

As soon as the amount required for Ramagiri was raised, my pupils wrote to me that they were pleased to have adopted the village and did the work in gratitude and were thinking of forming a committee.

My friends in India were coaxing them to take my village which might inspire them to work with greater force. I was sceptical at first because I thought that they might think that I was being selfish: but later I made up my mind to write to them to take up my village if they could. Immediately they came forward with suggestions and wrote back that I should have suggested my village in the beginning. With joy they adopted my village in March 1965. The ball started rolling to raise funds.

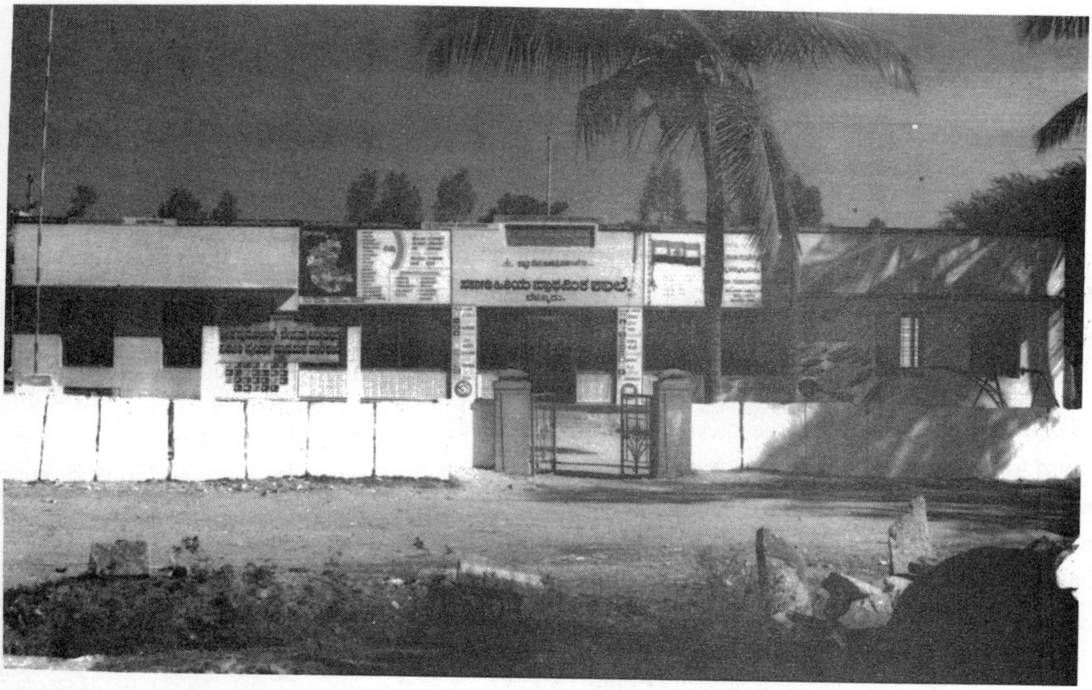

Plate n. 24 – Bellur School

IDEA OF THE SCHOOL

Now the responsibility of the inquiry into the requirements of the villagers fell on me. I went to the village for the first time in my living memory, though I was born there, to find out for myself what was essential. Different people offered different views. I was all the while thinking of the future generation. I asked them where the children might have a decent school to study in. I saw the present room and immediately made up my mind to take the school building in hand.

I started collecting information. The population of the place was 737, with 177 families. There were one hundred and fifty children under twelve, and the main occupation was agriculture. A living was earned by manual labour and working at the quarry. The people had insufficient production since there was a lack of manure and a shortage of animals. They borrowed at an interest of 10% to 18% to be cleared off in instalments which the majority never achieved. There were two wells for drinking purposes but unclean and therefore their health condition was very poor and unsatisfactory. About eighty children under twelve years of age were illiterate and idle.

Though my pupils agreed to help, it was not as easy as I had thought. Both *Sarvodaya* and War on Want were not in favour of encouraging school buildings. To channel the money and to send it free of taxes, we had to approach the internationally recognised organisations. First both were reluctant but my arguments convinced them that education is a necessary first factor to improve one's lot in life.

Field and research worker at War on Want, London, Owen Battersby appreciated my suggestion and agreed to forward the amount to Akhil Bharat Sarva Seva Sangha, Varanasi.

Bellur was not a Bhoodan or Gramadhan village nor was it in the list of War on Want villages for aid, but instead it was adopted by my pupils in Brighton, England, following the request to War on Want for assistance in channelling the money collected by them and allowing my pupils to form a branch for that specific purpose.

In order to gain support for funds, my pupils asked me whether any money could be raised from the village. After knowing myself the conditions of the people, I was hesitant to ask them to raise money. As the saying goes, "Charity begins at home"... we, the children of Bellur, Krishnamachar, myself and my brothers, came forward to donate a sum of Rs 1500/- and land for the building. We put this before the village *panchayat* on condition that the school be named after our revered parents. They agreed and passed a resolution to that effect. Later the village *panchayat* gave an alternative place but also promised to donate Rs 1000/-.

My pupils wrote me to inscribe these words on a stone: "A LASTING TRIBUTE TO B.K.S. IYENGAR FROM HIS EUROPEAN PUPILS IN APPRECIATION OF HIS GREAT TEACHING IN THE NOBLE ART OF YOGA". They wanted this so that it could be a constant reminder to all who enter the school, that a son of Bellur had risen to greatness in his life time and that it might be an inspiration to all the young people as they receive their education.

A total sum of 990/- pounds then equivalent to Rs.15,670/- was collected by arranging my yoga demonstrations in England and Switzerland, and through music and songs, jumble sales, Bellur bazaar, giving lifts in cars at bus rates, collecting in streets by standing for hours in the cold, moving sealed boxes at parties, singing carols at Railway stations and so forth.

Here I would like to mention one or two instances of selfless services rendered by my pupils.

Children of my pupils saved money from their lunch expenses, devoted endlessly by cleaning cups and saucers free of charge at several Bellur bazaars where refreshments were served in Indian style and donated the amount to the school building. A pupil of mine, instead of making merry in Christmas, went with a box to collect money and raised that day a sum of £ 9-2 shillings then the equivalent of Rs 175/-.

At Brighton station my pupils stood for hours in cold weather and sang songs on Christmas Eve and collected £14.10 shillings, the highest that day. This must inspire my Indian brothers to work for our national cause and imbue in them the service which alone is a way to know where God is.

Here is the account of money sent to Akhil Sarva Seva Sangha.

DATE	AMOUNT IN £	IN Rs.
April 1965	40.0.0	
June 1965	80.0.0	
July 1965	100.0.0	
September 1965	110.0.0	
September 1965	210.0.0	
October 1965	30.0.0	
March 1966	70.0.0	

	640.0.0	Rs. 8,320
After devaluation of the Rupee		
June 1966	100.0.0	
August 1966	50.0.0	
October 1966	200.0.0	

	350.0.0	Rs. 7,350
	-------	--------
TOTAL	990.0.0	Rs. 15,670[1]

Bellur Krishnamachar's children	Rs. 1,500
Village *Panchayat*	Rs. 1,000
Sri Sundarayya, school teacher in the village	Rs. 250

TOTAL	Rs. 18,420

Rs 18,420 is the total collection for the school building.

[1] As per the prevailing rate of exchange.

Last year, while I was in England, I discussed with a member of War on Want that I should be allowed to convert the amount Rs. 1,500/- into a trust as the amount collected in England was sufficient for the building. They agreed to my suggestion and now this amount of Rs 1,500/- will be deposited in the bank as a fixed deposit and whatever interest is earned, that sum will be given each year to two outstanding students of the school:

1) for first rank student, and

2) for an outstanding student in yogic performance, as the Bellur Krishnamachar scholarship. This suggestion was agreed upon.

Thus came about the most unbelievable achievement from a humble son of that soil.

PRACTISE TO HAVE DIVINE GRACE*

Friends,

I am very happy to be with you all and share this knowledge of yoga. Some of you have seen me before and some not at all. Sometimes you get a picture about me which may be contrary to my way of living, so I stand in your presence and you may see and perceive me directly now.

Yoga has become very very popular, particularly in Manchester, because when I came here for the first time (i.e. about thirty-six years ago), yoga practices were already going on. The seed of yoga was sown here before I came to this place, but it took a long time to realise that it was not a healthy seed. But now, I hear that about two to three thousand people are practising my method here alone. This is a grand success, and I am proud of you all for the simple reason that some of you have continuously pursued the subject for years without getting disheartened. In a way, you teach me that I should practise with that perseverance; for which I am grateful to you all.

I want you to continue the practice with this innocent mind for many years to come. The moment you lose that fragrance of innocence, you also lose the quality of humility. So friends, learn to maintain innocence, perseverance and humility and leave the goal of yoga to Almighty God or the Invisible Hands of Providence to bless and bestow the benefits of your practices. Practice culminates in divine grace, so continue your practice so that the divine grace, for which we have to wait, sometimes even for years, may fall on you. No doubt, without the grace of the Lord nobody can take this noble art to its culmination.

Yoga is not a religion but a religious subject which enhances the religiousness of mankind. Yoga is a subject which cultures the mind and the intelligence of the individual to develop

---

* Message given at the Free Trade Hall, Manchester, on the 18th July 1990. Published in the magazine of "The Manchester and District Institute of Iyengar Yoga", October, 1990.

religiousness through practice. It has nothing to do with the man-created religious order; yet, it is a religion of human beings, a religion of humanity, as it is filled with the message of good will to one and all.

Yoga is an art that associates the body with the mind and the mind with the soul and then surrenders the soul to the Invisible Hands of God. This is the yoga we practise. So it has nothing to do with religious denominations or man-made religions. Yoga is Supreme because self culture is the aim of every human being on Earth. Therefore, continue your *sādhanā*. What you achieve in your yogic discipline, savour that and continue with reverence the art of yoga to distill and savour further. I am sure the blessings of God will be on you all with your devotional *sādhanā*. God bless you all.

YOGA – AN EDUCATION COVERING HUMANITY*

Sri Mohan Dharia, Sri Shantilal Suratwala, Sri Azambhai Pansare, Sri Nana Chudasama, Sri Hastimal Firodia and members of the Residency Club.

I am indeed grateful to all of you for selecting me along with my esteemed friends Sri S.L. Kirloskar, Sri Suresh Kalmadi, Shrimati Shobhna Ranade and Pandit Bhimsen Joshi to receive this year's *Pune Pride* award.

I do not claim to be an intellectual, an academic, an educationist or a celebrity.

Hence I am surprised though not confused to find my name amongst Pune's persons of eminence, achievement and excellence in their respective fields.

I must confess that I am not an education specialist in the conventional method of education, but I am an educationist in my chosen field. In a way, I am an educator since I have been invited to give lectures by Harvard University, the University of Moscow, University of Philadelphia, University of London, University of Cambridge, University of Sydney, and just a fortnight ago I addressed the students of Seoul University on adoption of yoga in education. I am proud to say that I have been selected as a senate member of the University of Pune.

I have introduced my subject, yoga, in the educational scheme of Great Britain, community colleges of U.S.A., and other countries. As far as I understand, education means not only technology and general knowledge of the world, but also the culture of developing the power of reasoning and judgement. It is meant to aspire for better living and higher thinking. If this is considered as education, then I am an educationist.

I have developed skillful talents for one to unfold the hidden latent energy of the body and to come in contact with one's mind, intelligence and consciousness, all which is an education of the self.

---

* Message given by upon receiving the "Pune Pride" award in 1992.

I have taken my art, my science and my philosophy to all the six continents and I am proud to say that I have taken millions by storm towards yoga, transcending all barriers of religion to earn health, contentment and peace. It is surprising that six lakh copies of *Light on Yoga* have been sold in English alone, and they are in fifteen languages including Persian, Hebrew, Japanese, Korean, Hungarian, Ukranian, Georgian, Romanian and Bulgarian. I am happy to say that my culture of yoga has an effect on the civilisation of the world.

We are all endowed in one way or another with a keen sense of truth, justice, beauty or loyalty. Yet our natures differ from one to another. Some may be very intelligent but lazy, some may be indifferent, some may be pleasure-seeking, while some may be selfish. The yogic umbrella of self-culture gives shelter and protects everyone.

Yoga, being a science of self-culture, made me a healthy man even though I was born unhealthy; gave me emotional stability and intellectual clarity while I was a back-bencher in school.

What yoga gave me, I thought I should share with others and my mission to educate people for a healthy body, sound mind and contentment took shape 60 years ago and I am still carrying on the work to educate people for understanding their own dormant physical, physiological, psychological, mental, intellectual and spiritual wisdom and the ways to awaken them.

The end of knowledge is the realisation of the Self. The art of yoga makes one experience the serenity and the diffusion of the all pervading soul to be in touch or in contact with the trillions of cells in the body in order to feel just oneness of existence, without deviation in body, mind, intelligence and consciousness.

In short yoga makes an individual develop universality. As all religions believe in cosmic consciousness, yoga becomes the key to all religions.

Dr. S. Radhakrishnan said that Brahman means growth. Life in us is Brahman and hence it is dynamic, and so growth must be dynamic. This dynamism has motion, action, stillness and silence. As motion has vibration, so does action. In action stillness and silence flow. The vibration of action, stillness and silence have power, rhythm and movement without the feel of movement.

This is akin to the Chinese philosophy as conveyed by their masters as stillness in stillness or silence in silence. Is not real stillness or silence a rhythmic movement, in life-force and spiritual consciousness? This stillness or silence links and brings the union of life-force and spiritual consciousness making one experience heaven on earth in one's very existence.

My main aim in life is to take the values of yoga to one and all and to develop in them the philosophy of life which stands on three columns – word, work and worship. That is the path of *jñāna, karma* and *bhakti* through which the welfare of society, community and nation is built up with understanding and pliability in intelligence.

Hence I leave my sixty years of teaching for the coming generations to evaluate how I have put the heritage of India – the art of yoga – on the map of the world with a firm foundation to remain steady and stable in the coming years.

GURU – THE HUB, *ŚIṢYA* – THE SPOKES*

Our *Gurujī*, Shri T. Krishnamacharya's biography, is a touching story for all his students, past, present and future.

It was kind of Shri T.K.V. Deshikachar to ask for a foreword from me. I was amazed and at the same time hesitant because *Gurujī* was not an ordinary person, and my acquaintance with him was very limited even though he was my sister's husband.

It is impossible for a humble student like myself to measure his calibre and stature; a man of firm discipline, perseverance, and persistence in his precept and practice; a living yogi of the century, a versatile personality, a fountain of knowledge, an encyclopedia on all facets of the *Sṛti, Smṛti, Upaniṣad, Darśana, Itihāsa,* and *Purāṇa.* All subject matters were at his fingertips. His powerful memory never let him down, not even once.

Being an ardent seeker of *jñāna,* he would undertake journeys under all circumstances. His heart was always burning to read and to learn. His dire poverty became a garland for acquiring knowledge.

His is the shining example of a "Seeker of Knowledge", for all to emulate.

In his biography, it is said that he taught the *Veda* and revealed the secrets of our sacred knowledge to one and all. Maybe his pupils in Chennai (Madras) were extremely fortunate and clever enough to change his heart, and to milk his knowledge to the best of their abilities, or age must have mellowed him to impart his knowledge and experience to one and all.

This favour was not there when I was his student. I vividly remember that the *panditas* of Mysore would avoid meeting him, moving to the other side of the footpath if he was on that path. His mastery on almost all subjects made him proud intellectually, and left him isolated from friends and relatives.

---

* Foreword to *Śrī Krishnamacharya the Pūrnacarya,* by Krishnamacharya Yoga Mandiram, 10th March, 1997.

With all his intellectual prowess, his ways and moods were unpredictable. We were afraid even to talk to him, let alone question. Yet his conduct, his way of living, left an indelible mark on our lives.

As his first students, though we did not benefit from his knowledge, what little we got from him remains a great inspiration.

We all owe much to him, who made us take yoga to the masses. The popularity of yoga today goes to his credit and merit.

In our Wheel of Yoga, he was the hub, and we as spokes rolled the wheel without creating bends or dents in.

He sowed the seed of yoga and we nurtured it to grow slowly and steadily into a gigantic tree now covering almost all continents of the world.

With my respect and reverence to *Gurujī*, I feel that I am not worthy of this task. My association with him in yoga is just accidental, yet his grace turned out as a messenger in me to carry the subject of yoga everywhere.

It is a great honour to associate myself with such a great soul, and with humility I shall feel more than ever grateful if his works and words inspire and ignite the readers in the pursuit of the yogic discipline.

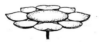

FRAGRANCE OF "MYSORE MALLIGE"*

Mr. Chancellor, Vice Chancellor, distinguished Chief Guest, Members of University Executive Council, members of the other University bodies, respected teachers, students, friends and the citizens of this distinguished city.

I am overwhelmed with gratitude for this great honour that has been conferred on me by the oldest University of Karnataka, the University of Mysore, in recognition of my contributions to yoga.

I studied in the Maharaja's high school from 1934 to 1936 and I had no chance of entering the premises of any college or University because I scored three marks too few in English to go in for college studies. Yet I had the occasion to address the Universities of London, Oxford, Munich, Harvard, Pennsylvania, Michigan, Sydney and Seoul on yoga through demonstrations.

I was under the tutelage of the late Vidwan Sri T. Krishnamacharya, the Director of *Shriyogashala* at the Jagamohan Palace patronized by the late Krishnaraja Wadiar Bahadur IV.

My Guru Sri Krishnamacharya sowed the seed of yoga in me as I was a weakling afflicted with malaria, typhoid and tuberculosis.

As there were no wonderdrugs in those days, destiny took me to him for yoga.

In 1935 His Highness had hosted an 'At Home' party for the international Y.M.C.A and he had arranged a yoga demonstration where my *guruji* wanted me to demonstrate and the Maharaja presented me Rs. 50 /- as a token of appreciation.

I learnt the alphabets of yoga in Mysore and now I am here to receive the most coveted award of D.Sc. from the University of Mysore after a lapse of 60 years.

---

* Speech delivered by the author when he received the degree of Doctor of Science from Mysore University, 21st April, 1997.

Though I have been conferred several honours both nationally and internationally including the *Padmashree* award, I cherish this honour the most because here, in the fragrance of my birthplace, the grace of goddess Chamundeshwari had entered into my yogic discipline. Without that grace I would have died prematurely as an unknown entity.

Barely at 16, destiny forced me to take up yoga as my career and I was called to teach yoga in Pune where I have remained ever since.

But it was not an easy task. After three years of teaching, my services were terminated and I was in the wilderness for years when even a meal was a luxury.

Trials and tribulations, insults and humiliation, poverty and hunger did not divert my mind from my yogic practices, nor was my mind ready for a job.

My *sādhanā* bore fruit when I married and set up a house with borrowed utensils and stove from friends and pupils.

Soon after marriage the grace of Godess Lakshmi dawned on us and my practice started attracting lovers of yoga, people with medical problems, and distinguished personalities.

I taught yoga to Lokanayak Jayaprakash Narayan, former Vice Presidents Dr G. S. Pathak, Shri B. D. Jatti, former chiefs of army staff, General Srinagesh, General B. C. Joshi, former chief minister of Karnataka, Shri Veerendra Patil, Rajamata Vijaya Raje Sindhia, Queen Elizabeth the late queen mother of Belgium, Shri J. Krishnamurthi, Prof. D. B. Deodhar, Sri Kiran More, Sri Javagal Srinath, Sri Lalgudi Jayaraman and many top class musicians of the West.

I gave a number of lectures and demonstrations before such distinguished personalities as Dr Rajendra Prasad, Marshall Bulganin, Mr. N. K. Krushchev of Russia, Dr. Mohamad Hatta - former Vice President of Indonesia, Shrimati Sarojini Naidu, former speakers Dr. G. V. Mavalankar, Sri B. G. Kher, Sri Anantashayanam Iyengar, and Shrimati Vijayalakshmi Pandit and almost in all Indian embassies abroad.

It was in 1952 that I met the world famous violinist Yehudi Menuhin who was invited by no other than *Pandit* Jawaharlal Nehru. He sought my help as he had problems with his playing.

My teaching helped him to such an extent that his playing improved considerably and he invited me to visit him in Europe in 1954. He presented me with an Omega chronometer watch inscribed "to my best violin teacher".

Since 1954 I have been visiting various parts of the world teaching and setting up centres. Now millions of people are practising at180 centres of the Iyengar Yoga Associations in all the continents.

All the credit goes to my country in general and Mysore in particular for I am not a learned man nor do I have a background of books. With my lack of education, poverty and struggle, my only book was my body and I worked on it to gain subjective experience and made use of the experience to attract people towards yoga.

Through my penetration and study of the inner body and the inner mind through the two *aṅga* of yoga, namely *āsana* and *prāṇāyāma*, I learned the functions of the skeletal body, the organic body, functions of the mind, attention, intelligence and awareness of the consciousness.

My devotion, dedication and application in yoga made me a hard task master, an ardent student and an intense teacher in order to take the pupils towards the goal of perfection and precision.

As *Īśāvāsyopaniṣad* says, *Īśāvāsyaṁ idam sarvaṁ yatkimca jagatyām jagat*, meaning "All that is moving and unmoving in this world is pervaded by divinity", I learnt to use my body as the only means to feel the divinity from my skin to the self and from the self to the skin.

Through trial and error, and experimentation, I developed experiential knowledge. I filtered this experienced knowledge repeatedly to taste the fragrance of life which is the wonder of wonders.

By this *rasātmaka jñāna* a semi-educated boy became the author of *Light on Yoga, Light on Prāṇāyāma, Art of Yoga, The Tree of Yoga* and *Light on the Yoga Sūtras of Patañjali* which are reviewed as classic works. In particular my book *Light on Prāṇāyāma* in Hindi won the National award for books (first prize) in 1987.

All these books have been translated into a large number of Indian as well as foreign languages which are reprinted every now and again.

I am saying all this with humility because the credit and the merit of my work goes to my birthplace Karnataka and mother Chamundi.

Sirs, I am:

- the first to promote yoga in schools and colleges in 1937;
- the first to introduce yoga in the National Defence Academy;
- the first to conduct mixed classes for boys and girls and men and women in the 30s;

- the first to introduce yoga in the adult education schemes of the U. K. and the U. S. A. in 1968 & 1974;
- the first to teach yoga to eminent heads of state!
- the first to give thousands of demonstrations all over the world as a solo artist;
- the first to make more than a thousand people do yoga together in the Euro Yoga Convention held at the Crystal Palace, London where the Olympics were once held;
- the first to promote yoga as an alternative medicine by inventing props to fit all patients;
- the first to present yoga in front of one of the wonders of the world - the Taj Mahal in 1970; and
- probably the first to keep Pope John IV waiting for an audience!

Again I may be the first to receive this honour from the University of Mysore as a yoga practitioner and a teacher for more than six decades.

Sirs, though this is not the time to dilate upon the physico-physiological, physio-psychological and psycho-spiritual aspect of yoga, whatever I experienced, I have imparted to my students and I have not ventured beyond the frame of my experienced knowledge.

In the evening of my life I am devoting my time to practise so that I do not become a *yogabhraṣṭan* consciously in this life. The dimension I gave to yoga has attracted people in the same way as our "Mysore mallige" – the Jasmine flower of Mysore.

On this occasion along with me D. V. Gowda has been honoured by a doctorate and I offer my deep felicitations to him. I also congratulate the budding educationists and scientists who have came out with distinction. For them the good has not ended but begun. This life's journey is not smooth, but I am sure that with persistent perseverance in their subject, they may light the lamp of *jñāna* in their hearts as an example to pass on to the future generations.

As a son of this soil, I once again express my deep sense of gratitude to the University of Mysore though it was Mysore which sent me out 60 years ago to make my base in Maharashtra and to be a non-resident Mysorian.

May God's blessing be upon you all.

YOGA : A GARLAND OF HEALTH AND KNOWLEDGE

Mr Chancellor Sri Shankar Raoji Chavan, Vice-Chancellor Smt. Hira Adyantaya, the Honourable Minister Sri Murali Manohar Joshiji, Executive Council Members of the Tilak Maharastra Vidyapeeth, respected teachers, students, friends and distinguished citizens of Pune city.

My heart is filled with this great honour that has been confirmed on me by this great Tilak Maharastra Vidyapeeth in recognition of my contributions in the art, science and philosophy of yoga.

As there is much closeness in the knowledge of yoga and *āyurveda*, I am proud of this honour.

If *āyurveda* is the view of knowledge on life and health, yoga too is filled with the knowledge of life and health but it shows the ways of acquiring these through the ingredient of the life force itself.

Patañjali says, *draṣṭṛdṛśyayoḥ saṁyogaḥ heyahetuḥ (Y.S.*, II.17) meaning, the cause of pain is the association or identification of the seer *(ātmā)* with the seen *(prakṛti)* and the remedy lies in their dissociation.

It is the conjunction of nature with the Self that causes disturbance in the five elements of the body, seven *dhātus*, namely *rasa, rakta, māṁsa, meda, asti, majjā, śukra* as well as *manas, buddhi, ahaṁkāra* with *puruṣa*.

Through its *aṣṭadaḷa mālā*, practice of yoga helps man to utilise this conjunction of seer and seen – *dṛṣṭā* and *dṛśya* – *puruṣa* with *prakṛti,* for balancing the *pañca bhūta* and *sapta dhātu*, for balanced physical, moral, mental, intellectual and spiritual health.

This is what I learnt in my uninterrupted *sādhanā* from the age of sixteen.

The only difference between yoga and *āyurveda* is that the practice of yoga needs sheer will power while *āyurveda* prescribes various herbal medicines, modern pills and tonics to gain confidence and will power, so that patients can take to yoga later. As health cannot be purchased in the market, it has to be earned with inspiration and perspiration, and yoga acts as a principle instrument to gain health.

If *āyurveda* and yoga are studied and practised together, maybe a new and fresh approach on health can be presented with which to live a better contented positive life. If *āyurveda* is a *darśana śāstra*, yoga is not only a *darśana śāstra* but also an *ānubhavika* (experiential), *bhāvanā śastra* (a scientific treatise for a conscious perception and conception of the seer).

If yoga defines diseases through the modalities of the *tri-doṣa*, namely: *vāta*, *pitta* and *sleṣma*, yoga too speaks of *tribhūta doṣa* through *āp*, *tej*, *vāyu* as *slesma*, *pitta* and *vāta*.

In addition to this *tri-bhūta doṣa* yoga speaks of *tri-guṇa*, namely; *sattva*, *rajas*, and *tamas*, which are also connected to the *tri-doṣa* and *tri-bhūta*.

Practice of yoga leads one from *tamōguṇa* to *sattvaguṇa* and balances *vāta*, *pitta*, *slesma* towards *svāsthya*, which means a sound state of health, prosperity, happiness, comfort, compliance and satisfaction. Here, the co-relation between yoga and *āyurveda* can help man to build up a sound body and a sound mind.

I was born during the time of the world influenza epidemic, later contracting malaria, typhoid and tuberculosis. As no wonder drugs were in existence, destiny took me to yoga to gain health, which later became my mission of service to humanity.

I learnt the alphabet of yoga in Mysore under the able guidance of Śrimān Vidwān T. Krishnamacharya who was well versed in *darśana* and a master of yoga.

Again, destiny unknowingly played its role by bringing me to Pune in 1937 through Dr V.B. Gokhale, a retired civil surgeon who had watched my demonstrations in Belgaum in 1936. He had contacted the educational institutions of Pune to depute 10 students from each college and school and then invited me to teach yoga in Pune, for a period of six months at the Deccan Gymkhana Club. These classes were extended every six months for three years.

Though the students showed great interest, the authorities of the institutions terminated my services for want of financial funds which was a paltry Rs.8/- per month from each institution.

As we say a known devil is better than an unknown devil, I stuck to Pune but faced problems of survival.

Here I learnt yoga in depth combining *jñāna saṁskāra kriyā*[1] and *kṛti saṁskāra jñāna*[2] with *anubhava* and am grateful to all those who helped me for my continuous practice and teaching whenever occasion arose.

Though I have been conferred several honours both nationally as well as internationally, I cherish this honour the most, because we often hear that a wise man is not honoured in his own country. In my case this adage has been proved wrong on many occasions.

Trials and tribulations, poverty and hunger acted as a garland of knowledge by which I continued my yogic *sādhanā* with zealousness.

If I had not received such encouragement from my fellow citizens in general and particularly my sisters and brothers of Pune, I would not have reached the status of receiving these honours.

My books *Light on Yoga, Light on Prāṇāyāma, The Art of Yoga, The Tree of Yoga, The Light on the Yoga Sūtras of Patañjali, Yoga – A Path to Holistic Health* and *Aṣṭadala Yogamālā* are considered as classic books and *Light on Yoga* as a Bible on yoga. All these books have been published not only in other foreign languages but also in many Indian languages.

Sirs, I share the merit of my art with you all as you were all responsible for me to maintain *sādhanā* with zeal throughout my life. Even now I practise four to five hours daily, simultaneously sharing my experiences with my students.

Sirs, in the eve of my life, I have only one ambition to be fulfilled. That is to take my experienced knowledge of yoga to my brothers and sisters of our villages, so that they too can drink the nectar of health, happiness and contentment, flavouring it as one takes the flavour of the Indian Jasmine flowers.

On this occasion, I am happy also for the presence of my friend and well-wisher and a worthy Son of Bharat, Dr Ragunath Mashelkar, Director-General, the Council for Scientific and Industrial Research, New Delhi, who fought on the patent of *basmati* rice and brought credit to my mother land.

Once again I thank you all. Thank you for this honorary Doctorate of Literature Award.

---

1 Knowledge that acomplishes clean and pure action.
2 Action that accomplishes clean and pure knowledge.

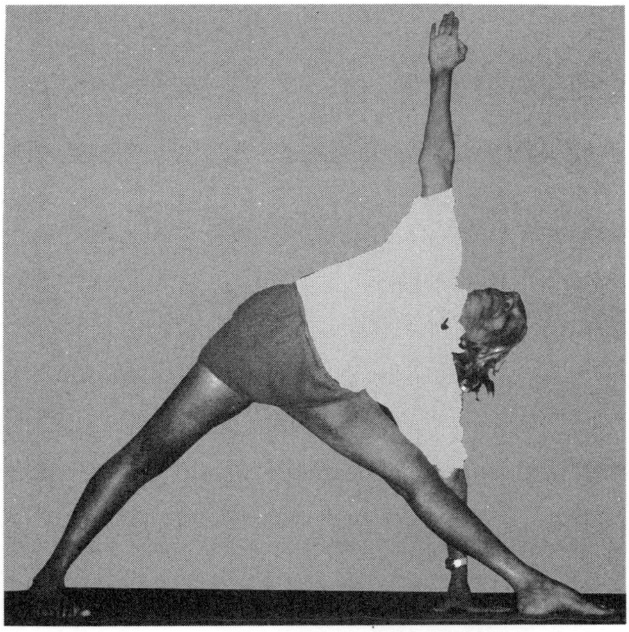

Plate n. 25 – *Utthita Trikoṇāsana*

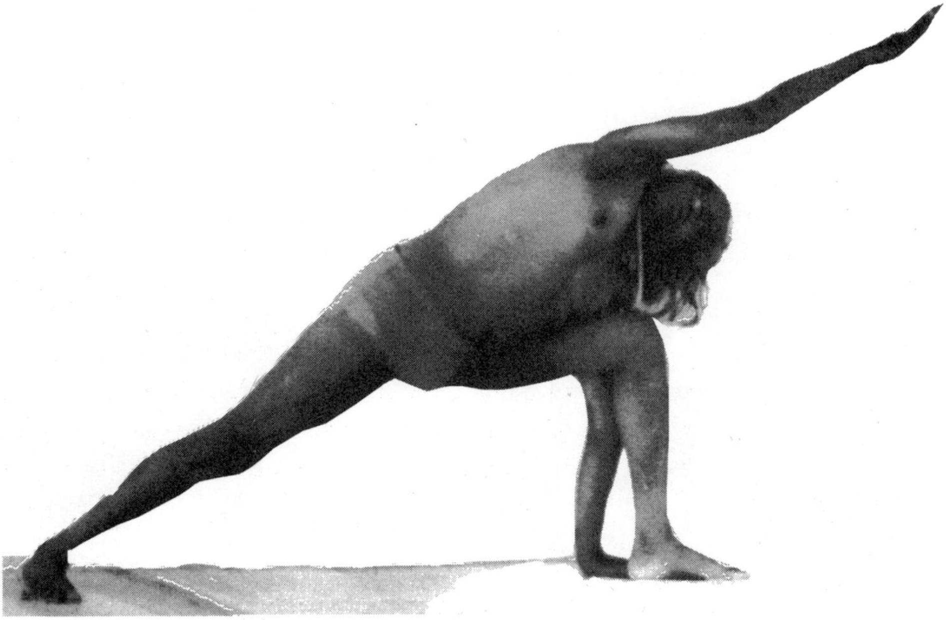

Plate n. 26 – *Utthita Pārśvakoṇāsana*

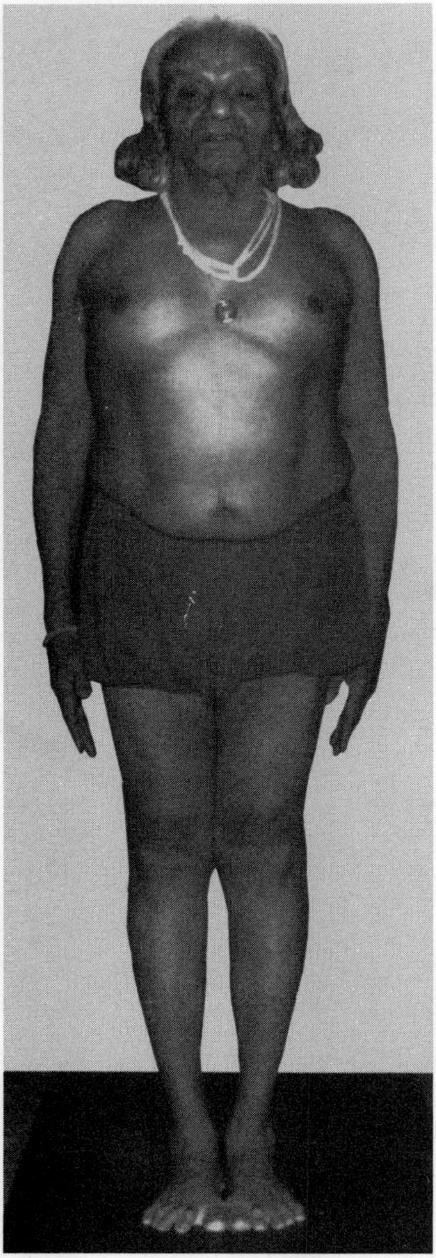

Plate n. 27 – *Tāḍāsana*

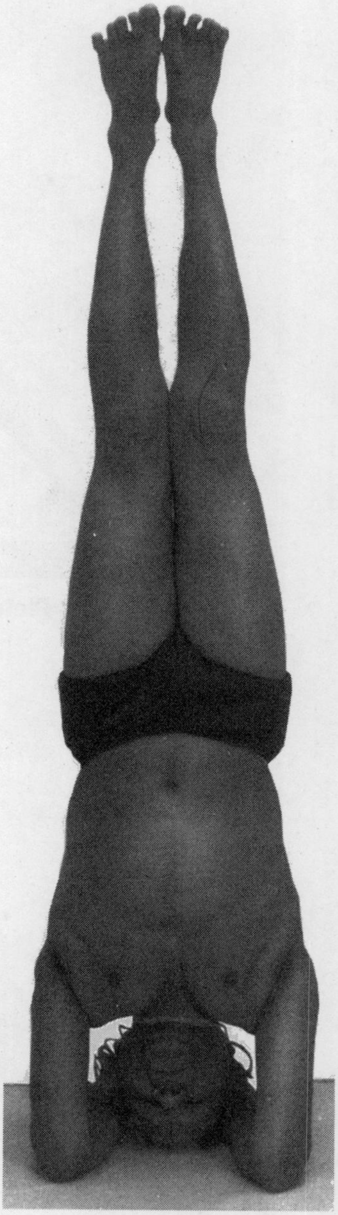

Plate n. 28 – *Sālamba Śīrṣāsana*